Care and Consequences

Care and Consequences:
The Impact of Health Care Reform

edited by Diana L. Gustafson

Fernwood Publishing • Halifax

Editing: Brenda Conroy
Design and production: Beverley Rach
Printed and bound in Canada by: Hignell Printing Limited

A publication of:
Fernwood Publishing
Box 9409, Station A
Halifax, Nova Scotia
B3K 5S3

Fernwood Publishing Company Limited gratefully acknowledges the financial support of the Department of Canadian Heritage and the Canada Council for the Arts for our publishing program.

Canadian Cataloguing in Publication Data

Main entry under title:

Care and Consequences

Includes bibliographical references and index.
ISBN 1-55266-033-8

1. Women's health services — Canada.   2. Health care reform — Canada.
I. Gustafson, Diana L.

RA184.C37 2000   362.1'082'0971   C00-950121-5

Contents

List of Acronyms

AMA	Alberta Medical Association
ASOG	Alberta Society of Obstetrics and Gynecology
BSF	Brief Solution Focused (therapy)
CCAC	Community Care Access Centre
CHST	Canada Health and Social Transfer
CIHR	Canadian Institutes of Health Research
CMG	Case Mix Groups
CNATS	Canadian Nursing Association Testing Services
CNO	College of Nurses of Ontario
CQI	Continuous Quality Improvement
CRIAW	Canadian Research Institute for the Advancement of Women
CUPE	Canadian Union of Public Employees
DRG	Diagnosis Related Groups
DSM-IV	Diagnostic and Statistical Manual, fourth edition
HIV / AIDS	Human Immuno-deficiency Virus / Auto Immune Deficiency Syndrome
HSTAP	Health Sector Training and Adjustment Program
LPM	Licensed Practical Nurse
NSGVP	The National Survey of Giving, Volunteering and Participation
OCHU	Ontario Council of Hospital Unions
OHIP	Ontario Health Insurance Plan
OMA	Ontario Medical Association
OMOH	Ontario Ministry of Health
ONA	Ontario Nurses' Association
PAHO	Pan American Health Organization
PCSYR	Palliative Care Services of York Region
PRN	Provisionally Registered Nurse
RHA	Regional Health Authority
RHPA	Regulated Health Professions Act
RN	Registered Nurse
RPN	Registered Practical Nurse
SACC	Sexual Assault / Rape Crisis Center
SAT	Sexual Assault Treatment
SBU	Strategic Business Unit
SSHRCC	Social Sciences and Humanities Research Council of Canada
TQM	Total Quality Management
UCP	Unregulated Care Provider
WHO	World Health Organization

to Debbie and Richard

Contributors

Jane Cawthorne is a mother, activist and instructor at Mount Royal College in Calgary, Alberta. She also serves as a trustee for the Calgary Board of Education.

Donna Denney is a collaborative associate faculty member in the School of Nursing, Dalhousie University, and teaches undergraduate students.

Gail J. Donner is a professor and the Dean at the Faculty of Nursing, University of Toronto, where her research and practice interests include health policy, career development and bioethics. She has been honoured by several organizations for her contributions to nursing and to the community. She is listed in Canadian Who's Who and in Who's Who of Canadian Women.

Douglass Drozdow-St. Christian is a medical anthropologist and assistant professor in the Department of Anthropology, University of Western Ontario. He spent the last decade studying health and illness among older women throughout southern Ontario and among street-based sex trade youth in Toronto and Buffalo. He has worked as a consultant for UNICEF and the governments of Western Samoa and Fiji and as a research contributor to the World Health Organization's annual report.

Elizabeth Esteves is a doctoral student in the Department of Anthropology, Social/Cultural Section, University of Toronto.

Suzanne Foster is a collaborative associate faculty member in the School of Nursing, Dalhousie University, and teaches undergraduate students.

Frances Gregor is a full-time faculty member in the School of Nursing, Dalhousie University, and teaches undergraduate and graduate nursing students.

Doris Grinspun is the Executive Director of the Registered Nurses Association of Ontario. Prior to that Doris worked for twenty-two years in the hospital sector in staff nurse, advanced practice, and management positions. A native of Chile, she received her nursing education in Jerusalem, Tel Aviv, and the University of Michigan in Ann Arbor. She is currently a doctoral candidate in the Department of Sociology, York University. For the past ten years, Doris has also worked on many international projects with the World Health Organization in Latin and Central America.

Sepali Guruge received her MSc in the Ethnic and Pluralism Collaborative Program in the Faculty of Nursing at the University of Toronto. Her research interests include immigrants' and refugees' health issues and their access to health services. Born in Sri Lanka, she was first educated there and later in the Soviet Union and Canada. She is now the manager of the Women's Inpatient Unit, Society, Women and Health Program at the Centre for Addiction and Mental Health in Toronto.

Diana L. Gustafson is dual enrolled as a doctoral candidate in Sociology and Equity Studies in Education and the Institute for Women's Studies and Gender Studies, University of Toronto. She worked as a nurse and a clinical educator for many years before turning her focus to research. Currently, she is studying gender and race equity issues in the educational preparation of nurses.

Barbara Keddy is a full-time faculty member in the School of Nursing, Dalhousie University, and teaches undergraduate and graduate nursing students.

Janet M. Lum is an associate professor in the Department of Politics and School of Public Administration, Ryerson Polytechnic University.

Lynn Morrison is a Medical Anthropologist specializing in the area of women and HIV/AIDS in Canada and internationally. She received her Ph.D. from the University of Toronto. Her interests include gender and health, sexual decision-making and inequities in accessing health care. For eight years, she has been an AIDS educator and activist in the City of Toronto.

Sheila Porte is a long-time resident of Georgina Island. She is a registered nurse with experience in the institutional and community health sectors. Sheila currently works as a community health practitioner in the Town of Georgina and is a member of the Chippewas of Georgina emergency response team. She is also an active Hospice Georgina visiting volunteer caregiver and is pursuing continuing studies at Lakehead University.

Farah M. Shroff, Ph.D., is an educator, researcher and activist—primarily in the health field. Her research interests include social justice issues, holistic health, women's health, child/family health. She edited and contributed to *The New Midwifery—Reflections on Renaissance and Regula-*

tion. She lives in Vancouver where she teaches medical/dental students and conducts health research.

Patricia E. Simpson is a long-time resident of Keswick in the Town of Georgina, Ontario, and a past executive director of Hospice Georgina. She is a doctoral student at the Ontario Institute for Studies in Education, University of Toronto. For the past ten years, Patricia has worked in the area of community and international development among diverse populations, including the Ojibwa and Cree Nations in Canada and the Romany people of Eastern Europe.

Denise L. Spitzer teaches women's studies at the University of Alberta where she is also Co-Director of the Centre for the Cross-Cultural Study of Health and Healing. Her primary academic and activist interests lie in the area of women's health and the health impact of social inequality.

Si Transken is a social worker with a private practice for women who have experienced trauma and oppression. She is listed in Who's Who of Canadian Women for her work as an activist in her Northern Ontario community. She identifies as an ecofeminist, almost-vegan, amateur Buddhist, bisexual, biclass (white trash recycled and now middle-class wannabe), person in love with progressive ideas—and in love with other persons who promote progressive ideas.

A. Paul Williams is an associate professor in the Department of Health Administration, University of Toronto.

Acknowledgements

Bringing together this collection has been a rewarding experience and there are many people to whom I owe my gratitude. In particular, I thank the contributors for their passionate commitment to this work and the collaborative spirit they brought to this project. I am honoured that Pat Armstrong, one of the outspoken critics of Canadian health care reform, agreed to write a forward to this collection. The thoughtful comments of many reviewers enhanced the chapters and I acknowledge the generosity of Cecilia Benoit, Marie Campbell, Carol Couchie, Keith Denney, Gail J. Donner, Frances Gregor, Jane Krilyk, June Larkin, Paula Maurutto, Susanne Nelson, Roxana Ng, Si Transken, Dorothy E. Smith and Pamela Wakewich. To my colleagues at OISE/University of Toronto and the new friends I have met during this journey, I thank you most sincerely for enriching my intellectual life. In particular, I thank Margrit Eichler for her wisdom and spirited encouragement as I negotiated this process. My thanks to Errol Sharpe who recognized the value of this collection and supported my efforts as a first-time editor, and to Beverley Rach, Brenda Conroy and Jackie Logan at Fernwood for their contributions to this book. I am also deeply indebted to Debra Bélanger for sharing her friendship and sage advice throughout the process and for her skillful review of the original manuscript. Finally, to my partner, Richard Kater, I offer my sincerest thanks for the love and countless acts of material support that helped make this work possible.

Foreword

Pat Armstrong

These are indeed revolutionary times. And nowhere is this revolution more obvious than in health care. It is a revolution in discourses and practices; in values and methods; in institutions and communities; in states and households.

The language of this revolution in health is seductive. There is talk of community and care closer to home; of evidence-based practices and evidence-based decision-making; of consumer choice and flattened hierarchies; of patient rights and patient-focused care; of team work and empowerment; of integration and continuity; of efficiency and effectiveness; of quality and accountability; of the determinants of health rather than the medical model; of report cards and gender-based analysis.

As is the case in most revolutions, the alternatives are set out as stark dichotomies. Either you are endorsing the way health care is being transformed or hopelessly supporting an outmoded system. Either you are in favour of hospital mergers or stupidly defending expensive old buildings that wastefully duplicate services. Either you embrace one-stop shopping for health care or you want to struggle on with a disconnected system that leaves gaping holes in services. Either you participate in managerial strategies to continually improve quality and remove wasteful practices or you represent special interests that stand in the way of lower cost, quality care. Either you love your mother and are willing to do the care work for her or you refuse to take the responsibility that goes along with citizenship. Either you defend equity as defined by formulas that treat everyone the same or you defend discrimination. Either you agree with deregulation that removes the monopolies from doctors and nurses or you are complicit in the perpetuation of rigid structures of power that interfere with efficient management. Either you believe in evidence of the sort provided and the way it is used or you reject evidence as a basis for decision-making.

The language of this revolution has a great deal of appeal for feminists. This should not be surprising, given that much of the language was first brought into currency by feminists. And many women find themselves on the revolution side of the dichotomies. This too should not be surprising, given that feminists have been among the most vocal critics of the public health care system and the services it provides.

This book is an excellent tonic for those who feel seduced by the language of health "reform" and forced to choose between the alternatives. In carefully documented and thoughtfully theorized ways, the articles demonstrate both the complexity of reforms and their contradictory nature. They reveal how the discourses and other practices of reform play out in women's daily lives as employees, volunteers, relatives, patients and decision-makers.

Placed within the context of the dominant business paradigm the articles focus on the details of particular aspects of reform in particular locations, often in terms of how they affect women from a particular community. At the same time, the articles move back and forth between the particular and the general or abstract, in the process making the personal political and the political personal.

What is revealed is how these new relations of ruling serve to further limit women's alternatives. Exposed as well are the specific impacts on the women who are already the most marginalized and the women who provide the paid and unpaid care.

After reading these articles, few will accept that the language of reform has the same meaning for feminists and reformers. And few will remain convinced that it is necessary to choose between this reform and no reform. The dichotomies no longer feel like clear alternatives. It is possible to be in and against the state; to support public care while seeking to change it; to resource communities while working to alter institutional care for those who need it; to critique the medical model while recognizing the need for expertise; to provide continuity without limiting access through a single point and to a single service; to seek both equity and equality; to struggle for women's collective interests while accommodating differences among women.

1

Introduction:
Health Care Reform and its Impact
on Canadian Women

Diana L. Gustafson

From coast to coast to coast, Canadian women as care providers and care recipients are responding to health care reform in the 1990s. Our stories and struggles are as diverse as we are. First Nations, Vietnamese-Canadian and Indo-Canadian women strive to be heard in a large western city hospital with too few staff and other resources to provide them with culturally and linguistically appropriate care during their childbirth experience. A group of older women in southern Ontario challenge traditional health resources, opting instead to shape and control their own definition of health care and what it means to age well. Nova Scotia nurses displaced by hospital restructuring implement a variety of strategies to maintain their economic viability and professional identity. These and other critical accounts in this collection illustrate how diverse groups of women in various social and institutional contexts are navigating through a changing health care system—a system that does not necessarily function in the best interests of women; a system upon which many women rely for their wellbeing as caregivers and care recipients; a system that operates by its own complex logic.

Health care reform may be understood as the dynamic interplay among economic changes, the role of the state, institutional discourse and practices, and social reproduction within the public and private spheres. The literature points to five fundamental political and economic forces taking place in Canada and globally over the last decade. These are:

- a general emphasis on advancing technology (Duffy and Pupo 1992, Menzies 1996) and, specifically, new medical technologies (Armstrong and Armstrong 1994b, Maher and Riutort 1998);
- changes in the nature and distribution of work (Armstrong and Armstrong 1994a and 1994b, Baines et al. 1998, Cameron et al. 1994, Glazer 1993);

- the Free Trade Agreement, closer ties to the United States and the unity debate (Armstrong and Armstrong 1994b, Badgley and Wolfe 1992, Maher and Riutort 1998, O'Neill 1998);
- evolving demographic shifts (Badgley and Wolfe 1992, Maher and Riutort 1998, McDaniel and Gee 1993); and
- economic trends toward growing consumerism, higher unemployment, transnational corporations and global economies (Cameron and Finn 1998, O'Neill 1998).

Collectively these political and economic changes are informing the assumptions, processes and outcomes of health care reform across Canada.

One assumption underlying reform is what Harley Dickinson calls "the neoliberal imperative of public sector health cost-containment" (1996: 187). Cost-containment is not a new theme in Canadian health care debates. In a study of 243 health policy documents from all regions of Canada dating from 1974 to 1994, cost-containment is the overarching theme (Shroff 1996). Indeed, since universal medical insurance was implemented, all levels of government have undertaken measures, at least rhetorically, to contain medical costs (O'Neill 1998, Shroff 1996). While the push to contain costs and improve care is not new, changes implemented in the 1990s swept through institutions and penetrated the everyday lives of Canadians.

Grounded in what Jan Angus calls the "discourse of scarcity" (1994: 36), strategic plans implemented at the federal, provincial and municipal levels were aimed at containing costs and improving efficiencies. These plans resulted in sweeping health sector reordering, hospital downsizing, amalgamations and closures, job displacement and work redesign, and rationalization and regionalization of service provision. Canadians who re-elected their provincial and federal governments were persuaded by the rhetoric about consumer involvement in decision-making and a realignment of priorities toward health promotion and disease prevention. The promises of more accessible, higher quality care are very different from the actual consequences of reform. The preoccupation with cost-containment and short-term deficit reduction coupled with minimal community consultation (O'Neill 1998) and inadequate long-range health planning (Storch 1996) is proving detrimental to the health of Canadians. And as this volume attests, it is especially detrimental to the health and wellbeing of many diverse groups of women.

While this volume was being compiled in 1999, the Social Sciences and Humanities Research Council of Canada (SSHRCC), an independent, federal research funding agency, issued a challenge to the academic community. They called on researchers in the social sciences, humanities and health sciences to develop new ways of understanding health and health care in "the increasingly complicated environment in which Canadians live." This new direction for funded research is intended to encourage collaboration across disciplines and with community groups in building richer, more layered knowledge about the health of Canadians and Canadian institutions. Investing in research partnerships signals a recognition that neither the current model of health care nor the recent health care reforms are serving the needs of Canadians. Sadly, this initiative also serves as a stark reminder of the marginalization of social scientific theory and the long-standing dominance of the biomedical model in the development of Canadian health policy and popular thinking about health and health care.

For years prior to this initiative, researchers in the social sciences and humanities have addressed SSHRCC's central theme of society, culture and the health of Canadians (Bolaria and Dickinson 1988 and 1994, Coburn et al. 1998). Some literature focuses on the health of specific Canadian populations, such as Aboriginal communities (Waldram et al. 1995), racialized minorities (Bolaria and Bolaria 1994), the aged (Marshall and McPherson 1995) and women at work (Messing et al. 1995). Other issues examined include the role of community nursing in promoting Canadians' health (Stewart 1995) and childbirth in the Canadian North (O'Neil and Gilbert 1990). Still other research explores the history of the Canadian health care system, its funding arrangements and the centrality of the biomedical model (Armstrong and Armstrong 1994a and 1994b, Armstrong et al. 1997, Stingl and Wilson 1996). Clearly, researchers in the social sciences and humanities have established their commitment to exploring various aspects of the historical, social, cultural and economic factors impacting on Canadians' health and health care.

This volume continues this commitment by exploring the link between the restructuring of health care in Canada and the restructuring of women's lives as health care providers and health care recipients. Until now, the small but important works that explore the link between women and health reform draw their explanatory power from a focus on capitalism and institutionalized patriarchy, or on the axis of male/female dominance/subordination. The use of gender as a category of analysis makes at least two assumptions. First, categories of female and male are not discrete but are constructed in relation to one another. Second, differences attributed to each sex are not neutral but contribute to unequal power relations (Pan American Health Organization [PAHO] 1997: 27–30).

This collection moves beyond a singular focus on gender to the use of a more integrated analytic lens that embraces three additional principles. First, women are not an homogenous group. Women's experiences of health and health care are varied, dynamic and historically and regionally located. How a woman thinks about health, perceives her own health and engages in health practices are interconnected. Furthermore, how women, individually and as members of social groups, come to understand health and health care is shaped by beliefs and social practices about gender, age, race/ethnicity and social class that are firmly embedded in our health care institutions, political processes and legislative policies. Consider the way that state institutional structures and processes embody and impart dominant beliefs about sex/gender, ethnoracial diversity, aging and other social differences. The historic and systemic nature of gender and racial inequalities is reproduced by legislated reform initiatives and enacted and experienced in various institutional and social settings (Bakker 1996, Connell 1990, Pettman 1992, Yeatman 1994). Thus, social differences including sex and gender shape each woman's experience of health, and, by extension, our responses to health care reform. Therefore, an integrated gender lens reflects the multiplicities of women's experiences, histories, and social and political locations.

This leads to a second principle underlying the integrated gender lens assumed in this volume—that is, a recognition that gender is context-specific (PAHO 1997). Age, race/ethnicity, class and a web of other social differences filter and organize women's everyday ways of thinking about and performing our health. By complicating women's location as the gendered subordinate in a male-dominated world, this volume reveals that some women more than others are disadvantaged by reform initiatives and these disadvantages are experienced in different ways. Attention to diversity is further reflected in the personal histories and disciplinary perspectives that the contributing authors bring to their work. Our various social locations as researchers, educators, health practitioners and activists organize how we come to think about health care reform, the kinds of questions we ask and the critical lens we use to make sense of the myriad social, economic and political consequences we observe. The result is a rich, multi-disciplinary resource for senior undergraduates, graduate students and academics in women's studies, health sciences, labour studies and the sociology of health. Additionally, this collection provides policymakers and health professionals with a lucid and accessible discussion of the issues affecting diverse groups of women and offers recommendations for responding to and influencing change.

Looking to the future and imagining woman-positive change calls attention to a third principle guiding the use of an integrated gender lens. Gender roles and relations are not fixed or static categories (Lather 1991). They are fluid and change from one political or historical location to the next. Examining historical changes in caregiving activities like midwifery, nursing and hospital volunteering provides insight into the ways that current reforms are shaping some women's participation in the health care system.

Considering Canadian health reform in historical and contemporary contexts draws attention to a second analytic dimension that frames this collection. In addition to the integrated gender lens, the element "time" is a thematic which emerges. Time may be understood as a process experienced biologically and socially as in the developmental process of human aging. As women mature, our bodies change in response to normal physiological processes, disease, injury and the social and economic context of our lives. Thus our health needs change and so does our relationship to the health care system. Women need adequate time to invest in our wellness as long-term projects. All women need time to meet, to share our concerns, to raise our political voices and to lobby effectively for change. Having adequate time is necessary to women's healthful living.

Time is also a vital tool in the paid and unpaid work women perform. Having enough time is as necessary as having any other material resource. Care providers need adequate time to assess health needs, plan and negotiate care options and provide care to their clients. Moreover, each day brings new ideas and new technologies. Care providers need time to educate themselves—to embrace new ways of thinking and develop new skills. Reform initiatives that cut staff and resources deny many women the time they need to work wisely and well and in the best interests of those they serve.

Market-driven strategies implemented in health care settings use time as a measure of efficiency and work productivity. The use of workload measurement tools is one of many strategies used to justify cuts to staff and resources. While the instrumental or technical aspects of caring labour are more easily quantified, the emotional aspects of care, which also take time, are not. Nor does each client have the same needs for the emotional aspects of care. Still, any given set of caregiving activities is associated with a standardized time allocation as if it were a task performed by an automaton on an object, rather than the human interaction that it is. Staffing and individual workloads are assigned in accordance with these abstracted time calculations. This cost-saving strategy is about task completion rather than care delivery. The focus is on the job, not on the caregiver and the care recipient involved in the activity. When a caregiver's time is squeezed to the margin, there is little time to provide care in a caring way—to be truly present in the moment. The time of homecare workers, nurses and social workers is managed by processes external to them and their professional decision-making.

Time is also understood as a flexible commodity used to organize a predominantly female workforce of caregivers. Health sector restructuring transforms caring labour into part-time, insecure work. For example, principles guiding agency staffing now resemble the principles of just-in-time delivery currently in vogue in industrial settings. Nurses and other care providers are called on short notice to work a shift with a heavier than usual workload. Conversely, part-time and casual workers can be sent home on short notice when demand falls. By providing just-in-time health care, the institution saves money on full-time wages and benefits. However, just-in-time health care sacrifices the quality of care and the quality of women's personal and professional lives.

Women's time may also be understood as personal property appropriated for the common good. Reform initiatives driven by economic considerations reassign work from the hospital to the home and from paid skilled labour to unpaid family members. Hospital and community volunteers and women engaged in unpaid caregiving work in the home complete labour processes begun by paid workers in the hospital. In this way, "work transfer" (Glazer 1993: 28), a process that rationalizes the use of labour, reduces labour costs, increases revenues in the private service economy and contributes directly to the wellbeing of the economy.

Time is variously understood by the authors as a vital tool, a scarce resource, a flexible commodity and appropriated personal property. Time is also a factor in the various stories that were left out of this volume. One woman withdrew her proposal following the premature birth of her tiny son, anticipating the hundreds of hours she would need to devote to her role as primary caregiver. Another woman withdrew because her own health problems prevented her from adding this project to her considerable workload as wife, mother, researcher and community activist. There are no accounts in this volume about the impact of reform on women with disabilities and chronic illnesses. As Sally A. Kimpson points out, few have time left after caring for their basic daily needs to enrich their health in other substantive ways or to undertake writing and research projects (personal communication, Oct. 24, 1998). Absent, too, are the stories of homeless women and those living in subsistence housing. One author intended to contribute a follow-up story on a nurse displaced by hospital downsizing who was living with her daughter in a series of cheap hotels and homeless shelters. The initial story documented this woman's daily struggle to acquire the basic necessities to sustain their physical and mental wellbeing (Gadd 1997). Despite an exhaustive search, the woman and her daughter were not found—disappearing from the system and from this account of women's lives under health care reform.

Overview of the Chapters

The integrated gender lens and the analytic dimension of time frame the overview of the chapters in this anthology, which begins with a critical examination of the shift from the cure-care paradigm to the business paradigm and its impact on hospital management, patient care and care providers. Doris Grinspun traces the historical development of management theories that inform current health reform initiatives. In what she refers to as "the race to the bottom line," Grinspun argues that there is little empirical evidence supporting the cost-effectiveness or quality outcomes promised by business models. There is, she points out, evidence that market-driven strategies impact negatively on women care providers and care recipients. The political-economy framework used in this chapter to examine the business paradigm provides the foundation for discussions advanced in subsequent chapters.

Hospital downsizing, amalgamations and closures are having a profound impact on a labour-intensive health sector largely comprised of women and nurses. Janet M. Lum and A. Paul Williams show how these cost-cutting initiatives combined with the introduction of the *Regulated Health Professions Act* (RHPA) resulted in unanticipated and negative consequences for women health providers. Initially, the RHPA was considered a progressive piece of legislation. It was intended to remove barriers among health disciplines and promote autonomy and more equitable status and participation among the various (and emerging, female-dominated) health professions. While some gains were realized, the RHPA also intensified historical divisions among and within health professions and reinforced complex hierarchies among caregivers. Analyzing the response of the Ontario nursing profession illustrates this point. Registered nurses pushing for greater professionalization are divided against other categories of nurses and unregulated care providers, all trying to defend their jobs and caregiving terrain. These divisions are further complicated by race/ethnicity, class and country of origin, as minoritized women are concentrated in the lower paid, less prestigious positions most vulnerable to staffing cuts.

Frances Gregor, Barbara Keddy, Suzanne Foster and Donna Denney continue the discussion of hospital restructuring and changing employment patterns in their qualitative study of Nova Scotia nurses. Displaced nurses, uncertain about short- and long-term employment, use a range of strategies to secure both nursing and non-nursing work and make themselves accessible to employers. For nurses with childcare responsibilities, this often means depending on the help of other women—family and friends. This study illustrates that organizing a workforce of women based on the assumption that time is a flexible commodity has short- and long-term economic and political implications for nurses and the institutions who employ them. The authors speculate that the poor treatment of nurses by governments, hospitals and health agencies during this period of restructuring may be a factor in the so-called nursing shortage some institutions now face.

Time is also a scarce resource for the obstetrical nurses in Denise L. Spitzer's qualitative study of the childbirth experiences of First Nations, Indo-Canadian and Vietnamese-Canadian women. Spitzer examines the efforts of these women, in a large, culturally-diverse, western city hospital, to assert their needs and create more positive childbirth experiences. Frustration and anger are common to the stories of these new mothers and their nurses. The new mothers are generally dissatisfied, noting a lack of responsiveness from nurses and a lack of adequate and appropriate support both in hospital and at home. The nurses are generally distressed because staffing cuts and higher patient care loads mean they have too little time to provide even basic care, to perform a thorough assessment, to follow through appropriately and to follow-up in a timely fashion. Some admit to avoiding patients with whom they anticipate communication problems—patients who need more time and attention than they feel they can give.

Time to be with women during pregnancy, labour and birthing is also a theme in Jane Cawthorne's chapter on maternal care delivery in Alberta. In May 1998, Alberta's obstetricians and gynecologists began a lengthy job action in which they refused to accept new patients. These specialists were hoping to highlight a growing concern within their profession, but their actions left pregnant women in the province feeling they were without options or advocates. Cawthorne argues that a lack of options is at the heart of the problem with maternal care delivery, a fact that the job action and the dominant voices in health care obscure. She situates the job action within this wider context by incorporating the voices of midwives into a more comprehensive view of the goals of health care and health care reform. The author recommends sweeping changes to the delivery of maternal services—changes that will improve conditions for both midwives and pregnant and birthing women, especially those living in poverty and in rural or isolated areas.

Social workers are another group of health professionals fighting against the dominance of the biomedical and business models. Drawing on extensive interviews with social workers in sexual assault treatment (SAT) programs and sexual assault crisis centres (SACC), Si Transken examines the effects of cutbacks to services for women who have been sexually violated. Women's options and access to caring services are shrinking and so is the time in which they are expected to heal physically, emotionally and spiritually from sexual assault. Agency workers are increasingly operating within a system that compartmentalizes and quantifies women's pain and limits the amount of time they have to give their clients. Central to Transken's analysis is the way that responses to victims' needs are being reshaped away from a grassroots and feminist social justice model toward a depoliticized, business-oriented model of care. This includes the trend toward Brief Solution Focused therapy, a therapeutic model which is expected to reduce health care costs by accelerating treatment time. Transken asserts that limiting time for giving and receiving care negatively impacts on social workers, their clients and the community at large.

Elizabeth Esteves' chapter examines the work of hospital volunteers historically and in the context of current health care reform. This anthropological study examines changes in volunteering, an important and largely unexamined topic in Canadian health care. Once the work of white, English Protestant, middle-class, middle-aged and older women, volunteer participation is changing. Now membership is younger, includes both females and males and is more diverse in terms of class and race / ethnicity. Changes in volunteer work, like paid work, are aimed at increasing productivity and intensifying task-based activities through greater administrative control. Esteves argues that the hospital volunteer, with less time to *give* care, is being reconstructed as a wageless worker.

Diana L. Gustafson examines how women's time is being appropriated for the public good through the restructuring of home care services. This chapter explores one way in which government goals of cost-containment and efficiency penetrate the actual work processes of women working in home care agencies. She compares two administrative procedures: one in place prior to and one in place after major restructuring of home care services. Her analysis illustrates how the process of coordinating home care services has been reconstituted so that health care workers come to act in business-oriented ways that may not be consistent with their knowledge and perspective, and that contribute to the downloading of caring labour onto other women who are unpaid and often untrained and unprepared to assume this burden.

As in the preceding chapter, Patricia E. Simpson and Sheila Porte also use everyday experience as the standpoint from which to explore institutional practices. This chapter documents the efforts of local organizers to respond to the needs of both Native and non-Native residents by designing an integrated community-based health service. Central to the gaps in health service delivery in this northern community is the reduction of multiple, complex identities and differences in places of residence into two monolithic groupings—"white / mainland resident" versus "Chippewa / island resident." Simpson and Porte show how the historical and contemporary factors shaping these groupings further complicated efforts to negotiate the fragmented and increasingly complex bureaucratic maze ushered in by health care restructuring.

Negotiating a complex health care bureaucracy is also a problem for women who are recent immigrants and refugees and who also face discrimination, marginalization and difficulties with language and cultural adjustment. Sepali Guruge, Gail J. Donner and Lynn Morrison identify three areas where changes to the health care system are most deeply felt by this group of women: the shift to increased patient participation in care; the shift toward health promotion and disease prevention; and the shift toward community- and home-based care. The authors propose practical ways for improving health care for immigrant and refugee women that will ultimately benefit all Canadian women as care providers and care recipients.

Attention to alternative strategies effecting woman-positive change continues in the next chapter. Douglass Drozdow-St. Christian examines how a diverse group of aging women actively resist being victimized by shrinking health care resources. Based on a long-term ethnographic study of gender and aging among women in several urban centres in southern Ontario, this chapter explores the emergence of a "contestatory ground of engagement" between older women and a health care system characterized by political expedience. In a period of diminishing access to traditional health resources, older women are devising strategies for healthy aging. Whether taking on new political responsibilities through activism, building new social networks for shared caregiving or exploring alternative health models, aging women are responding to a collapse of the expectations with which they prepared for their old age.

In the concluding chapter, Farah M. Shroff questions the utility of reforming a health care system that is centred on the male-dominated, biomedical model. She proposes, instead, a "revolutionary agenda for transforming health care in Canada." This would require a shift away from the dominance of allopathic medicine enshrined in federal, provincial and municipal legislation toward an entirely new approach to health care that is based on social justice principles and holistic principles and practices. Combining proven aspects of allopathic medicine with the valuable aspects of other health systems practised around the world, a "holistic-multiparadigmatic health care" has the potential to improve the health of all Canadians.

2

Taking Care of the Bottom Line:
Shifting Paradigms in Hospital Management[1]

Doris Grinspun

Introduction

The management of North American hospitals has experienced in the last decade a shift from a cure-care paradigm to a business paradigm. The shift has been promoted through a re-conceptualization of hospitals as financially competitive enterprises and implemented through a series of management and marketing strategies, of which the most transformative has been re-engineering. These trends in hospital management follow very similar ones in the corporate world. The increasing emphasis on the measurement of cost outcomes above health outcomes does not serve the interests of care recipients. Furthermore, it protects the interests of some categories of care providers (physicians and administrators) at the expense of others (nurses). This chapter explores the new management paradigm, its application in hospitals and its possible implications. The chapter also puts into a broad context the remaining chapters in this book by tracing the evolution of management theories on which health care reforms in Canada are advanced.

A paradigm is a set of universally recognized guiding principles (Kuhn 1962). Paradigms are central models that provide direction to policy formulation and guide the given responses to internal and external needs or pressures. The goal of the business paradigm ranges from reaching balanced budgets to creating profitable enterprises. In the field of health administration, this means finding efficient and cost-effective ways to organize hospital operations. It also means introducing a discourse that changes the way we think about, and act, during our day-to-day encounters with patients. With the business paradigm, the emphasis is on achieving a competitive edge by using specific management tools such as product-line management, program management and re-engineering. The cure-care paradigm, in contrast, emphasizes the service aspect of hospital management. The traditional focus of this approach was the pursuit of curative excellence. Throughout the 1980s, the focus expanded to include curative and carative excellence.[2] The goal of this paradigm is to gain a competitive edge through excellence in medical and psychosocial services. It is important to note that neither paradigm completely ignores the curative-carative or the business aspects of its operations. It is the significantly higher relative weight given to each of these imperatives that characterizes one paradigm from the other.

This chapter examines the shifting power relations in hospital management, a critical outcome associated with the shift toward the business paradigm. A select group of physicians and administrators—traditionally male—have gained greater power to influence, direct and control the decision-making process. At the same time, the power base of nurses—traditionally female—has been eroded and so has their influence over decisions. Nurses play a key role as gatekeepers of quality and resource utilization. There are many ramifications of weakening nurses' presence and power as decision-makers. Caring, a central aspect of nursing practice, suffers from the race to the bottom line. The fragmented and rushed approach to nursing care promoted by the business paradigm does not allow for the human connectedness which is necessary for caring relationships to flourish. Furthermore, heightened power imbalances between physicians, administrators and nurses translate into a weakened position for patients within the hospital structure. As structural changes diminish nurses' ability to influence decision-making, nursing's role in patient advocacy is similarly compromised.

Theories of Change in Organizational Design and Regime of Production

The conceptual underpinnings for the business paradigm in health care can be traced to theories of change in organizational design and regime of production. The current debate on hospital and health care restructuring relies heavily on sociological, economic and industrial engineering discussions. In particular, the paradigm shift within the hospital sector in North America is informed by three movements to develop new forms of organizing production. The first one originated in the late 1890s under the heading of "scientific management"; the second one was the growth of "Fordism" in the early twentieth century; and the third one involves "post-Fordist" and "flexible specialization" regimes of production and management.

Scientific management or "Taylorism" (following its main proponent, F.W. Taylor) is a set of rules for the design of production in the workplace that entails separating mental from manual labour, subdivision of tasks, deskilling, close managerial control of work effort and incentive wage payments. This management strategy aims for tight pre-set specifications of tasks embedded in a high division of labour. It embodies three main principles: fragmenting work into simple, routine operations; standardizing each operation to eliminate idle times; and separating conception from execution—i.e., the design and control of work remain a management prerogative.

Taylorism assumes that individuals are, by nature, lazy and instrumental in their attitude to work. This view is consistent with neo-classical economics and individualistic theories in psychology. An engineer by training, Taylor conceptualized work as measurable tasks that could be broken down into constituent parts. Various physical motions were precisely timed with a view to reorganizing jobs to achieve the most efficient use of effort and to maximize productivity gains. Closely monitoring time and motion characteristics of work required a hierarchical management organization with clear lines of authority and spans of control. Thus, Taylorism, as a work design, legitimated management control over workers and the workplace.[3]

The term Fordism relates to Henry Ford's innovations in the production process and their associated social and political consequences. Fordism refers to the introduction of mass production of a standardized product and is characterized by capital-intensive large-scale plants, inflexible production processes, rigid and hierarchical managerial structures and the use of semi-skilled labour doing routine and repetitive tasks (subject to the discipline of scientific management). Ford's innovations in the production of cars in the interwar period were readily shifted to other sectors of manufacturing and served as the organizational basis on which the industrialized economies grew after World War II. The provision of services under the growing concept of the "welfare state" was directly related to the Fordist concepts of scale of production, central control, standardization and mass consumption. Thus, in simple schematic form, until the 1970s, the North American way of organizing production and management was based on this joint application of Taylorist and Fordist methods.[4]

Starting in the mid-1970s, there were dramatic changes in the forms of organization and practice of manufacturing activity. These changes represent a shift from a Fordist to a post-Fordist regime. Bernard (1994: 216) summarizes the main components of post-Fordism as involving: small-batch production of a variety of products; the use of flexible machinery; a physical reorganization of the factory to reduce inventories and defects; a decentralization of manufacturing-related decision-making to workers on the shop floor; and the application of microelectronics to product and process design and to production machinery. Post-Fordism is an offspring of the computer revolution and is deeply dependent on the intensive use of microchip technology, computers and robotics in the production process. The ability to produce a larger variety of specialized goods and services in smaller batches using flexible machinery and workforce is sometimes called flexible specialization—a term synonymous with post-Fordism.

Management structure also shifted from the integrated corporation to a network of firms, and thus, to a less hierarchical and more decentralized structure of management. Each smaller unit caters to a specialized market. To conform to the flexible work organization, the labour process became more flexible and decentralized. The labour market was reorganized into a skill-flexible core of employees and a time-flexible periphery of low-paid insecure workers performing contract labour. The traditional unionized blue-collar working class declined while a segmented labour force grew. On one side were white-collar, professional, technical, managerial workers and on the other side were low-paid, easily dispensable and mostly unskilled workers, often women (Jary and Jary 1991).

A shift toward post-Fordism and the characteristic "lean production" regime in the general industrial area is part and parcel of the internationalization of production, the growth of a corporate culture of globalization and the impact of Japanese management techniques. The keywords of this management trend have become ubiquitous: efficiency, cost-effectiveness, elimination of duplication, flexibility, clear processes, etcetera. Of particular importance to lean production and flexible specialization is the multi-skilling of workers. Indeed, these keywords of post-Fordist approaches serve as the intellectual grounding and discourse for the new business paradigm in hospital management.

Hospital Management: Shifting to a Business Paradigm

This section describes the new models of organizational design as they are applied to the hospital environment. The move from departments and divisional design to product-line management, program management and re-engineering are explored within the theories of change in organizational design and regime of production.

During the 1980s and 1990s, American and Canadian hospitals faced a changing economic and political environment. This included the move toward free-market economic policies and the spread of a predominant ideology of corporate globalization. The American approach toward the privatization of public services soon placed pressure on, and encroached upon, the autonomous role of the Canadian public sector. Canadian hospitals became increasingly threatened in terms of their financial support from governments. Their traditional ideology of caring and public service lost legitimacy in the face of a corporate offensive to redefine the public sector.

Several developments coalesced to promote this transformation: a drastic reduction in federal transfer payments (through the 1995 Canada Health and Social Transfer Program), continuous budget cuts to hospitals at the provincial level, and changes to the way by which hospitals receive funding. The growing pressure to promote a corporate perspective in hospital management was accompanied by a proliferation of management consulting firms marketing the "right solution" and the forceful introduction of a "health care industry discourse" emphasizing corporate goals, products and outcomes. Alongside persisted an intense and consistent message promoted by politicians and the media that fiscal deficits and a growing national and provincial debt means we cannot afford our health and social programs anymore.

This new economic and ideological environment was the foundation for a shift in management paradigm. Hospital administrators, seduced by the rhetoric or convinced by its ideology changed the way they run their organizations. "Organizational survival," a well-known slogan that embraced the myths and realities of economic pressures, meant hospitals refocused on cost-containment and achieving a competitive edge. The traditional focus on balancing the cost-quality equation was soon replaced by the search for "innovative solutions." One such solution was a paradigm shift in hospitals' management and operations. Tertiary care hospitals moved away from the traditional cure-care paradigm to a business one.

The shift in management paradigm is closely linked to new forms of hospital organizational design. The traditional paradigm driving the management of acute care hospitals can be viewed as functional or divisional or a combination of the two. In the functional design, the organization is divided into departments that deliver specific functions (i.e., departments such as: nursing, social work, laboratory, housekeeping and others). Leatt, Lemieux-Charles and Aird (1994) state that this type of organizational design is best suited for small organizations which have few goals and operate in a simple environment. A functional design does not respond to the needs of more complex organizations in which functions and goals are numerous. Within functional organizations, management activities such as budgeting, resource utilization and productivity, quality assurance and performance are organized according to key departments (Stuart and Sherrard 1987). Care delivery is divided into specific activities delivered by specialized individuals working within the given departments. This type of organizational design is most commonly found in nursing homes, long-term care facilities and small community hospitals (Leatt et al. 1994).

The divisional design, typically found in teaching hospitals and large community hospitals, is comprised by a number of medical units (i.e., divisions of surgery, medicine and obstetrics) that are semi-autonomous under the overall direction of the hospital. In the departmental/divisional model, elements of a functional design persist in the larger divisional design (i.e., if divisions such as surgery and medicine coexist with departments such as nursing, social work and occupational therapy). The guiding paradigm of the departmental/divisional model is the cure-care one. The decentralized design allows for greater specialization and expertise and greater control over resource use at the local level. However, according to Leatt and colleagues, a drawback of this type of decentralized management is that "semi-autonomous units can be difficult to coordinate, often behave competitively with each other, may develop goals that are not compatible with the corporate mission, and may produce duplication of services and activities" (1994: 2).

Diagnosis Related Groups (DRGs) provided the impetus for shifting from a cure-care paradigm, operationalized through functional departmental and divisional models, to a business paradigm, operationalized through product line and program management models (Stuart and Sherrard 1987). DRGs are a mechanism for hospital reimbursement introduced in the United States in the mid-1980s, following enormous pressures from the insurance industry. Under DRGs, hospitals are reimbursed a set fee for specific groups of diagnoses. Thus, there is a clear incentive to decrease the cost of service, which is most often achieved through streamlining processes and decreasing length of hospital stay. In Ontario, a similar shift occurred with the introduction of Case Mix Groups (CMGs) and its impact on funding formulas for hospitals. CMGs imposed new performance indicators geared towards improving efficiencies and reducing cost variances amongst similar hospitals. Thus, CMGs served to propel the shift from the cure-care paradigm to the business one. As is noted later, one of the outcomes of this shift toward the business paradigm is the decreasing weight, or the outright elimination, of some professional departments from the organizational design. Although the proponents of such transformation forecast clear benefits, there are pitfalls to this approach.

Product-line management, an innovation introduced in 1973 at the Johns Hopkins Hospital (Heyssel et al. 1984), expanded during the 1980s as the new management paradigm that could respond to the challenge represented by the implementation of DRGs. The basic premise of product-line management is that hospitals should be managed as a portfolio of businesses or what Leatt and colleagues call Strategic Business Units (SBUs). They state that "each SBU produces a defined product or service and it plans strategically to meet its own competitive needs while maintaining consistency with the organization as a whole" (Leatt et al. 1994: 2).[5] As Stuart and Sherrard write:

> In the United States, where hospitals typically are viewed as private sector institutions and where a competitive environment requires definition and promotion of hospital products to respond to various market demands, discussion has centred on the notion of product-line management. (1987: 54)

Product-line management was seen as a model that would provide the necessary structure, tools and direction to be able to respond to the new budgetary demands.

Program management is a related approach, which focuses on a set of activities addressing the needs of a particular group of patients (e.g., high-risk obstetrics). While some argue that program management is a more appropriate approach for the Canadian scene (Stuart and Sherrard 1987), in general, both product-line management and program management have been used interchangeably (Smith et. al 1989). Indeed, there are no fundamental differences between these two models, which are, in fact, complementary elements of the broader application of a business management paradigm. In product-line management the entire organization is divided into specific types of products. In program management the organization decides upon priority areas on which to focus, and products are defined only for these areas. Clearly, these two models are entirely congruent with one another. As if this barrage of technical jargon were not enough, it is noteworthy that in Canada product-line management was introduced with the much more appealing title of *patient-centred* or *patient-focused care.*[6]

Promoters of a business approach to hospital management appear imbued by a deep sense of the benefits of such approaches. Their perspectives derive from the wider discussion of a shift from Fordist to post-Fordist regimes of production and the emphasis on flexible specialization. They follow trendy fashions in the management literature produced by the latest gurus and business schools. Such has been the movement from Total Quality Management (TQM)/Continuous Quality Improvement (CQI), to re-engineering, to re-tooling, to branding and more to come.

Not surprisingly, the idea of product-line management came from the manufacturing industry, where there is a clear and well-defined line of products. Some controversy, though not sufficient, has risen as to the appropriateness of applying an industrial model to the health care system. Those few dissidents that raise their voice have stated "the product here [in health] is not cars or computer chips, but people"

(Registered Nurses Association of Ontario 1995). Unaware of the potential pitfalls or more likely ignoring them, management consultants rapidly conquered the health care environment. In the process, they are making huge profits and changing the conceptualization, discourse and service of health care.

The most transformative tool put to use by health care consultants and administrators in recent years has been the re-engineering one. Hospital re-engineering emulates the wider management trend by the same name. Its author is consultant Michael Hammer from Cambridge, Massachusetts (Bergman 1994). Kralovec, vice president of First Consulting Group in Long Beach, California stated: "the underlying premise of re-engineering is that business processes should be designed around related and interdependent tasks that together produce an outcome that fulfils a defined costumer need" (as cited in Bergman 1994: 28). Although it is difficult at first to discern how this definition differs from product-line management or program management, its underpinning values do reveal fundamental differences. While both product-line management and program management assume work re-design within a *given* context, re-engineering assumes the position that the key to success is *starting over*, or, as Hammer said, "beginning again with a clean sheet of paper" (as cited in Bergman 1994: 28). Thus, re-engineering, in its concept and in its practice, moves away from any existing context. As a result the re-engineering principles and practices can be readily transported from one organization to another with little variation. Indeed, re-engineering has moved as a mantra from one health care organization to another across North America and to other parts of the world.

Comparing re-engineering with previous initiatives such as Total Quality Management shows substantive differences. A common thread of TQM is worker-team problem solving. The process owners and stakeholders (line managers, workers, customers and suppliers) use the approach to continuously streamline processes that will enhance quality and efficiency. Re-engineering differs from TQM in two respects: first, while TQM is focused on continuous improvement (an incremental approach), re-engineering insists on the need for discontinuous improvement or breaking away from "outdated operations." Second, re-engineering breaks from previous approaches by requiring the introduction of state-of-the-art information technologies to achieve desired outcomes. Keywords of the re-engineering movement are efficiency, cost-effectiveness, elimination of duplication, flexibility and clear processes—concepts directly drawn from the broader post-Fordist literature. Of particular importance are elements of flexible specialization achieved through the multi-skilling of workers.

Under the retrospective payments of CMGs and related case costing formulas, similar hospitals have identical procedures reimbursed according to the same pay scale; thus, the most efficient hospital (the one having the lowest "cost per case") wins. Clearly, costing of hospital products and obtaining a competitive edge become the new rules of the game. New management trends epitomized by re-engineering are explicitly oriented to prepare the hospitals to thrive in this competitive environment. What began as a small shift when Johns Hopkins Hospital adopted the product-line management approach back in 1973 (Heyssel et al. 1984), culminated in a full-blown paradigm shift with the introduction of re-engineering. The most important landmark of the new paradigm is the a-contextual nature attributed to it. In other words, it is touted as universally transportable and applicable around the globe, despite vast cultural differences, societal needs and values in other contexts. Consistent with the new economy of flexible specialization and globalization this new paradigm attempts to close the chapter of the cure-care paradigm.

Impact of the Business Paradigm

To date, most ideas about product-line management, program management, re-engineering and other related strategies come from consultants who translate concepts from the general management field into the health care environment. Unfortunately, there has been insufficient systematic research done to evaluate the effects of these approaches on health care (Bigelow and Arndt 1994), and with few exceptions (Leatt et al. 1994: 2), these models have not been critically examined. Despite the lack of evidence, these approaches are presented as the ideal paradigm in which all is good and there are no possible pitfalls. However, significant gaps exist between their marketed claims and reports from those experiencing their impact in practice. This section looks at the impact of the business paradigm on organizational structures, power allocation and decision-making, clinical outcomes, caring encounters, costs and the community.

On Organizational Structures
Hospitals have re-engineered themselves by adopting program management structures, introducing flexible specialization, reducing inventories and significantly intensifying the use of information technology.[7] Organizational structures moved from a functional approach (departmental/divisional structure) to a programmatic approach organized around specific product-lines. As Leatt and colleagues state, strategic business units (SBUs) are set to plan and meet the needs of a defined product or service which represents usually groupings of alike patients.

To accomplish these goals, health care providers, professionals and others work for a specific SBU and report to the chair of that business unit. A consequence of this new structure has been the dismantling of professional departments such as nursing, occupational therapy, physical therapy, respiratory therapy and social work. In stark contrast, physicians have been exempted from this move by keeping their medical divisions intact. The special status of the medical profession is greatly due to their gate-keeping role. As the entry point of patients to the health care system, physicians have ultimate control over patients' admissions and discharges.

Regrettably, there is no available documentation detailing the rationale for the dismantling of professional departments or its possible effects on patient care.[8] Most literature discusses the dismantling of professional departments simply as one of the steps or components of program management (Nackel and Kues 1986). Cole and Brown (1988) state that decentralizing service and management to specific profit centres allows managers to manipulate resources within their particular services in a more dynamic way. However, there is no empirical evidence of cost-containment outcomes resulting from this approach. Thus, it is unclear whether dismantling professional departments positively contributes to cost-containment of hospital budgets, or if it is mainly used to re-allocate funds (and power) to other managerial structures (i.e., program chairs and administrative support).

Based on anecdotal accounts and a cursory review of various models in use in Ontario hospitals, it appears that hierarchical levels have not been reduced but rather reorganized around a program management structure. For example, within the traditional model, a staff nurse reported to a nurse manager who reported to a director of nursing who reported to a vice-president (four hierarchical levels). Within program management, a staff nurse reports to a unit administrator (from any health care discipline or from a business background), who reports to a program director (in general from a health care discipline), who reports to a vice-president (also four hierarchical levels). Deleted in the program management model are the discipline-specific managerial positions. Added, in their place, are managerial positions at the program level. Therefore, in practice, structural reorganization means a change in who assumes a managerial role rather than the creation of less hierarchical or less expensive administrative structures.

At the conceptual level, it is unclear how the move from functional departments or divisions to a programmatic approach will allow more cost-effective resource management. Consider, for example, the traditional departments of nursing, respiratory therapy and social work. In the functional model, each department was responsible for departmental budget targets. To achieve these targets, they might have changed clinical practices, adjusted staffing patterns or adjusted supply expenses in their own areas. In the programmatic approach, the program directors respond to budget targets set for the program by changing clinical practices, adjusting staffing patterns of one or more disciplines or adjusting supplies expenses. In both cases, targets are achieved by making adjustments congruent with clinical priorities. However, with the traditional approach, each professional discipline has more control over choosing the best strategy for achieving the required savings. With the programmatic approach, decisions are made at the program level where it is doubtful that strategies would result in more cost-effective outcomes.

Some might argue that the cost-effectiveness of the programmatic approach results from enhanced coordination among health care providers. In other words, consensual decision-making among the various disciplines allows for a better response to budgetary requirements while at the same time respecting patient needs. This argument emerges from post-Fordist literature on the team concept where the team (i.e., the program) is presumed to find better responses to challenges than individual workers (or segregated professional groups). The argument is linked to two critical conditions. First, it assumes that patients' needs drive decisions. Second, it assumes that the process of decision-making is truly participatory and that all disciplines have a similar relative weight in terms of their power and authority to influence decisions. No doubt, if these two assumptions existed in reality, programmatic decision-making would be ideal to achieve what is best for patients. Neither of these conditions is a priority of the business paradigm as the following discussion illustrates.

On the Allocation of Power and Decision-Making
The new organizational structure clearly strengthens the physicians and administrators' span of control while that of nurses and other health care disciplines diminishes.[9] These results are congruent with a strategy of program management, that is, to increase physician involvement in resource utilization with the goal of improving cost-effectiveness (Ellis and Gaskin 1988). As Patterson and Thompson point out:

> The initial business strategy must be built upon a real need to achieve a closer relationship between operations, the hospital's physicians, and the markets they serve. To achieve this relationship, medical and management must perceive product line management staff as a mutually beneficial tool. In short, it must be perceived as a 'win-win' proposition. (1987: 70–72)

Indeed, in business models such as program management, physicians are positioned in strategic roles within formal structures of organizational power where they have more control over resource allocation and cost-containment. As a result, physicians have gained even greater influence within the hospital system. However, the growing power differentials brought about by the shift to the business paradigm may ultimately have a negative impact on the relationship between physicians and other health disciplines and on the planning and implementation of patient care.[10]

The literature is already saturated with theoretical as well as descriptive accounts of power imbalances amongst health care professionals (Abbott and Claire 1990, Rachlis and Kushner 1989). The particular way in which program management has been implemented exacerbates the existing power imbalance by the general tendency to place physicians as chairs, or at least as co-chairs, of programs. Moreover, the chosen physicians tend to be the ones that hold the highest hierarchical status within their divisions and the organization as a whole. The outcome is that a select group of physicians and administrators gain greater power to influence, direct and control the decision-making process. While program management is supposed to decentralize the process of decision-making, in reality, when increased power and prestige are allocated to those already enjoying a higher status within the organization, the opposite result is achieved.

One reason that program management appears to increase participation is that it entails greater team involvement, through, for example, interdisciplinary program meetings. However, a meeting may or may not be a participatory environment, depending on the power structures that underlie the groups represented in the meeting and the nature of the decision-making process. Consider a context where the so-called allied health disciplines have lost power within the organization through weakened or dismantled professional departments and where the program itself is managed in a non-participatory fashion. In this case, a meeting can serve to assert dominance rather than diffuse hierarchical power bases and promote a participatory approach.

Flexible specialization further adds to the complexity of power differentials and ability to influence amongst physicians, health care administrators and nurses. Flexible specialization entails replacing full-time staff (who have sick time benefits) with casual and/or non-unionized part-time employees. This strategy is compatible with some post-Fordist tendencies to weaken labour unions and increase the flexibility of the workforce. This contributes to the creation of a segmented labour market with a primary market for a minority of highly paid, full-time and secure jobs and a much larger secondary labour market characterized by short term contracts, part-time, casual, often lower skill, low wage and low benefit jobs.[11] Such segmentation will inevitably contribute to further deterioration of staff morale, stress related to job insecurity, lack of risk taking initiative and entrepreneurial spirit, disincentives to specialization and skilling and absence of loyalty and commitment to the workplace. Clearly, this type of workforce loses its ability to influence both because of lower status and limited opportunity for engaging in any kind of participatory initiatives. Collectively, these shifts in power allocation and decision-making impact on patients' clinical outcomes.

On Patients' Clinical Outcomes

Re-engineering and patient-centred care can be described as a lived contradiction. Two key tools heavily used in re-engineering, "flexible specialization" and "multi-skilling," negatively impact on the ability to provide patient-centred care.

Flexible specialization requires a skill-flexible core of employees who work on a full-time permanent basis and a time-flexible large proportion that work on a part-time or casual basis. In the case of Ontario nurses, over 50 percent belong to the "time-flexible" category—that is, 36.2 percent of the province's nurses self-report part-time employment and 14.2 percent self-report casual employment (College of Nurses of Ontario 1999a). The implications for patient-centred care are enormous. It means that patients receive nursing care every day from a different nurse. And lack of continuity in caregivers means that continuity of care is compromised.

Multi-skilling, or cross training as it is sometimes called, is another key component of re- engineering and one which has been forcefully promoted by program management advocates. As discussed earlier, the idea of multi-skilling is not a new one but can be traced back to post-Fordist concepts of flexible specialization. It is of critical importance to analyse the impact that multi-skilling has on patient care and on health care professionals.

George Whetsell, a specialist on re-engineering and total quality management says: "In theory, the ideal would be if every employee would have the knowledge and skills to do every job" (as cited in Bergman 1994: 33). This, he believes, would allow for total interchangeability and flexibility. The first impact of cross training in the hospital sector during 1993 to 1997 was the epidemic trend to replace registered nurses (RNs) with lesser-educated professionals, such as registered practical nurses (RPNs) and unregulated care providers (UCPs). This is referred to as "lowering the RN ratio." This strategy was implemented despite published evaluations that presented disturbing implications for health outcomes.

Studies from various disciplines have indicated for over two decades that hospitals using a higher percentage of RNs experience decreased adverse clinical outcomes. Dating back as far as the mid-1970s, these studies show that RN staffing levels correlate with patient outcomes such as mortality and morbidity rates. For example, using a measure of surgical care quality based on death and severe morbidity for 8,593 high-risk surgical patients in seventeen hospitals, Scott and colleagues (1976) found the higher the qualification of nursing staff, the lower the mortality and morbidity rates. Knaus, Draper, Wagner and Zimmerman (1986) reported that in a sample of 5,030 patients from thirteen hospitals, lower mortality rates were positively correlated with RN staffing levels as well as positive RN-physician communication. Hartz and colleagues (1989) found that the hospital characteristic most strongly associated with a lower mortality rate was related to the training of medical and nursing personnel. Both a higher percentage of physicians who were board-certified specialists and a higher percentage of RNs were associated with a significantly lower mortality rate. Mitchell et al. (1989) reported a positive correlation between RN staffing ratios and survival of patients in critical care units. Aiken et al. (1994) found a lower mortality rate at hospitals that met certain characteristics, which made them attractive places for nurses to work. One of these characteristics was the number and percentage of RN staff. Schultz et al. (1998), using a sample of 373 hospitals studied the relationships of eight hospital structural and financial characteristics to mortality rates and length of stay in patients with acute myocardial infarction. They found that as the percentage of RN care hours increases the mortality rate and the length of hospital stay significantly decreases.

The claims regarding the benefits of flexible specialization and multi-skilling are dangerously misleading. The actual impact of this shift on quality of care is negative and the claimed financial advantages remain unproven. Moreover, with increasing pressures to discharge sicker patients faster, retaining only the most acutely ill, it is puzzling how personnel with less depth of knowledge can be justified.

On Caring Encounters

Not only are measurable clinical outcomes suffering from the flexible specialization approach, patients and nurses are also suffering from inferior caring encounters as a result of the new business paradigm.[12] Caring, a central theme in nursing discourse and practice, is profoundly compromised by the introduction of flexible specialization and multi-skilling.

Care, in nursing, has been variously described as: nurturing and skillful activities to assist people on their own terms (Leininger 1978 and 1980); as the moral ideal of nursing, which entails, above all, concern for the dignity of patients (Gadow 1985, Gaut 1984, Watson 1985) and more. Historically, society has attributed the responsibility of caring for those in need to unpaid women in the home and community and to professions such as nursing and social work.

Nurses' caring as well as the caring of other health care professionals is grounded in a context of human connectedness, bonding and attachment (Gadow 1985, Gilligan 1982, Noddings 1984). It is through this human relationship that nurses develop a comprehensive understanding of individuals that allows them to respond to patients' needs in a way that is relevant for them. Caregiving requires detailed, everyday understanding of a patient's present needs in order for the caregiver to devise appropriate strategies. Caregiving requires knowledge, skills and judgement. To enact their skills, caregivers also require what Abel and Nelson call "basic resources" (1990: 43). These can be material resources or resources such as time and access to bureaucratic structures.

Although the expectation exists that nurses will respond to the caring needs of patients, little thought has been given to the impact of the business paradigm on the ability of nurses to care. Three aspects within the re-engineered workplace negatively impact on this ability. The first is the fragmentation of the nursing care amongst various care providers. Such was the case of team nursing, in which different types of care providers performed segments of the nursing care required by patients (i.e., bathing, medications, health teaching, emotional support). This method of delivering nursing care was abandoned in most work settings over two decades ago, due to its negative impact on nurses' clinical decision-making and patient satisfaction. With the introduction of un-regulated care providers, we are regressing to the team concept of nursing care. The trend entails assigning professional nurses to coordinate patient care while leaving the so-called less complex activities to other, less skilled, health care providers—including UCPs. Extensive use of UCPs spells direct danger to the public health, and most nurses are concerned about accepting responsibility for patients' responses when expected to supervise unqualified personnel. This represents a return to the Taylorist model where mental work is separated from manual work.

A second factor that influences the ability of nurses to care is their diminished power within the organization and resulting decreased ability to influence what Graham would call "the transaction of goods and services" (1983: 16). These goods and services are pivotal to carrying out the process of caregiving. The dismantling of professional departments impacts dramatically on the power base that nurses have to influence decisions favouring quality and human concern over cost (e.g., length of hospital stay). The decreased power base undoubtedly influences other "transactions of good and services" which impact on labour conditions and on clinical outcomes (e.g., staffing levels, support for ongoing education).

There is a large body of literature on caring, which is only briefly mentioned here. The intent is to point out that no attention has been given to the effects of a business paradigm on patients' experience of caring and nurses' ability to enact caring practices. Some argue that as long as we have a woman doing the caring work, caring will automatically occur. Others argue that caring is good as long as we do not pay too much for it. However, if caring is not well attended to, there are human as well as financial prices to pay. Caring does not occur in a vacuum. Even assuming that the basic motivation of caregivers is the wellbeing of care recipients, one cannot forget that caring, as other human services, is historically and socially constructed under particular conditions, values and power relations (Graham 1983).

A third, and less considered factor, is the exacerbation of already existing power differentials between physicians, administrators and nurses and how this is likely to further weaken patients' positional status within the hospital system. These power imbalances arise from highly hierarchical organizational structures and from entrenched power imbalances among health care professions and between health professionals and patients. It is unfortunate that, despite our rhetoric about patient-centred care, patients are the most disenfranchised individuals within the hospital structure. And, it is naive to assume that the allocation of more power to those that are already the most powerful players in the organization will result in greater patient empowerment. This is not the context that will position patients as full partners in their care; nor will it result in greater responsiveness to their needs.

On Costs

One of the most emphasized benefits marketed by the program management gurus is the improved cost-effectiveness realized through increased physician involvement in resource utilization (Cole and Brown 1988, Ellis and Gaskin 1988). Yet, because proponents of this theory have disregarded the system of incentives that guides physicians' behaviour, their optimism is not warranted.

A requirement for successful results is that there be compatibility of interests between organizational cost-effectiveness on the one hand and physicians' earnings and self-interest on the other. This compatibility does not exist when physicians' remuneration is fee-for-service based. In most Canadian hospitals, physicians are not hospital employees who earn a salary but, rather, are reimbursed directly by government according to the number of patients they see and the procedures they do.

Moreover, physicians' increased influence may in fact strengthen the conflict of interest that exists at times between hospital goals and physician needs. Such is the case when hospital cost-containment requires a limit on certain types procedures. Physicians resist this strategy as it affects their earnings. Resource utilization is also compromised by physicians' preferences in favour of, for example, invasive procedures such as caesarean sections over more conservative (and cheaper) interventions. The failure of most business models to address such a key area as the structural conflict of interest between physicians' remuneration and hospitals' needs is certainly noteworthy.

There are ample anecdotal data to support the claim that program management has indeed increased physicians' involvement in hospital decision-making. What remains to be proven is that physician involvement leads to better accountability for resource utilization and improved overall organizational cost-effectiveness. The question becomes: Is program management the best model for achieving physician's contribution to cost-effectiveness? Other approaches, such as joint practice committees have existed since the 1970s and are known to promote interdisciplinary work, joint decision-making and enhanced resource utilization. Similarly, sociological models, like the one implemented at the renowned Beth Israel Hospital in Boston have improved participation and cost-effectiveness (Rabkin and Avakian 1992). Unlike program management, that increases power imbalances, these alternative models have achieved cost-effectiveness improvements while decreasing power imbalances. From the quality of care and the cost-effectiveness perspectives, it is essential that all health care professionals be better positioned.

Published evaluations are also of limited value when considering the financial benefits of re- engineering as it relates to flexible specialization and multi-skilling. Some reports suggest that decreasing RN staff ratios is an efficient and cost-effective strategy (Abts et al. 1994, Hancock et al 1984, Hesterly and Robinson 1990, Shukla 1983). However, these studies do not account for indirect expenses related to lowering RN staff ratios. These indirect expenses include higher levels of supervision related to working with lesser qualified nursing staff, increased absenteeism and decreased efficiency related to low staff morale and inappropriate use of nurses' knowledge, skill and time.

Other studies show that a higher RN staff ratio is more efficient and cost-effective. For example, Halloran (1983) reports that the cost of operating a ward with a predominantly RN staff (72 percent) was actually lower than operating a similar ward comprised of 40 percent RNs, 20 percent LPNs (Licensed Practical Nurses) and 40 percent nursing aides. Donovan and Lewis (1987) note that from 1972 to 1985 the percentage of RNs to lesser-qualified staff increased from 36 to 94 percent while the nursing salary budget decreased from 17.8 to 14.7 percent of the corporate budget. They went on to say that transformation to an all RN staff resulted in a significant increase in output per dollars spent, with twice the patient care being given in the same amount of time. An important study conducted by the American Hospital Association (1991–1992) reports that while hospitals *increased* the number of RNs within their skill mix, hospital labour as a percentage of total hospital expenditures *declined*. Another study of an acute surgical ward notes that a staff comprised of 80 percent registered nurses and 20 percent enrolled nurses is more costly than an all-RN staff (Pratt et al. 1993).

Some researchers attribute the cost-effectiveness of a higher RN ratio to an increased productivity of RNs. Halloran (1983) notes that a nursing unit predominantly staffed by RNs spends more time in direct care aimed at meeting patients' physical and psychosocial needs and is more cost-effective than a similar ward comprised of a much lower nursing staff mix. Mineyard, Wall and Turner (1986) report that RNs spend less time in non-productive activities than LPNs. Specifically, the RNs spend 11.4 percent of their time in non-productive activities; level II LPNs, who are certified to administer medications, and at times, act as team leaders, spend 17.4 percent in non-productive activities; and level I LPNs, who have less skills than level II LPNs, spend 23.4 percent in non-productive activities. They go on to say that the cost of a level higher staff mix may actually be considered cost-effective when the amount of productive time contributed by each staff level is taken into account. Another study found that productivity, as measured by time spent in direct nursing functions, increased by 210 percent when a higher RN ratio was utilized (Donovan and Lewis 1987).

Absenteeism is an unacknowledged cost associated with the shift to the business paradigm. In her study of the U.S. hospital sector, Shindul-Rothschild (1996) found a significant increase in absenteeism directly related to the level of stress that nurses are experiencing in the workplace and to the absence of senior nursing leadership. She supports these claims with other studies showing that absenteeism is related to stress-related illnesses caused by excessive workloads. Motivational and morale factors and poor supervision also play a role in levels of absenteeism. Since absenteeism is a well-documented factor influencing hospital costs, an increase in absenteeism impacts negatively on hospital finances.

Absenteeism is only one of many hidden costs of moving toward a segmented caring labour force. Those who loudly proclaim the benefits of multi-skilling and cross training have not taken these costs into account. A singular focus on the bottom line ignores the impact of re-engineering on the wellbeing of a predominantly female, casual and part-time workforce, and the compounding effect of a more temporary workforce on the already compromised quality of care that patients receive in institutions guided by a business paradigm.

From the above discussion it is clear that claims of cost-effectiveness put forth by the business paradigm are highly speculative. Many of the so-called cost-savings of a business paradigm are really a shifting of the costs somewhere else. For example, this paradigm focuses purely on one episode of treatment—the hospital—while ignoring completely the before and after effects. For example, the focus on direct hospital costs may obscure overall costs related to shorter length of stay. One expression of this deterioration is the "revolving-door syndrome" already documented in the United States where those discharged early from the hospital who have little access to community services are soon re-admitted to the hospital with complications related to the previous hospitalization.[13] This results in increased costs to the overall health care system. The increased social (and health care) costs involved in transforming well paid, permanent and secure jobs into lower paid, part-time, casualized and insecure jobs have also been ignored. In all these cases, there have been no real savings. Although the proponents of the business paradigm may be able to show how they have successfully improved their bottom line (by shifting the costs somewhere else), they have also contributed to a less humane and less healthy society.

Even if one accepts a very narrow approach to cost-effectiveness, that is, one focused strictly on the hospital's bottom line, the cost-saving claims are doubtful. The savings from the dismantling of professional departments and the introduction of business models may in reality be just hidden expenditure shifts. Examples include: the shifting of managerial costs from dismantled professional departments to expanding program management structures; the hidden costs incurred by the need to increase supervision when replacing registered nurses by less qualified personal; the not-so-hidden cost of increased rates of mortality and morbidity and the costs resulting from giving more power to the main cost-producers and users of resources in the hospital—the physicians— while those other professions which could serve as gatekeepers for hospital costs are weakened.

In general, the arguments presented in favour of the introduction of a business model tend to be weak, unproven and flawed. One such argument emphasizes the competitive environment encouraged by the business paradigm—an environment that is purported to increase over-all cost-effectiveness (Flynn 1991). Associating competition with cost-effectiveness should be regarded with healthy scepticism. At the very least, this claim demands a specific explanation of *how* more competition leads to real cost savings, not just a shifting of costs. No strong explanation is available in this case. It is revealing that the American health care system, which emphasizes more than the Canadian the role of private enterprises and free-market competition, is more expensive and wasteful of resources.

On The Community

The impact of the business paradigm on the community has been understated. Business models in conjunction with hospital funding formulas aimed at reducing costs will undoubtedly continue to drive down the length of hospital stay, shifting the burden and costs of care to the community sector. Patients will stay for shorter and shorter periods of time in the hospital, completing the recovery process at home or somewhere else. This is the reality in the United States and similar trends have emerged in Canada (Anderson 1990, Morris et al. 1999, Neysmith 1998). Acute in-patient length of hospital stay in Ontario was reduced from an average of 8 days per patient in 1990–91 to an average of 6.5 days per patient in 1998–99 (Ontario Ministry of Health 1991 and 1999). There has been a 26 percent decrease in average length of stay, in acute care beds, over the last nine years! Although a significant portion of this reduction can be attributed to the introduction of advanced technologies that allow for less invasive procedures, there is no doubt that length of hospital stay has been impacted also by performance measurements set to reduce hospital costs.

This trend is congruent with health care reforms which aim to move care into the community (Armstrong 1994). It is also congruent with broader goals set by the World Health Organization that emphasize primary health care. Although noble and desirable, this goal requires a community that is well prepared to address the needs of those discharged quicker and sicker from the hospital setting. The availability of adequate and qualified resources in the community will assist individuals to further their recovery.[14]

Unfortunately, community health services in Ontario have increased disproportionately less than demand for them. In the absence of adequate public investment to develop accessible health care resources in the community, private for-profit community services have and will continue to proliferate (Armstrong 1997). Patients who are discharged early and who need health care services in the community will pay for these services, if they can afford them. Others, the poor, the elderly and the disenfranchised, will have to devise alternate strategies or do without. Most likely we will witness a regression in health conditions, particularly for those less privileged social groups that cannot afford to pay for private providers.[15]

Those who promote a business paradigm in the hospital setting seldom take into account the overall social cost implied by a worsened health status of the poor and the elderly (Morris et al. 1999). In the absence of well-developed health care services at the community level a shorter hospital stay means the social burden is shifting to the private pocket and to caregivers at home, most of whom are women. Thus, the adoption of business models in hospital management has contributed to the creation of a two-tier health care system by generating greater demand for privatized services in the community. This seems to be an outcome that is congruent with a business paradigm!

Conclusions

The need for improved cost-efficiency within the hospital sector is necessary. However, a business paradigm is not the answer to resolve this challenge. This chapter argues that the shift from a cure-care paradigm to a business paradigm in hospital management fails to achieve cost-effectiveness. Moreover, the models that have been implemented have detrimental effects for the quality of hospital care and potential harmful cost and social implications for the overall health care system and for those in need of health care services. It is imperative that any restructuring initiatives be measured and evaluated in terms of quality of care, cost-effectiveness and social burden. The empirical evidence to date does not support the cost-effectiveness or quality outcomes of business models. Moreover, it indicates that the social burden, especially on marginalized groups and on women, is great. There are several reasons why business models (program management, re-engineering and other variations) within the hospital sector should be closely scrutinized:

- The focus is mainly on financial bottom-line performance. Thus, there needs to be close monitoring of downfalls in quality of patient care and staff morale.
- Hospital restructuring further increases physicians' allocation of power and influence in decision-making and exacerbates existing power imbalances amongst all health care professionals.
- These models ignore a pivotal factor that impacts on health care costs, physician remuneration.
- The dismantling of professional departments pushes aside important gatekeepers to resource utilization, such as nurses, social workers and others. Thus, the business model could prove to be more expensive and wasteful than previous models.
- Replacement of well-trained professionals by less knowledgeable ones impacts negatively on quality of care, as well as

clinical, financial and system outcomes.
- A decrease in hospital length of stay without community readiness for follow-up results in the revolving-door syndrome, which, as the American experience shows, is a very expensive outcome in human and financial terms.
- Business models originated in the United States, embracing private for-profit provision of health care, and have resulted in a more expensive and less accessible a health care system than our Canadian one.
- These models are likely to advance the shift to a two-tier system of health care. Until the contradictions inherent in Canada's previous and current models are resolved, lasting cost-effectiveness and quality outcomes based on a truly patient-centred approach will not be achieved.

A set of tentative recommendations can be extracted from the analysis in this chapter:

- Hospital (and other agencies) using the business model must identify the specific areas to expect cost-savings and clear mechanisms to measure quality and financial outcomes.
- A decreased utilization of unregulated care providers is recommended. There is sufficient evidence to indicate that registered nurses contribute to a decrease in hospital costs by lowering mortality, morbidity, length of hospital stay and re-admission rates.
- Ensure that a sufficient number of nurses work on permanent full-time status to ensure continuity of caregiver. This is essential to enable nurses and patients to experience caring encounters.
- Evaluate other organizational models such as the matrix model set by some tertiary teaching hospitals in Ontario. The matrix model institutes program management while maintaining professional departments. This combination may avoid the problem of escalating power differentials and thereby respond better to the cost-quality equation.
- Examine the remuneration scheme for physicians. No effective control of health care costs will ever be feasible unless the system of incentives embedded in physicians' remuneration is made compatible with other health care interests.
- Focus on introducing evidence-based practice, i.e., practice guided by principles of intervention that have proven effective. This approach would serve to significantly decrease the

current procedural and treatment variation (and related cost variation) that exists amongst different practitioners today. It would also assure the public that they are receiving the best practice known to date.
- Substantially accelerate publicly funded health care services at the community level. To ensure proper utilization of our hospital sector and contain its associated escalating costs, we must have a fully implemented service of primary health care, home care and long-term care for all.

Notes

1. All opinions, errors and omissions expressed in this chapter are the author's alone.
2. See the studies on Magnet Hospitals (Kramer 1988a and 1988b).
3. The summary of Taylorism is drawn from the work of Jary and Jary (1991: 432–33).
4. The description of Fordism is based on Jary and Jary (1991: 173–75).
5. It is unclear how this claim is consistent with the criticism made by the same authors in reference to semi-autonomous units in the more traditional "divisional design."
6. Whether this model is really patient-centred or whether such terminology simply represents clever marketing techniques is discussed later in this chapter.
7. It is worth noting that, in the U.S., the impetus for the intensive use of microchip technology, computers and robotics is significantly higher than in Canada. This is most probably a result of the different funding structures.
8. Si Transken in this volume looks at the impact of organizational restructuring on social workers and the women they treat in hospital-based sexual assault treatment programs.
9. Janet Lum and Paul Williams in this volume explore the ways that health care restructuring is exacerbating the long-standing internal factionalization of various categories of nurses and unregulated care providers.
10. Jane Cawthorne in this volume examines the midwives and obstetricians' differential access to resources, power and decision-making in the case of maternal care in Alberta.
11. Thousands of nurses across Canada lost their full-time jobs as a result of hospital downsizing, thereby becoming part of this flexible labour force. Gregor, Keddy, Foster and Denney in this volume examine the strategies used by some Nova Scotia nurses to retain their economic and professional viability.
12. Denise Spitzer in this volume examines the negative impact of restructuring on the caring encounters between nurses and Aboriginal and immigrant women during and after childbirth.
13. Diana Gustafson in this volume describes a case illustrating the human and

financial costs associated with brief hospital stays and poor access to community services.

14. Guruge, Donner and Morrison in this volume explore some ways that an underdeveloped community infrastructure impacts negatively on recent immigrant and refugee women.

15. In this volume, Douglass Drozdow-St. Christian, in his study of aging women, and Simpson and Porte, in their study of a Chippewas community, describe how different groups of women are addressing the rationing of community services.

3

Professional Fault Lines:
Nursing in Ontario after the Regulated Health Professions Act

Janet M. Lum and A. Paul Williams

Introduction

In Ontario, as in other provinces and jurisdictions, the health system is undergoing major restructuring. Years of reform proposals have been aimed variously at enhancing consumer choice and participation; achieving cost-effectiveness in care delivery; assuring quality of care; strengthening access to care; and shifting from a bed-based, "illness" system to a community-based, health promotion and social support model. Now Ontario, under the Harris Conservative government, is engaged in a massive restructuring process to reduce the number of acute care hospital beds and shift the focus of care to the community. Led by the Health Services Restructuring Commission, an arms-length expert panel, the province is implementing large scale hospital mergers, amalgamations and closures resulting in significant reductions in in-patient hospital days (Ontario Health Services Restructuring Commission 1998).

In the heavily labour-intensive health sector, restructuring has profound implications for health care workers, the majority of whom are women. As health care systems are restructured to meet the policy imperatives of cost-containment and labour market flexibility, it is women who bear the brunt of massive job cuts, reduced wages, underemployment and professional deskilling. It is women who are pitted against employers, governments and each other in an often desperate battle to defend professional terrain and keep a declining number of well-paid, full-time jobs. It is also women who, as health care professionals and family caregivers, face the double burden of providing greater levels of care to patients with progressively higher needs and to family members who are being pushed out of hospitals "quicker and sicker."

In this chapter we examine the status of the nursing profession in Ontario in the wake of this latest round of restructuring and in the wake of the *Regulated Health Professions Act* (RHPA) of 1993 which set the stage for many of the changes now taking place in health human resources (Statutes of Ontario 1994, McKelvey and Bohnen 1998). This Act, introduced by Ontario's former New Democratic Party government, marked a watershed for the health professions in that it established a greater degree of equality between them, and particularly between nursing—an historically female-dominated profession—and medicine—which was historically male-dominated. Presented as a step toward health reform, the RHPA aimed to increase public participation in professional governance, reduce the historical control and dominance of medicine over the other health professions and increase consumer choice among alternate, safe providers. For instance, the Act again legitimized the profession of midwifery which had been politically marginalized in Canada by the rise of allopathic medicine prior to the turn of the twentieth century,[1] and made possible subsequent legislation to recognize nurse practitioners as independent primary caregivers (Armstrong et al. 1993: 22, Statutes of Ontario 1997). Thus, under the RHPA nursing, along with other female-dominated health professions, gained an important degree of professional legitimacy and autonomy.

In addition to levelling the regulatory playing field, the RHPA also provided for greater labour market flexibility with consequent challenges for nursing. By moving away from a monopoly licensure model of professional regulation to one which specified overlapping areas of professional competence, employers and policymakers gained increased flexibility to mix health care providers and to substitute less expensive, unregulated care providers (UCPs) for their regulated, better trained and better paid counterparts. While under the RHPA, nursing did achieve greater professional autonomy *vis-à-vis* medicine, it has increasingly found itself subject to employers and governments pursuing an agenda of cost-efficiency and cost-cutting (Coburn 1993: 133). We argue in this chapter that with the RHPA and as a result of health system restructuring, nursing in Ontario now experiences two contradictory tendencies which have exacerbated its historical internal factionalization. One is toward greater professionalization, autonomy and status, reflected in the drive toward a baccalaureate degree as a compulsory requirement for entry to practice. The other is toward deprofessionalization, fragmentation and deskilling. This latter trend, precipitated by the rise of generic workers performing routine nursing tasks such as bathing and feeding, is also reinforced by the profession's own insistence that it should continue to control such (unregulated) tasks. In contrast to physicians, who continue under Medicare to be virtually guaranteed full employment and full payment for every service which they deem to be medically necessary, nurses have no similar guarantees. They fight uphill battles to defend their jobs in hospitals and other service provider organizations, with cost-savings almost inevitably achieved at their expense. As a consequence, nursing now faces intensified internal conflicts which undermine its political power to act cohesively on behalf of the collective interests of the profession.

There are a number of reasons to focus on nursing. First, with approximately 144,000 members, it is the single largest health profession in Ontario, as it is in most other jurisdictions, and it is the largest female-dominated profession, accounting for a majority of all women health professionals. Second, nursing's development raises many issues common to other female-dominated health professions which emerged from the division of labour in the modern hospital, and which, in the wake of the RHPA in Ontario, have now emerged "from under the thumb of medicine" (Coburn 1993: 133). Third, nursing continues its evolution into a mature and highly differentiated profession. In addition to being racially and ethnically diverse, nurses are characterized by a broad range of educational qualifications and distinct occupational statuses. Of course, this is also true of other professions, like medicine, which itself is characterized by growing internal stratification as well as by increasing gender and ethnoracial diversity. In contrast to medicine however, nursing lacks the political power to protect and extend its professional status in an increasingly competitive and conflictual policy environment. This leads to magnified internal differences and cleavages and to a further erosion of nurses' ability not just to make gains *vis-à-vis* medicine, but to maintain political status and jobs as restructuring proceeds.

In the following sections, we begin by highlighting key features of the *Regulated Health Professions Act*, focusing on those which most directly affect the professional and political status of nursing in Ontario. We then examine the impact of health system restructuring within the context of the RHPA on patterns of nursing employment and analyze nursing's often conflicted professional and political response. In a concluding section, we assess implications for the future direction of nursing and other historically female-dominated professions.

Nursing and the Regulated Health Professions Act

Prior to the RHPA, the regulatory system for health care professionals in Ontario consisted of a patchwork of multiple pieces of legislation. Six professions (pharmacy, medicine, optometry, dentistry, dental hygiene and nursing) were covered by the *Health Disciplines Act;* chiropractic, physiotherapy, osteopathy and massage therapy were regulated under the *Drugless Practitioners Act;* and seven more (including dental technology, ophthalmic dispensing, psychology and radiological technology) were regulated by other statutes. Professions such as midwives, occupational therapists and respiratory therapists that are today regulated under the RHPA were not recognized at all under previous legislation.

Under this non-system, a small number of health professions had an exclusive licence to perform services that fell under the scope of their practice. Historically, male-dominated health professions such as medicine and dentistry with broadly-defined scopes of practice, effectively controlled other (female-dominated) professions such as nursing and dental hygiene, which had more restricted scopes and could perform medical procedures only under the direct authority and supervision of physicians. This created both a monopoly for medicine (and dentistry) that appeared broader than could be justified by the need to protect the public and a hierarchy of unequal relations among the professions.

In November 1982, the Minister of Health for Ontario announced the creation of the Health Professions Legislative Review (Ontario Ministry of Health 1989). The Review was the result of a range of converging forces for change, including: public demands for a choice of health care providers and a more open, responsive and accountable regulatory system, especially in relation to complaints and discipline; demands from excluded and marginalized providers for regulation and legitimacy; and a desire by government to include all health disciplines under a single legislative umbrella in order to facilitate policymaking. In addition, the rise of the women's movement put women's health issues directly on the public agenda, along with demands for greater access to women care providers. Perhaps most importantly, from a health services management viewpoint, there was a growing perception that the existing regulatory environment inhibited new ways of mixing the various health professions and substituting less costly for more costly providers. This made it difficult to achieve cost-efficiencies in an era of rapidly increasing health care costs.

More than seventy-five groups and occupations requested regulation. In the end, the *Regulated Health Professions Act*, introduced in 1991, and proclaimed into law in 1994, covered twenty-four health professions,[2] including eight that would be self-regulating for the first time: audiologists, dental hygienists, dietitians, medical laboratory technologists, occupational therapists, midwives, respiratory therapists and speech-language pathologists.

A key goal of the RHPA was:

> to ensure that the health professions are regulated and coordinated in the public interest, that appropriate standards of practice are developed and maintained, and that individuals have access to services provided by the health professions of their

choice and that they are treated with sensitivity and respect in their dealings with health professionals, the Colleges and the Board. (Statutes of Ontario 1994: c18, s.2)

The Act set out legal principles common to all the professions. For example, Schedule 2 of the RHPA established self-governing colleges for each of the professions, although some, such as chiropodists and podiatrists, share a single college. It outlines provisions relating to the operation of colleges, patients' rights and remedies, the rights and obligations of college members, and the duties of employers of health professionals. It details the functions to be performed by college councils, college committees and registrars. To strengthen public accountability, the Act increases lay participation on councils and committees and opens to the public, council meetings and hearings. Further, the Act established a Health Disciplines Board and a Health Professions Regulatory Advisory Board, both consisting of all lay members (Statutes of Ontario 1994: c18, s.2).

As stated earlier, the RHPA takes a new approach to professional regulation. Rather than controlling who does what by granting professions exclusive licences over entire areas of endeavour, the RHPA gives professions the authority to perform specific controlled acts, with most acts falling within the authority of more than one profession. In all, the RHPA identifies thirteen controlled acts considered to be potentially harmful if performed by unqualified persons.[3] The performance of a controlled act is prohibited unless a person is a member of a regulated profession specifically authorized to perform that act or a person who has been properly delegated authority. For instance, three controlled acts are authorized to nursing: performing a procedure on tissue below the dermis or mucous membrane; administering a substance by injection or inhalation; and putting an instrument, hand or finger into a body orifice or artificial opening into the body. It is important to note that all of these same acts are also authorized to medicine, which can legally perform twelve of the thirteen controlled acts (with the exception of fitting or dispensing a dental prosthesis), as well as to other professions, including midwifery, medical radiation technology and respiratory therapy. Activities not specifically identified as controlled acts (e.g., counselling) are in the public domain and may be performed by any individual.

There are several exceptions described in section 29 of the RHPA which directly affect nursing (Statutes of Ontario 1994: c18, s29, 1). These allow unregulated care providers (UCPs) to perform controlled acts when treating a household member or when assisting a person (even if not a household member) with routine activities of daily living such as dressing, bathing and personal hygiene. For example, UCPs may give medication by injections, administer a substance by inhalation, suction a client with a permanent tracheotomy or catheterize the bladder if these are routine daily activities.

Thus, on the asset side of the ledger, the RHPA puts nursing on a more equitable footing with medicine as well as the other professions. Nurses are authorized not only to perform but to initiate certain acts historically under the control of physicians and are accordingly legitimized as an independent profession with a recognized area of expertise and knowledge. On the debit side of the ledger, however, nurses, physicians or any other health profession authorized to perform nursing's controlled acts can delegate authority to UCPs. Moreover, any individuals in the so-called exceptional circumstances described in section 29 of the RHPA are permitted to perform such acts even without delegation. Such exceptions may become more commonplace as the focus of care shifts outside of hospitals to home and community and as family and volunteers take up a greater burden of care. In an increasingly competitive health care marketplace characterized by a declining number of full-time, well-paid hospital jobs, nurses find themselves confronted by each other, by other professions and by both paid and volunteer unregulated care providers, all attempting to render the same services. Under conditions of massive health system restructuring, the RHPA may provide employers with powerful tools for hollowing out nursing's professional gains.

Challenges and Responses

Health System Restructuring and Nursing Employment Patterns
Data compiled by the College of Nurses of Ontario (at the request of the authors) revealed substantial changes in the employment patterns of nurses even before the full impact of the latest round of health system restructuring was felt. They also suggest potential fault lines within the profession as such changes differentially affect the two categories of nurses.[4]

In 1992, there were 112,599 RNs, of whom 65.6 percent worked in hospitals, 6.9 percent in nursing homes and 10.1 percent in the community. By 1997, the total number of RNs in Ontario declined to 109,098, while the proportion of RNs working in hospitals decreased to 61.5 percent. At the same time, the percentage working in nursing homes increased (to 8.6 percent), as did the percentage of RNs working in the community (to 12.7 percent). These changes also affected employment status: in 1992, 55.7 percent of Ontario RNs worked full-time while 31.5 percent worked part-time and 12.3 percent worked on a casual basis. By 1997, the proportion of full-time jobs had declined to 49.8 percent, while the proportion of part-time jobs had increased to 33.3 percent and casual jobs to 14.2 percent.

Similar impacts are documented for RPNs. In 1992, the number of RPNs stood at 35,516, with 61.1 percent working in hospitals. By 1997, the total number declined to 34,623, with 56.5 percent working in hospitals. Between 1992 and 1997, the proportion of RPNs employed in nursing homes increased from 18.5 to 24.3 percent, and from 3.5 to 8.4 percent in community-based agencies. RPNs employed full-time in nursing in Ontario went from 55.2 percent in 1992 to 47.9 percent in 1997, while the percentage of part-timers increased from 29.6 percent to 33.6 percent.

According to the college, more nurses are looking for full-time nursing positions today than six years ago. For those who reported employment information in 1992, only 120 RNs (0.12 percent of 99,124) sought nursing jobs. In 1997, this number climbed to 4,321 of 101,281 nurses or 4.3 percent. The overall unemployment level was even higher for RPNs: 6.6 percent were looking for work in 1997.

Job dislocations are likely to increase as health system restructuring proceeds and more hospital beds are closed. Recently released statistics from the Health Sector Training and Adjustment Program (HSTAP) (1997) show that from 1994 to 1997, almost 21,000 health sector employees in Ontario were laid off or faced some other form of job displacement such as early retirement, voluntary exit, a significant reduction in working hours or a change in employment status (i.e., from full-time to part-time or part-time to casual). In 1996–97, a record number of employees (11,340) were laid off or displaced. Layoffs represented the majority (65 percent) of employees displaced in 1996–97, with most of the displacements (90 percent) occurring in the hospital sector. Most of the displaced workers (85 percent) were women (HSTAP 1997; Grayson 1997: 7). HSTAP (1997) further projects close to 30,000 layoffs of health workers over the next two to three years. The Ontario Nurses' Association (ONA) estimates that 10,000 RNs will lose their jobs in the next few years in addition to the 5,000 who have already been displaced (Ontario Nurses' Association 1997c: 12).[5]

How do these figures compare with unemployment rates for the historically male-dominated profession of medicine? Unemployment has generally not been a significant issue for physicians. In addition to guaranteeing universal access for Canadians to all medically necessary services, government health insurance guarantees physicians payments for virtually every service they determine is "medically necessary." Canadian physicians have few restrictions as to where or how they practice, and most work as self-employed entrepreneurs, not as employees. Although it has been suggested that health system restructuring may make it difficult for some specialties, such as surgery, to access hospital facilities, with potentially negative implications for professional earnings, to this point, there is no documented case of a physician being forced to seek employment outside of the profession.

A recent agreement between the Government of Ontario and the Ontario Medical Association (OMA) reinforces medicine's political dominance and intensifies the fear that physicians' share of the health budget will be preserved or increased at the expense of nurses and other health professions. This agreement was negotiated after a series of highly publicized job actions by physicians directed against a government-imposed cap on total physicians' payments, which had increased more rapidly than inflation or population growth over the previous decade. These actions included a refusal on the part of many orthopaedic surgeons and obstetricians to accept new patients. Faced by growing public concerns about deteriorating access to medical care, the government backed down and removed the cap on physicians' incomes. This meant that total physician payments would increase by approximately $1.14 billion in a health budget of about $18 billion (Mahoney 1997: A1, A12). The agreement also gave the profession an effective "veto" over proposed reforms which could potentially allow nurses, among other health professions, to take on primary care functions now controlled by physicians.

For example, the agreement includes the creation of a Physician Services Committee with a mandate to advise both the Ontario Ministry of Health (OMOH) and the OMA about: changes to the delivery of health care; new organizational, economic and physician distribution issues; changes in doctors' roles in the health care system; alternative models of service delivery; compensation for services; possible delisting of insured services; and questions such as what happens if physicians as a whole bill above authorized ceiling (Coutts 1997: A2). It also prohibits a transfer of funds out of the physicians' payment pool to finance payments to other professionals such as midwifery or nurse practitioners providing primary care (Williams et al. 1997).

The implications of this agreement were not lost on the Ontario Nurses' Association, which expressed shock at the increases given to doctors and declared that the "deal is a gender issue," to be paid for by the nursing profession, 95 percent of whom are women (Mahoney 1997: A12). In addition to job losses, this agreement, along with ongoing attempts to cut health costs, put increasing pressure on nurses to shift to part-time employment, to accept underemployment and to accept work in direct competition with unregulated care providers in the community. How many nurses have been displaced from well-paid, unionized hospital jobs to community agencies where some of the jobs are not unionized or unionized at a lower rate of pay? How many nurses have been pushed to work for private provider agencies where they may not have benefits or be covered by employment legislation? How many RNs are working as RPNs and how many of both categories of nurses are working as unregulated care providers? According to the Executive Director of the Registered Practical Nurses Association of Ontario, the Riverdale Hospital in Toronto (before its closure in 1998 was confirmed by the recommendations of the Ontario Health Services Restructuring Commission) laid off 240 RPNs who were to be rehired as health care aides (B. Thornber, personal communication, March 24, 1998). Although now standing on an equal legislative footing with medicine, nursing has not been able to mobilize politically as medicine has done to defend its interests.

The Rise of Unregulated Care Providers

Unregulated care providers (UCPs) are also known by names such as health care aides, unit assistants, personal support workers, personal attendants or patient care assistants. Although there is little publicly available documentary evidence of the extent of their use across the health care system, anecdotal accounts, including some provided here earlier, suggest that they are being employed more frequently and that they are displacing nursing jobs. This is a sensitive issue for nurses who see their work being taken up by UCPs with less training (training can range from a few weeks to several months) at lower rates of pay. Given the cost-cutting imperatives of restructuring and the ability under the RHPA to delegate work to unregulated providers, UCPs have become attractive alternatives for hospital administrators.[6]

For nursing, the rise of UCPs threatens jobs and cuts to the core of the profession. Nursing leaders argue that their professional knowledge consists of a complex and integrated set of cognitive and clinical skills which constitute more than the sum of its parts. Because nursing is not merely "a grocery list" of specific tasks, it cannot be subdivided, prioritized and parcelled out to minimally trained personnel without serious risk to public safety (Niblett 1997: 26–7). Assigning nursing tasks to UCPs is seen to undermine the philosophical foundations of a profession which considers the whole patient in the care process. From the viewpoint of nurses, when UCPs are asked to perform direct care services for patients, public safety is jeopardized. Although UCPs are accountable to employers and the clients to whom they provide care, they are not governed by the RHPA and are not accountable to the public through the same mechanism as regulated health professionals. According to nursing unions and associations, these are critical moral and ethical concerns which go far beyond mere turf battles for jobs. The key message, they assert, is that preserving nursing as an autonomous and viable profession is synonymous with the assurance of public safety (Zimmerman 1995).

Despite a fairly unified and coherent response against UCPs as a threat to the nursing profession, nursing associations and unions have adopted often conflicting and internally divisive political strategies in the struggle to preserve jobs, strategies which leave less well-positioned nurses feeling sold out by better-positioned colleagues. For example, one strategy has been to stress the higher qualifications and capabilities of RNs not just to plan and manage patient care but to perform routine nursing functions such as bathing and feeding which, it is argued, also give RNs the opportunity to apply their more developed patient assessment skills. This makes RNs better qualified to deal with the challenges posed by hospital restructuring, decreasing hospital resources, higher patient acuity and shorter hospital stays. There is support in a number American and Canadian studies that suggest that hospitals which increase RNs as a percentage of total hospital labour, can reap productivity gains (Shamian 1996, Prescott 1993).

Such arguments in support of the superiority of RNs, while aimed, in the main at UCPs, also tend to redound negatively on RPNs, thereby reinforcing rifts within the profession. A corollary to the above line of reasoning is that if hospitals resort to UCPs as a cost-saving measure, the use of unskilled workers should be matched by the use of highly skilled RNs. In comparison to RPNs, RNs are portrayed by their leaders as better able to teach, delegate, assign and supervise UCPs. Supervision, they argue, is part of the basic entry level competency for RNs but not for RPNs. In response, RPNs maintain that additional professional development courses include ones that teach supervisory skills, as well as that everyday practical experience enables them to supervise and provide leadership to members of multi-disciplinary teams. RPNs make the additional claim that they are willing to do many of the lower-level skills which, in their view, RNs are increasingly unwilling to do, all at a more cost-effective rate (B. Thornber, personal communication, March 24, 1998). In short, RPNs present themselves as a reasonable and safe compromise between more expensive RNs and lower-paid, but minimally trained, UCPs. The political reality is that RPNs are squeezed between the competing pressures to demonstrate skills comparable to RNs, while maintaining cost competitiveness with UCPs.

The RHPA produces other dilemmas for the nursing profession. As detailed above, it specifically recognizes that UCPs may perform acts not specifically prohibited by legislation and that they may also perform controlled acts when properly delegated authority to do so. The College of Nurses of Ontario (CNO) has had to address the fact that nurses are more frequently working with UCPs, whether they like it or not, and that in the course of their duties, they will often be responsible for monitoring acts conducted by UCPs under their delegated authority. The *Communiqué* (1996), the official publication of the CNO, set out guidelines for RNs and RPNs to follow when teaching, delegating, assigning and supervising

UCPs. This "Guide to Working with Unregulated Care Providers" was justified as an expression of the CNO's mandate to protect the public interest and to ensure public safety. Nevertheless, in the minds of some nurses, it was interpreted as "condoning" and "promoting" the use of UCPs, thereby putting the public at risk (ONA 1997b: 10).

The Ontario Nurses' Association, which represents Registered Nurses in contract negotiations with Ontario hospitals, was particularly critical of the College. The ONA (1997b) argued that, by outlining common conditions which must be met by either RNs or RPNs working with UCPs, the College failed to recognize the superior capacity of RNs compared to RPNs to teach, delegate and supervise UCPs. Additionally, the Professional Standards for Registered Nurses and Registered Practical Nurses in Ontario implemented by the College of Nurses in September 1996 failed to recognize the superior training and abilities of RNs. While the College emphasized professional accountability and common standards for all members of the profession, the ONA, with its mandate to protect RN jobs, saw such documents as a potential tool which employers could use to dilute RN complements in favour of less expensive RPNs and UCPs. The standards set out by the college were said by ONA to,

> totally muddy the waters with respect to the differences between RNs and RPNs. ... In the current economic climate, these standards will support employers who are trying to save money by using less-qualified care providers.... [T]he proposed Standards open the door for practice settings to position RPNs in roles that will prove dangerous to the public. (1997a: 9)

These words recognized the wedge that had been driven into the profession.

As can be seen, these sorts of internal responses detract from a unified professional identity and cohesion. Not only that, from the public's point of view, the polemics which elevate some nurses over others may often appear self serving. When both sides—RNs and RPNs—argue fervently in the interest of patient safety, the debates surrounding the assurance of public safety can be seen to obfuscate real tensions within and among groups as they contend to preserve their professional domain against perceived encroachment.

Race, Class and Country of Origin
The occupational tensions between RNs, RPNs and UCPs are complicated by the increasing diversity within the profession along the lines of race, class and country of origin. In the wake of the RHPA and as a result of health system restructuring, there is a growing concern that a negative

cycle of competition and displacement between categories of nurses, and between nurses and UCPs, has been established, and that the fallout from this cycle disproportionately affects visible minority workers.

Currently, the College of Nurses does not compile data on the racial background of nurses. Ontario's employment equity legislation passed by the New Democrats in September 1994 and repealed by the Conservative Party as one of its first moves after its election in 1995 would have provided the legal framework to ensure that hospitals gather employee background information as part of the employer's internal workforce survey. Presently, there are no publicly available data or systematic ways of tracking the pattern of dismissals or job reassignments by gender or racial background, either for individual health facilities or the health sector as a whole. Moreover, as part of the reversal of employment equity legislation, the Ontario Conservative government's *Job Quotas Repeal Act* ordered employers to destroy any previous data generated in compliance with the legislation. There no longer exists any base line data for analysis.

There are, however, other sources which suggest that visible minorities tend to be among those most vulnerable to cutbacks. For example, Head's 1985 study revealed that visible minority women were more likely than others to work in the areas of cooking, cleaning, laundering and in the lower levels of nursing. According to ONA (1996), visible minority nurses are rarely found higher in the nursing hierarchy, even in hospitals where 30 to 40 percent of staff nurses are racial minority group members. They tend not to become charge nurses, assistant head nurses, nurse managers, supervisors, or directors. Instead, they tend to be over-represented in such sectors as chronic care, rehabilitation, long-term care and geriatric units. Nurses in these units, more so than in other units, are being replaced by generic workers (ONA 1996). Furthermore, chronic care nurses are often seen by employers as lacking the skills to transfer into other areas of the hospital, even if they have the seniority to do so (Congress of Black Women of Canada 1995a and 1995b). Opportunities in these units for professional training and development are usually limited, since management perceives little need for such education. This further decreases the possibility for transfers or promotions. The situation differs greatly in high-tech, high status areas, such as intensive care or transplant units, which often have a much lower proportion of visible minority nurses. Opportunities for ongoing education in these areas are usually far greater and nurses are encouraged to attend courses. Predictably, nurses from less desirable units are passed over for promotions and transfers. Not only are they seen to be unmotivated because they have not moved to more dynamic areas, they are also perceived to lack the skills, ability, qualifications and experience for more responsible positions. In a period of downsizing, the implication of these employment patterns is that racial minority nurses may be disproportionately affected by layoffs and other forms of job displacement.

The literature also suggests that discriminatory practices in the labour market and in other related areas, such as education and immigration, have excluded visible minority women from better paid, secure, more desirable jobs, and that the pattern has been no different in nursing. Calliste, for example, describes the requirement of Black nurses to have nursing qualifications "over and above those required for white nurses" (1993: 95) when, between 1950 and 1962, immigration authorities started to admit limited numbers of Caribbean nurses to meet a nursing shortage in Canada. Many found employment in psychiatric hospitals, sanatoria, chronic care units, or long-term care facilities, where there were fewer chances or demands for training and rare or non-existent promotional opportunities. More recent evidence suggests that discriminatory practices continue to marginalize and inhibit the mobility of racial minority nurses (Das Gupta 1996, Gray 1994). In a highly publicized case at Northwestern General Hospital, an investigation by the Ontario Human Rights Commission (1994) concluded that there was sufficient evidence to support allegations of differential treatment of visible minority nurses as compared to white nurses. Examples of harassment and differential standards for visible minority nurses included over-supervision, more severe disciplinary measures, more difficult work assignments, less desirable shifts and more strictly enforced standards of work performance, all of which culminated either in dismissals or "forced resignations." The Congress of Black Women of Canada claims that such practices are not exceptional and exist in other health facilities for visible minority nurses (1995b).[7]

The pattern shows that hospital closures and mergers will hit the nursing profession hardest and will in particular affect visible minority nurses who are concentrated in rank and file positions in units most vulnerable to cuts.

Provisionally Registered Nurses
Declining jobs also adversely affect the employment opportunities of provisionally registered nurses (PRNs), a category of health providers who have been practising as nurses for up to twenty years. In the push to professionalize nursing, the category, PRNs, is no longer used.

In contrast to UCPs, who may not be professionally trained nurses, provisionally registered nurses, called graduate nurses before the RHPA, are nurses trained outside Canada, who were hired to fill nursing positions in Canadian hospitals and long-term care facilities during the nursing shortage of the late 1960s and early 1970s. As in other areas of nursing human resources, there are no firm figures for the number of graduate nurses in Ontario, although estimates range from a low of 170 to a high of 600.

Few of these foreign accredited nurses saw reasons to write the Canadian Nursing Association Testing Services (CNATS) examination or to be registered with the College. In their minds, they had been trained as nurses, and they held nursing positions where they practised essentially as RNs, performing all the procedures now identified as controlled acts for nurses. With the advent of the RHPA, graduate nurses could no longer perform these controlled acts unless they became registered with the College of Nurses, which also meant passing the CNATS. Alternatively, they accepted a reduced status as UCPs and performed controlled acts under delegation. The RHPA thus increased the vulnerability of graduate nurses; as hospitals attempted to trim costs, they were targeted for layoffs on the grounds that they could no longer provide essential nursing care.

The scramble prior to the RHPA about how to deal with graduate nurses ignited heated debates within the profession over a number of issues. Some of those issues, like discussions around public safety and the integrity of nursing as a holistic and evolving profession, resembled concerns presently being raised about unregulated care providers. Other issues, like human rights violations and systemic discrimination, were particular to this case. The ONA, which represented graduate nurses because they performed many of the same functions as RNs, advocated extending the time frame for passing the CNATS to ten years from the proposed three years. This would have allowed most graduate nurses to work until the early retirement age of 55, since most were in their 40s and 50s. As well, the ONA proposed that, rather than writing the whole CNATS exam, which covers all areas of nursing, PRNs might be required to write an exam in their own field (e.g., med-surg, obstetrics, gerontology). College staff discussed the possibility of registering working graduate nurses subject to certain restrictions, such as limiting their practice to their current employment setting. This suggestion was based on CNO statistics (1994) which showed that the average length of employment for graduate nurses was eighteen years, with two-fifths working for twenty or more years, often at the same institution; only a sixth have been working for fewer than ten years. Then Health Minister Ruth Grier also weighed in to support an extension of the three-year provisional registration to ten years.

In the end, Council members at the College of Nurses of Ontario rejected all of these grand-parenting proposals. Instead, graduate nurses were given provisional registration and a so-called window of opportunity of three years to achieve registration. This decision must be understood within the context of the push to professionalize through formal accreditation. The focus on establishing criteria consistent with other health professions under the RHPA ultimately overshadowed human rights considerations. At the crux of the issue was the idea that a category of nurses have been practising and could continue to practise without having passed the definitive credentialing hurdle of the CNATS. That many graduate nurses, according to CNO statistics (1994), had tried to pass the CNATS several times (averaging 2.6 attempts without success) and that some had never even attempted the examinations was perceived to reflect negatively on nursing as a profession. Plainly, the college could not conclude that the CNATS was defective as a definitive indicator of competence. Rather, it was argued that if graduate nurses had practised for years without jeopardizing patient safety, this was more a measure of longevity and luck than competence, quality and a capacity for self-reflective learning. In this conclusion, the college was supported by nurse leaders, associations and educators.

The ONA initially stood alone in raising concerns about systemic discrimination (1998: 24–25). The union argued that the form and content of many of the CNATS examination questions contain cultural biases which pose systemic barriers to graduate nurses, many of whom are older, foreign born, foreign trained and members of racial minorities. For example, almost 50 percent of the questions test psychological and social appropriateness, containing meanings and nuances derived from a domi-nant Canadian mainstream culture. It was further argued that multiple choice type questions required a higher level of proficiency in English than the working knowledge of English required to deliver hands-on, safe patient care. Since few graduate nurses have English or French as their first language, they would be disadvantaged.

Evidence gleaned from the CNO *Annual Report* (1993) lends support to this argument. The report compared the number of examination rewrites by nursing students graduating from Ontario to those graduat-ing outside Ontario. It noted that although 29 percent of all those who wrote the CNATS in 1993 failed, only 8 percent of Ontario students who wrote for the first time failed, in contrast to a failure rate of 67 percent of applicants from nursing programs outside of Ontario. The ONA (1996) argued that a significant proportion of those in programs outside Ontario were racial minority applicants from countries which were culturally very distinct from Canada. Furthermore, 44 percent of "Ontario repeats" failed while 64 percent of "other repeats" were unsuccessful (College of Nurses of Ontario 1993: 40).

The issue of systemic discrimination has since moved to another level. In October 1997, the Ontario Human Rights Commission initiated a complaint against the OMOH and the College of Nurses of Ontario concerning their treatment of graduate nurses. It is likely that the nature of the CNATS examination will play a key role in this case. On January 1,

1996, the three-year limit lapsed and those PRNs who had not passed the CNATS and were still working as nurses lost their jobs. In the meantime, there is little follow-up data tracking where graduate nurses are working and whether they are competing with RPNs for underemployment in unregulated care provider positions.

Diploma Nurses

The minimum educational requirement for Registered Nurses in Ontario has been either a three-year college diploma or a university degree in nursing (BScN). As of 1997, the highest level of educational attainment for most RNs (74.4 percent) was a college diploma; only 15.9 percent of RNs had BScN degrees; 1.3 percent had a master's degree in nursing; 0.1 percent, a doctorate in nursing; and 6 percent had degrees in other than nursing (CNO 1999b). In December 1998, the Council at the College of Nurses unanimously passed a motion making a university degree in nursing (BScN) the minimum entry requirement to practise nursing in Ontario by the year 2005. For almost three decades, the College of Nurses of Ontario, the Canadian Nurses' Association and other nurse leaders and educators had pushed for this decision but were invariably resisted by the Ontario provincial government, even though the baccalaureate has been the minimum entry-to-practise requirement for nursing in other Canadian provinces for a number of years. Aside from the equity consideration of erecting new barriers to accessing the profession, the provincial government appeared to be sensitive to the interests of the overwhelming majority of non-degree nurses and was unwilling to risk the political fallout should a nursing shortage in the health system result from imposing higher entry requirements.

Two interrelated factors may have tilted the balance in favour of the baccalaureate decision. The first was the publication of the *National Nursing Competency Project* released in 1997. This report identified entry-level competencies across Canada for registered nurses, registered practical nurses and registered psychiatric nurses. Thereafter, each provincial regulatory body undertook to articulate the competencies in its own jurisdiction compared to those at a national level. The CNO took the lead in coordinating a broad-based umbrella working group consisting of representatives from among educators, employers, nursing professional associations and unions. The CNO (1998) further validated the findings and conclusions of this group through questionnaires to 2,500 RNs, seventeen focus groups across Ontario and a series of key informant interviews.

A second related factor was health system restructuring. With hospital downsizing, it was recognized that nurses had fewer supports, less opportunity to learn on-the-job, heavier workloads and less time to make critical decisions around more acutely ill patients who were leaving hospitals after shorter stays. If nurses were expected to hit the ground running, it was argued that they needed essential skills like critical thinking, research-based practice and reflective practice, which were identified as key components of a degree, but not a diploma, education.

Not all nurses agreed. In interviews conducted by the authors, many diploma registered nurses resented this decision which, in their minds, diminished their opportunities for professional growth, status and mobility. They pointed to the hiring practices of a number of hospitals in the Greater Toronto Area, which, they claimed, preferred degree nurses for permanent positions even prior to the CNO's baccalaureate announcement. Diploma nurses conceded that these hospitals ensured that the diploma nurses already employed were equitably treated as far as salaries and benefits were concerned, but they alleged that degree nurses were preferred for management and supervisory roles. According to diploma nurses, if such promotion patterns became widespread, the breadth and depth of their long-term clinical experience would be undervalued; their hands-on supervisory and leadership experience would be underrated; their participation in committees and broader hospital activities overlooked; and their participation in professional workshops, training programs, courses and certificate programs, discounted. In their minds, the baccalaureate decision solidified their status as second-class practitioners as compared to their degree counterparts.

In an attempt to mend a potentially widening rift between diploma and degree nurses, the CNO urged employers, together with collective bargaining units, to work out supports to facilitate continuing education for diploma nurses. Among the recommendations of the *RN Entry to Practice Competencies Project Report* was "developing and implementing a plan, in concert with employers and educators, to expand access to postbasic nursing education for those diploma prepared RNs who choose to pursue such education" (CNO 1998: 14). In addition, the CNO attempted to assure diploma nurses that they would not lose their status as RNs should they choose not to obtain a baccalaureate. The Report also recommended that ongoing renewal of registration remain subject only to fulfilling quality assurance obligations and maintaining professional standards of practice.

While some hospitals did in fact provide supports, including funds for conference participation, scholarships to help pay for tuition fees, flexible schedules to accommodate studies, or time off to encourage degree completion, many diploma nurses still believed that the baccalaureate decision would result in discriminatory treatment. In interviews, diploma nurses expressed concern that professional training opportunities would be restricted to degree nurses if training was seen as a precursor to promotion to positions open only to degree nurses. Furthermore, they questioned whether their opportunities for transferring from casual or part-time positions to full-time positions would be limited if management preferred to hire degree nurses in permanent positions. Would they be increasingly pushed into part-time or casual positions? Diploma nurses perceived that within the current context of hospital closures, higher patient-nurse ratios and faster turnover of sicker patients, the requirements of higher formal credentials could very well translate into fewer jobs and promotion opportunities for them.

Dually Registered Nurses

While in a relatively stronger position than RPNs, RNs are also feeling the downward pressures of health system restructuring. Evidence of this is seen in the growing number of RNs seeking dual registration as RNs *and* RPNs. In 1993, there were 465 dually registered nurses. This figure increased steadily so that by 1997 the number of RN/RPNs stood at 1,177. While dual registration is not yet common, anecdotal evidence suggests that more nurses may take this route in order to make themselves more competitive in increasingly restrictive job markets. It is reported that a number of hospitals in northern Ontario are requesting dual registration in an effort to decrease organizational costs. Seasoned RNs who are near the top of their salary scale are encouraged to be dually registered. They are then laid off as full-time RNs and rehired as newly registered RPNs, who can be paid at the bottom of the salary scale. In unionized hospitals, RN salaries range from $17.94 per hour to a maximum of $27.80 per hour after ten years. The range for RPNs averages between $16.66 per hour and a maximum of $17.66 per hour after ten years. RPN rates in community settings are even lower: from $13.70 per hour to $16.39 per hour. There is no way of tracking accurate figures in non-unionized facilities where RNs can work as RPNs as long as they do not use the RPN title. Such employment arrangements may mean that the number of RNs underemployed as RPNs is actually under reported.

Dual registration is not a direct result of the RHPA. However, while this option has always been open to RNs, it is only recently that some RNs are resorting to this strategy in a heightened environment of work insecurity. Where the RHPA *is* relevant is in the intensification of professional responsibility and accountability when nurses are pushed to choose underemployment. As discussed in the next section, while RNs may choose to be registered as RPNs and to accept lower levels of occupational status and pay, they have less choice over their professional obligations. Under the RHPA they continue to be treated as RNs and remain responsible for standards of practice as RNs, including responsibilities with respect to delegation, education, supervision and so on. Thus, the

RHPA ensures that under conditions of dual registration employers get the best of both worlds: high levels of professional expertise and accountability at the lowest possible price.

Into The Future

As noted earlier, nursing has struggled since its inception as a profession to move from "under the thumb" (Coburn 1993: 133) of medical dominance. There is no question that the RHPA does much to strengthen a new kind of autonomy, especially for health professions that were recognized for the first time and for nursing. The Act recognizes nursing's capacity to make authoritative decisions based on an established area of expertise; to control the direction of the profession; and to ensure accountability to clients, society and the profession through quality assurance programs and ethical guidelines (Norris 1995: 59, Schutzenhofer 1988: 93). Autonomy is said to be the hallmark of professionalism, part of the "bargain" which health professions "strike" with society in which "competence and integrity are exchanged for client and community trust, and relative freedom from lay supervision and interference" (Rueschemeyer 1983: 41).

As we have also emphasized in this chapter, the RHPA and the new degree of autonomy it establishes for nursing do not come without costs. Under conditions of massive health system restructuring, motivated in large part by the goal of cost-containment, the RHPA also sets the stage for the displacement of professional nurses with generic health care workers and for increased tensions within the profession between different categories of nurses all vying for a declining number of well-paid jobs.

There are some significant gains. A concrete example is Ontario's *Expanded Nursing Services for Patients Act* (Statutes of Ontario 1997). Passed in April 1997, this Act gives legislative recognition to a specially trained, extended class of nurses, commonly referred to as nurse practitioners, to perform some acts previously controlled by physicians. These include the capacity to autonomously diagnose, treat and prescribe medications for common illnesses in primary health care, and, under certain circumstances, order ultrasounds, x-rays and laboratory tests.

This marks a sharp contrast to the status of nurse practitioners up to this point. Nurse practitioners gained support in Canada in the 1970s as a relatively quick solution to a shortage of physicians; they were to provide primary health care, especially in under-serviced areas, outpost settings, community health centres, and more recently, in neonatal intensive care units. Their distinctive role as para-physicians was never explicitly supported by legislation or regulation. Instead, they worked under medical protocol, at the discretion of physicians, who were ultimately accountable. After graduating approximately 250 nurse practitioners, most nurse practitioner programs were cancelled in 1983 when the number of doctors climbed. The shutting down of these programs was indicative of the dominance of medicine within the hierarchy of health professions. When push came to shove, nurses lost.

The dominance of medicine persists to this day. While nursing is legitimized as an autonomous profession under legislation, it continues to lack the political power to consolidate its gains. First, nurse practitioners continue to be hemmed in by a lack of funding. Not only have nurse practitioners in Ontario not been given dedicated resources, the recent agreement between the Ontario government and the Ontario Medical Association specifically prohibits any transfer of funding from physicians to other health professionals. Thus, instead of providing a safe, lower cost alternative to physicians' services, nurse practitioners become a potentially expensive added cost to the health system. The Ontario government agreement with the OMA also gives physicians a direct role in determining the direction of health reform. Given the medical profession's historical resistance to any measure perceived to erode its clinical and economic dominance, it seems safe to assume that the broader deployment of nurse practitioners, potentially in direct competition with primary care physicians, will continue to be hotly contested.

In addition to these external political factors, debates *within* the nursing profession provide an added cautionary note. For instance, some nurses continue to argue that the promotion of nurse practitioners as mini-doctors who are trained to do what doctors do, at a fraction of the cost, does not serve the interest of nursing, which as a profession attempts to carve out a role that is distinct and separate from medicine. Such a course, it is claimed, will blur nursing and physician roles, rather than optimize nursing knowledge and skills. Any successes in health outcomes will be attributed to medical knowledge and skills, reinforcing "old stereotypes of nursing as a second-rate, 'simpler' form of medicine" and obfuscating nursing's "unique role" in the health care system (Gottlieb 1994: 3–4). This perspective argues that the cost-containment gains by governments and health facilities will be paid for by undermining nursing as an independent and distinctive profession.

While the RHPA provides mixed benefits for the professionalization of nursing, there are also considerable costs at the professionalization end of the continuum. Most notably these are increasing pressures for RNs to compete with RPNs and the increasing substitution of unregulated care providers for professional nurses. Such developments not only put extreme pressure on nursing jobs and pay, but they also increase internal divisions and fragmentation within nursing, which undermine the profession's ability to consolidate gains in professional autonomy. As discussed earlier, under conditions of restricted labour markets, relatively stronger categories of nurses have engaged in strategies to defend their interests at the expense of relatively weaker categories of nurses, while the latter have been pushed to accept the duties and pay scales of unregulated workers. Nevertheless, even under conditions of underemployment and lower pay, nurses remain accountable at their level of registration. For instance, if there is an emerging condition, i.e., a medical emergency, RNs working as RPNs are obliged by legislation to perform as registered nurses until another RN is available.

As fewer nurses face busier hospitals where numbers, acuity and complex patient care profiles are increasing, emerging conditions and emergencies may become more the norm than the exception. The likelihood that nurses will be performing above their "formal job descriptions" may also become the norm (Armstrong et al. 1994: 54–92).

Similarly, the increasing use of UCPs presents a real challenge to the profession. Guidelines established by the CNO clearly differentiate the responsibility of regulated nurses from that of unregulated care providers. Regulated nurses are accountable for deciding whether it is appropriate to teach a procedure; whether the conditions for teaching can be met in a particular situation; and, how best and how frequently to monitor continuing competence. Nurses are not responsible or accountable for unsafe actions by unregulated workers. For example, if a UCP demonstrates competence to a nurse while a procedure is being taught but does not follow the procedure in actual practice, the UCP is personally accountable. Frontline reality is not nearly as clear cut. Where nurses work with UCPs, they may be faced with difficult dilemmas. For instance, a decision by a nurse not to delegate will result in a heavier workload for that nurse; a decision to delegate may, in the nurse's view, jeopardize safe care.

The professional accountability dimension of the RHPA, which is the appropriate flip-side of professionalism, combined with the downward pressures of health system restructuring, produce many such dilemmas for nursing. The above examples describing the circumstances of working with UCPs or the acceptance of lower occupational positions illustrate the worst of two worlds: professional accountability and responsibility, but lack of control over decisions affecting care. As well as leading to the underutilization of nurses and to underemployment and lower pay, these contradictory forces exacerbate longstanding hierarchical tensions within nursing which detract from the capacity of the profession to make advances *vis-à-vis* dominant professions like medicine. This is consistent with Coburn's (1993: 139) view that even with self-regulation, the nursing profession never achieved the professional status and autonomy accorded to other professions like medicine and dentistry, but continues to fight its political battles on turf which it does not control.

Where does this lead nursing? As discussed earlier, one path chosen by nursing is credentialism, in the form of increasing the entry-to-practice requirements for the profession. As Pat Armstrong and colleagues (1993) point out, the use of certification as the path to professional autonomy was critically important to counter false notions that the caring responsibilities of nursing were based primarily on the intuitive knowledge inherent in women's genetic make up. Formal accreditation sends out a strong message that nursing is skilled work based on a discernible body of knowledge that requires education and standards of practice. However, this path to power and prestige, which supposedly imitates doctors, will not likely solve current challenges facing the profession because it fails to understand that "doctors' power and respect did not come mainly from their credentials," but "because doctors worked hard to maintain their own dominance" (Armstrong et al. 1993: 37). In other words, the path was primarily political. The lesson for nursing is that current strategies by different categories of nurses worsen the fault lines within the profession and undermine the viability of political solutions. The strategy of seeking professional power through credentials may increase the power of some nurses over others, but more importantly, it reinforces inequities within nursing and prevents solidarity among nurses to challenge the hierarchical system of health professionals.

Removing barriers among the different health disciplines was seen to promote a fuller and more equitable participation among different health professionals. This analysis shows that barrier removal alone is ineffective and that the RHPA incorporates the value of equity without considering what equity looks like in its specific implementation. At the end of the day, the RHPA, within the context of health system restructuring, has created conditions that threaten the professional autonomy and increase the internal fragmentation of a politically weaker, female-dominated profession.

Notes

1. Cawthorne in this volume for a discussion of the status of midwifery in Alberta.
2. The following health professions are covered by the RHPA: audiology and speech-language pathology, chiropody (including podiatry), chiropractic, dental hygiene, dental technology, dentistry, denturism, dietetics, massage therapy, medical laboratory technology, medical radiation technology, medicine, midwifery, nursing (registered and practical nurses), occupational therapy, opticianry, optometry, pharmacy, physiotherapy, psychology and respiratory therapy. (Statutes of Ontario 1994: c18.)

3.   These include: communicating a diagnosis; performing a procedure below the dermis or mucous membrane; setting or casting a fracture or dislocation; moving the joints of the spine beyond the usual physiological range of motion using fast low amplitude thrust; administering a substance by injection or inhalation; putting an instrument, hand or finger into a body orifice or artificial opening into the body; applying or ordering the application of a form of energy; prescribing or dispensing, for vision or eye problems, subnormal vision devices, contact lenses or eye glasses; prescribing a hearing aid; fitting or dispensing a dental prosthesis, orthodontic or periodontic appliance; managing labour or conducting the delivery of a baby; and allergy challenge testing of a kind in which a positive result of the test is a significant allergic response.

4.   The CNO recognizes two categories of nurses. Registered Nurses (RNs) have a minimum of three years of college or university training. Registered Practical Nurses (RPNs, previously called Registered Nursing Assistants) take a twelve- to eighteen-month college program.

5.   Gregor, Keddy, Foster and Denney in this volume discuss the impact of job displacement among nurses in Nova Scotia.

6.   Grinspun in this volume challenges the notion that replacing registered nurses with UCPs is a cost-effective strategy.

7.   Guruge, Donner and Morrison in this volume propose strategies for addressing systemic discrimination against visible minority caregivers and care recipients.

4

Nova Scotia Nurses
and Health Care Restructuring:
Strategies to Manage Job Displacement[1]

Frances Gregor, Barbara Keddy, Suzanne Foster
and Donna Denney

Introduction

For the past decade, provincial governments in Canada have been restructuring the health system. All Canadians have felt the impact of this process but none more so than nurses. In an address to the Canadian Nurses Association in June, 1998, the federal Minister of Health, the Honourable Allan Rock, admitted as much when he said, "No professional group has borne the brunt of health care restructuring more than have Canada's nurses...." (Canadian Nurses Association 1998). Three aspects of restructuring have had enormous significance for registered nurses (RNs), most of whom are women and most of whom still work in hospitals (Statistics Canada 1998b). The first is the shrinkage or downsizing of the hospital sector, leading to nursing job loss and job displacement. The second is the move to establish a flexible nursing workforce through a process of casualizing nursing workers. The third aspect is the substitution of less qualified nursing workers and/or volunteers for RNs.

In Halifax, in the spring of 1996, in the midst of yet another round of hospital bed closures, we decided to investigate the problem of job displacement among Nova Scotia nurses. As faculty members in the School of Nursing at Dalhousie University, we were appalled by the silence surrounding the layoff of nurses in the tertiary care hospitals close to the university campus. The silence of nurses and nursing organizations extended across the province and across the country (Shamian and Lightstone 1997). There were little data available on the number of nurses actually losing jobs, but each of us was hearing stories from our students of nurses working as grocery store cashiers and nurses' aides in order to survive financially. We decided to give voice to the situation of these nurses by describing, first, the variety of job displacements they were experiencing and, second, the ways in which displacement affected their personal, work and family lives (Keddy et al. 1999). A third goal, and reflective of our own critical stance towards health care reform, was to give light to nurses' own analysis of the deteriorating job situation in nursing and specifically to their understanding of health care reform (Gregor et al. 1998).

However, in the course of our conversations we also learned how these nurses were managing to survive economically under conditions of job displacement. At the time of the study, only two of our participants were without paid employment of any kind, although virtually all were working fewer hours than they desired and some were not working as RNs. Most of the nurses reported they were anxious, felt hopeless and experienced feelings of insecurity, yet most of them were engaged in paid nursing work of some sort. A few nurses also worked in non-nursing jobs. The purpose of this chapter is to report in detail on what these nurses did to secure work in the face of health care restructuring. Nova Scotia contains just 3.7 percent of all practising RNs in Canada; yet we believe neither their employment situation nor their response to it is unique. This chapter adds to the knowledge of how public-sector service workers respond to employment restructuring.

Additionally, this chapter aims to bring a note of caution to policymakers considering health care reform today. Three years after we gathered the original data for this chapter, a nursing shortage began looming in Nova Scotia. We will refer to this later. But suffice to say now that not only is this latest development ironic, it is also a lesson in the fallacy of restructuring health care on the backs of nurses.

Methodology

Our intention in carrying out this study was to interview enough nurses from all regions of the province to generate a comprehensive account of their experience and analysis of job displacement. Following ethical approval, we set out to find nurses who identified themselves as displaced or under threat of displacement. Finding them proved more of a challenge than we first thought. We contacted the president of each of twenty-one local chapters of the Registered Nurses Association of Nova Scotia and asked them to announce the study at chapter meetings. We notified the two unions in Nova Scotia representing nurses and posted notices on bulletin boards in Halifax hospitals. We also used our own connections to get word of the study out into the nursing community. Nurses who agreed to participate were asked to pass on word of the study to other nurses experiencing job displacement.

When we received the name of a potential participant, we sent the nurse a letter of information, a consent form, a demographic data sheet, a card on which to indicate where to call for an interview and an envelope to return relevant forms to us. In addition to the demographic sheet, we developed a semi-structured interview guide to ascertain expectations for employment in nursing, past, present and future, and the impact of present employment status on personal, family and work life.

While the guide provided some structure, discussion with partici-pants was open and informal and followed many paths. Towards the end of the interview each participant was asked to describe their understand-ing of health care reform. All interviews were tape recorded and tran-scribed. All personal and institutional identifiers were removed from the transcripts. Analyzing the interviews involved the entire research team, working first individually, then as a group, to identify and confirm the major themes.

The Study Participants

In approximately nine months of seeking out displaced nurses, we were able to solicit participation from forty, thirty-eight females and two males. Fourteen of the participants were from the Halifax Regional Municipality, which is the major urban area in the province and includes the cities of Halifax and Dartmouth. The remaining twenty-six were from towns and villages in rural Nova Scotia. Participants ranged in age from 21 to 55 years, with a mean age of 36.8 years, somewhat below the average age of a nurse in the province, which, in 1998, was 46 years (M. Muise, personal communication, April 1, 1999). Twenty-two had an RN diploma, fifteen a bachelor's degree and three a master's degree. Thirteen partici-pants had additional preparation, such as a certificate course in a clinical nursing specialty. Their years of work experience ranged from less than a year to over twenty years. Three participants identified that they had less than a year's experience and six said they had more than twenty-one years. The remaining thirty-one participants were in between, with the greatest number (ten) having one to five years of experience.

Their employment status varied considerably and participants were free to place themselves in more than one category of displacement. While no participant said she or he had never been employed in nursing, eleven volunteered they had been displaced though layoff, seven had been bumped from one nursing area to another and nine reported that they expected to be bumped or laid off. Six participants said they were working in less than an RN role, for example as a personal care worker or practical nurse; eight reported they were working at several part-time positions and twenty said they were working at several casual positions. Of the forty nurses we interviewed, fourteen said they were the sole wage earner in the family. Twenty-four reported they belonged to a union.

We were surprised by the very few nurses in our study with less than one year of work experience; only three out of the forty were in this category. When we began to recruit nurses, we understood that new graduates were having an especially hard time at finding full-time employment. This was confirmed by a study of employment patterns within the first year of graduation carried out by the professional nursing association in Nova Scotia (Registered Nurses Association of Nova Scotia 1996). On examining registration statistics for the years 1990 through 1995, the Association found a marked decrease in the percentage of new graduates finding regular full-time employment, from 61.6 percent to 14.6 percent, and a corresponding increase in new graduates finding casual employment, from 24.3 percent to 67.9 percent. There was also an increase in the percentage of new graduates seeking work in other non-RN nursing roles, such as licensed practical nurse and personal care worker. The number of new graduates looking for work in areas other than health care also grew from 2 percent in 1990 to 24.2 percent in 1995. Thus, new graduates seemed to be especially affected by the move in hospitals to a flexible nursing workforce but we were unable to recruit them in large number. Perhaps these new graduates either did not know about our study or felt too threatened to participate.

Nurses' reaction to the job situation tended to be affected by how long ago the participant entered the nursing workforce. Those who began nursing in the 1960s and early 1970s expressed disbelief at the erosion, if not evaporation, of full-time employment. They had expected, they told us, to hold full-time jobs for as long as they wanted to work. Participants graduating after 1980 were much more likely to report that they had been warned by their teachers on graduation from nursing school that the job situation was tight.

Surviving Restructuring

All of the nurses in our study had suffered job displacement or threat of displacement, yet the majority were still working as RNs, albeit as casual staff. We identified two major themes in the actions nurses took to secure nursing work: being accessible to employers seeking casual nursing staff and being available to respond to a call for work. We named the first theme "Being Easy to Reach" because the essence of this theme was conditions, some directly influenced by the nurse's accessibility to an employer. We named the second theme "Being Willing and Able to Work" because the focus was the nurse's efforts to put in place the personal arrangements necessary to respond to a work call. In the world of flexible staffing of health care facilities, the strategies within these two themes were the key to getting nursing work.

We identified two other sets of actions that seemed to be related to, or a precondition of, the two main themes of accessibility and availability. Nurses who were easy to reach were more likely to be rewarded if the people making the staffing decision knew their face and name. Thus some nurses employed actions which we organized under the name "Staying in Touch." In various ways they stayed in contact with those whose job it was to decide whether a nursing unit needed extra staff.

Being available to work when you are the mother of young children, and especially a single mother, depends on being able to hand over care of your children to another person and to make other needed domestic arrangements. The nurses in our study with childcare responsibilities made flexible arrangements with their mothers, neighbours and babysitters to take their children when they were called for a shift. We called these actions "Back-up Planning with Family and Friends."

Being Easy To Reach
Nurses, like many people, use cellular phones, beepers and answering machines to communicate. For a nurse looking for work, owning one of these devices can mean the difference between getting a shift and not getting one. But some devices are better than others at linking a nurse to an employer urgently searching for nursing staff for the next work-shift. The device that increases nurses' chances of receiving calls for work, no matter where they are, and that enables them to respond before other nurses are called, is the cellular phone. One nurse told us, "I bought a cell phone so I can be reached anywhere." When asked to explain her decision to buy this device she said,

> I talked to a couple of nurses during orientation and they carried beepers. So I thought, well, if I get a cell phone it would give me an edge because I wouldn't have to call them back. I would have the shift right then.

The response of this savvy nurse points to the competition that occurs among nurses when work is scarce.[2]

Another dimension of accessibility is exemplified in the comment of a nurse in a small town in rural Nova Scotia. She did not carry a cell phone or beeper, she said, because the nurses in her local health facility would know where to find her. They were her friends, the community was small, and they would know where in the community she was likely to be if she was not at home. Her response displays a dimension of accessibility related to social network.

Maintaining and nurturing employment related networks was a strategy some nurses used to enhance accessibility. This "Staying in Touch" strategy took the form of nurses who wanted additional shifts maintaining friendly relations with unit managers and head nurses and, if possible, responding positively when called to work a shift. The nurse who bought the cell phone said this,

> I've become friends with these people, and I wouldn't want to let them down. I appreciate so much that they phone me, as opposed to phoning another casual. I certainly wouldn't want to make them, you know, call someone else when they call.

A second strategy we learned of was the practice of checking out the potential for work from a position both inside and outside the institution, sometimes in combination with work, to nurture a professional relationship. One nurse told us,

> I go over to City Hospital[3] about once a week. I've got four floors I'm kind of concentrating on. And I try to seek out the head nurse, just to say "Hello, anything changed from last week?" The time can vary, because they may not be around. So then I come back. Just when I get five minutes. It's "Hi, how are you doing?" kind of thing.

Another nurse who was habitually called by the same unit to come to work, nevertheless scouted new opportunities for work in the hospital during breaks from the unit. He would go to other units to determine their pattern of demand for extra staff. This strategy was not without risk, we learned, as one's loyalty to the unit that usually called could be questioned if it became known one was hunting for work on other units.

A third strategy we placed in the category of "Staying in Touch" was to do volunteer nursing work. We learned of two interesting examples of volunteering. A nurse in a small town in Nova Scotia who could find minimal amounts of casual work in her field of community health nursing, volunteered several times a month at an adolescent health clinic. The clinic was operated by one full-time paid nurse working on an Employment Insurance grant. The remaining ten staff were all RN volunteers, like our participant, who had only bits and pieces of paid work. Their volunteer responsibilities at the clinic included drawing blood to test for HIV/AIDS and crisis counselling.

The other example was from a nurse living in a rural area of the province. This nurse had been laid-off from her small community hospital but returned on her own time to act as the education coordinator for the remaining nursing staff. She arranged training opportunities and brought journal articles into the hospital for the other employed nurses to read.

It was clear to us that both these nurses wanted to do this work, even though they were not paid for it. It seemed to be important to them to continue to make contributions as nurses either to patients or to other nurses. For one of these nurses, however, the strategy of volunteering appeared to be related to the possibility of finding paid work. She said,

> Volunteering, where I am, is very enjoyable for me and it holds the same responsibility as an RN even though it is a volunteer position. I guess that.... I do think it will benefit me as I go to apply for more jobs, as well as in the community nursing area.

Being Willing and Able to Work

Being accessible to an employer makes sense only if you are also willing and able to come to work. Nurses in all parts of the province told us the same thing about availability. Work comes first: personal and family plans are at the mercy of the telephone call that says a work-shift needs to be filled. Family and friends have to understand that plans for a night out evaporate in the event of such a call. One nurse we interviewed felt compelled to respond to a request to work for fear of not being called again. This fear is evident in the words of this nurse who said to us,

> I go whenever I possibly can, so you have to have an understanding family and friends. Sometimes you are interrupted in the middle of a meal.... I have had to flip back and forth from being scheduled for two twelve-hour nights and then having an eight, being home until 3 o'clock in the afternoon, and being called in again. Feeling that you have to take these shifts even though you are dead tired because you don't know when you will get them.

The requirement for a nurse to be available for casual work affects the entire family and plays havoc with plans for family activities. This is evident in the words of this nurse from rural Nova Scotia, who said,

> Before I was laid off, I used to have a schedule. Like I had every second weekend off or so. And so I'd be able to make plans with my family, you know, according to my schedule. But now, its more like a last minute thing. And more often than not it's weekends that I work when my husband could be off. So, when

he's off I'll be working, and I'll be doing most of my work in the summer time which is when people usually do some vacationing. And he's going, he'll have time off but that's when I'll be working.

For another nurse in rural Nova Scotia, availability meant, in some cases, long drives, perhaps as much as an hour to and from work. This is not an insignificant matter when it means driving in the dark in winter on isolated county roads and on highways with few other vehicles. But it was made clear to us by this nurse, that in the job situation that prevailed at the time, the price one paid to work included just such personal time, effort and dollars.

When a nurse has childcare responsibilities, availability for work depends on a set of flexible arrangements for care. A flexible nursing workforce which includes mothers with small children (and which nursing workforce does not?) must be backed up by an equally flexible network of care providers and caretakers. In this regard we heard that mothers of these nurses were often backup care providers in addition to babysitters who were prepared to be flexible (including ex-husbands). A nurse from a rural community in southwest Nova Scotia told us,

> I have a couple of really good babysitters who are quite flexible. Sometimes I have to juggle them around. I have to take the children to their dad's [this nurse was a single parent] or sometimes I don't go. Sometimes I have to turn down a shift. I'm fortunate because I get more days than nights And at this hospital there are quite a few casuals who prefer to do the nights, I suppose because they have families and they have back-up at home. The nights are difficult for me but I make whatever arrangements I have to.

Another single mother in rural Nova Scotia was available to work only on weekends when she could take her children to her ex-husband.

It is worth noting that all the nurses in our study with male partners told us these men were helpful and understanding about the work demands they faced. This "family response" to the work situation of the nurse reflects, we think, both the fact that more than 25 percent of our participants were the sole wage earners in the family and an accommodation to the reality faced by many Canadian families that two incomes are essential for economic survival.

Other Strategies to Survive Restructuring
Being accessible and available to an employer were the major, but not the

only, strategies these nurses used. Three other employment strategies were: increasing the number of hours worked through seeking additional nursing opportunities in other facilities; working in a non-nursing position; and improving chances for work by bettering qualifications, that is, by obtaining more education. This last strategy had both a short- and a long-term dimension.

With respect to increasing the number of hours worked, we heard from one nurse who worked in two different facilities, and every day of the week, for a total of 110 hours in a two-week period. During the week, she worked in a long-term care facility in rural Nova Scotia and was paid $10 an hour. During the weekend she worked in the regional hospital and was paid considerably more. Explaining this to us, she reported that the nursing home did not hire her into a designated RN position even though they called her an RN and gave her the responsibility of an RN, including giving injections. She said, "They called me an RN and they paid me more than a nursing assistant, but they only paid me $10 an hour." After six months of full-time work at this rate she called a friend who was a nursing unit manager at the regional hospital and was able to get casual work on the weekend at a better rate, as well as holiday and vacation shifts. She told her nursing supervisor at the long-term care facility she was doing this, and this individual started doing the same thing, we were told. Apparently she made less money in her administrative post in the nursing home than she did working casual shifts Friday nights and weekends at the regional hospital.

Working outside of nursing was a further employment strategy nurses used. We spoke to one RN with a first degree in biology who was in the process of completing her post-RN nursing degree and who worked part-time in a supermarket. She had done so throughout her science degree and returned to this work while finishing her nursing degree because she could not get enough casual nursing shifts. Two nurses from a small rural community in Nova Scotia worked on a casual basis as ambulance attendants. They maintained their certification in life-support skills in order to respond to calls to transport critically ill patients to the regional hospital or to Halifax.

Compared to the dominant strategies of accessibility and availability, obtaining more education as a way to improve job prospects played a minor role as a response to job displacement. In general, the uncertainty of both short- and long-term employment seemed to narrow the job horizon for these women and men, constraining their professional aspirations and impelling them to make market-driven career choices. Some nurses reported obtaining extra training in technical skills, or of intending to do so, as a way to make themselves more attractive to a potential employer. Like the possession of a cellular telephone, skill training, some nurses reported, might provide the competitive edge to a nurse seeking work. From those nurses whose only credential was an RN diploma, we heard talk of trying to get a baccalaureate degree at some future point. But plans for study were usually vague and hostage to the need to earn a wage in order to survive financially.

In concluding our description of the measures these nurses took to survive restructuring, we want to make clear we are not claiming that every nurse used every strategy, nor that they constitute all these nurses did, or other nurses do, to manage job displacement. They are the strategies we heard about in the course of a study whose chief aim was to map the experience of job displacement.

Discussion

In 1997, of the almost 230,000 practising RNs in Canada, almost half (47.3 percent) reported working part-time (Statistics Canada 1998b). This figure suggests that the job displacement and economic insecurity that our Nova Scotia participants experienced is the lot of many Canadian nurses. Indeed, it is the lot of many Canadian women. Schellenberg (1997), in a report to the Canadian Council on Social Development on part-time work, stated that 18 percent of all jobs in Canada are part-time and that 50 percent of part-time jobs are held by women aged twenty-five years and older.

Members of professional occupations are experiencing an increase in part-time work along with other workers. The incidence of "involuntary part-time work," as Schellenberg (1997) describes the state of wanting full-time work but not being able to find it, rose from 11 percent to 35 percent between 1975 and 1994 and included all sectors. The desire for full-time work is in part related to the disadvantages associated with part-time status: most part-time workers have no access to workplace benefits such as pension plans, medical and dental plans and paid sick leave.

Part-time workers experience a higher rate of casual employment than full-time workers, regardless of occupation. The Canadian Council on Social Development report cites the example of education, a female-dominated occupation like nursing, where 54 percent of part-time workers compared to 12 percent of full-time workers, said their job was not permanent (Schellenberg 1997).

The experience of and response to the casualization of work appears to be similar across service occupations. Broad (1997) in a study of Saskatchewan part-time private sector service workers, mostly women, reported a pattern of response to casualization very similar to that which we identified among professional nurses in Nova Scotia. Workers in the retail food, hotel, banking and telemarketing industries reported they had to be accessible and available to their employer if they wanted to get work. They had what Broad termed an "on-call" relationship with their employer. Scheduled for only a minimum number of work shifts per week, these workers were compelled to take on-call shifts and be available to respond to a call to come to work. Like the nurses in our study, they too struggled to make childcare arrangements. And, as in the case of our participants, family plans often had to be set aside in favour of employer demands.

One response that Broad (1997) did not report among the private sector workers he studied was volunteering to work. Two nurses in our study responded to job displacement by volunteering their labour. At first we reacted with cynicism to their decision to contribute their nursing knowledge and skill for free. But upon reflection, we believe it is not difficult to see why they did so. Volunteer work, when it includes professional tasks, keeps a nurse's skills current. And it lets others, such as nurse managers or others who might need to employ a nurse, know that a nurse is keen to keep up-to-date and is committed to nursing. At the time of the study, the nursing regulatory body in the province allowed volunteer nursing hours to be counted towards the annual required minimum number of practice hours. This was important for nurses in retaining their licence to practice as registered nurses. Finally, job layoff can disrupt important social networks, especially in a small or isolated community, as is typical of many communities in Nova Scotia. Volunteering labour provides a nurse the opportunity to be with work friends, or make new ones. This aspect is not insignificant for a nurse who can experience unwanted solitude after job layoff or when paid work is unavailable.

The casualization of labour that nurses and other female workers have experienced in recent years is a consequence of the move by private and public sector employers to establish workforce flexibility. Connelly and MacDonald (1996) describe three strategies of flexibility that are touted in the social science and management literature as necessary for increased competitiveness in the global marketplace: functional flexibility, or flexibility in the allocation of labour across tasks; numerical flexibility, or flexibility in the amount of labour; wage flexibility, or flexibility in compensation. These authors are highly critical of this literature because it fails, they say, to take into account the gendered nature of restructuring and the differential impact on men and women of flexibility strategies. To quote them:

Much of women's work, whether on the line in manufacturing

plants or in service jobs ranging from nursing to social work, is being made more routinized, sped up and degraded, and made more non-standard in terms of hours and the rewards of work. Flexibility strategies create marginalization for the majority of women. (Connelly and MacDonald 1996: 84)

We believe our participants' situation illustrates the marginalization that Connelly and MacDonald (1996) claim is a consequence of restructuring in the service sector. Despite their years of experience in nursing and their willingness and efforts to secure work, these nurses were denied both a meaningful career and compensation structure in their chosen occupation. At the mercy of employers' often quixotic demands for casual nursing staff, they used both traditional job search methods (Payne 1997) and the latest in communication technology to cobble together enough work to survive. For a significant number of these nurses, survival meant accepting work at less than an RN level and outside of nursing.

Jenson (1996), in a recent discussion of part-time work, describes the emergence of good jobs and bad jobs, the former characterized by full-time work, benefits and a career structure, the latter by low wages, precarious employment and a stunted or absent career ladder. Glenday (1997) observed that in "yesterday's economy" examples of good jobs included a factory worker in an automobile plant, a registered nurse, a high school teacher and an administrative secretary with government or a large private company. In "today's economy" good jobs are held by brokers, bankers, doctors, entertainers and consultants of all kinds. The author notes that these and other good jobs he describes require advanced education or specific post-secondary credentials and are available to relatively few working Canadians. The large numbers of RNs working part-time in this country at the time of the study and at the present time, appear to herald the emergence of "bad jobs" in nursing. Compared to many service sector workers, RNs cannot be described as low-waged workers yet. However, as a consequence of health care restructuring, they have begun to experience the precariousness of work and truncation of career characteristic of the "bad job."

Post-Script

We gathered this data in the spring and fall of 1996. Three years later, in April 1999, a nursing shortage is looming in Nova Scotia and across the country (Ryten 1997). The shortage is of such magnitude that it has been called a "public safety issue" by the Canadian Nurses Association, the official voice of nurses in Canada (Sibbald 1998). Advertisements for nursing jobs fill the classified sections of many Canadian newspapers and the Canadian Nurses Association offers electronic job searching through its web page. At the same time, nurses in Newfoundland, Saskatchewan and Quebec have withdrawn their services (and in some instances, been legislated back to work) to press home the point that working conditions in hospitals must improve if new nurses are to be recruited into vacant jobs. A prominent feature of nurses' demands is the return of full-time jobs with benefits. A further dimension of the problem is the lack of applicants in relation to future demand for university nursing programs, now the only way in most provinces to enter the profession. To hasten the "production" of more nurses there is even talk in some quarters of reopening hospital diploma programs (B. Downe-Wamboldt, personal communication, April 21, 1999).

As researchers, we think of the forty nurses we interviewed for our study and ponder their fate and that of their families. As nurses, we consider the apparent old-fashioned values of loyalty and service which are at the heart of nurses' commitment to care under difficult conditions, and we think of the absence of these values in employer's relations with nurses. In our more cynical moments, reflecting on the impact of health care restructuring on nurses and the spectre of too few nurses for too many patients, we are tempted to observe, "What goes around, comes around."

Notes

1. An earlier version of this paper was presented at the Annual Meeting of the Canadian Sociology and Anthropology Association, Ottawa, Ontario, June 3, 1998.
2. Lum and Williams in this volume discuss some ways that health system restructuring is pitting Ontario nurses and other health care providers against employers and each other.
3. Pseudonyms are used to protect the anonymity of participants.

5

"They Don't Listen To Your Body": Minority Women, Nurses and Childbirth under Health Reform

Denise L. Spitzer

> I think if somebody needs help to stay in the hospital, they should keep it. When you go to the doctor, they always tell you, you should listen to your body. When you're in the hospital and you tell them, I'm listening to my body and they'll tell you, no, you can go home and take a rest—they don't listen to your body again.

Michelle,[1] the thirty-four-year-old mother and recent immigrant from India quoted above, suffered from a massive postpartum hemorrhage following childbirth at a Canadian hospital undergoing health care restructuring. Policies established under health reform demand that new mothers and their infants are to be discharged in twenty-four to thirty-six hours following childbirth, although women in extraordinary circumstances may remain in hospital for up to three days. Michelle, weakened by her massive blood loss, knew what her body was telling her: she would be incapable of caring for her new baby, husband and household while in this condition. Moreover, family members closest to her spoke little English and would have difficulty contacting health personnel should an emergency arise. The nursing and obstetrical staff—coping with the effects of health reform—was unable to listen to what Michelle's body was telling her. She was discharged three days after a birthing experience that was nearly fatal. In the end, Michelle was lucky. Her extended family rallied around her, providing in-home care; other members of her community, however, have not always been so fortunate.[2]

This story of health reform looks at the relationships between minority women and nursing staff in hospitals and community-based health programs as they undergo dramatic shifts in obstetrical and postnatal care. Commissioned by a coalition of community-based organizations and health care institutions, five First Nations, six Indo-Canadian and five Vietnamese-Canadian mothers were interviewed about their experience of birth at one of three hospital sites in a large culturally-diverse Western Canadian city. Three low-income Euro-Canadian women, whose partners were of either First Nations or African-Canadian status, were invited by one of the First Nations participants to a group interview. As their experiences were informed by their position as economically and socially marginalized women, the original research objectives were expanded to include their commentary. This paper, however, will focus primarily on the experiences of the visible minority women as mandated by the originators of the research project. Community health workers from each of the communities served as co-researchers, helping recruit participants, conducting interviews with me, providing on-going feedback and validating research findings. In the second phase of the study, eleven nurses from two of these sites were interviewed to discuss their perceptions of their interactions with minority women within the context of health reform. This paper examines the impact of health reform on nurse–minority patient interactions during pregnancy, childbirth and postpartum.

I begin with a review of the development of obstetrical care in Canada and turn to the nurses' testimonies to assess the impact of the most recent changes on nursing staff and patients. Next, I present background information regarding pregnancy and childbirth that informs the expectations of the three groups of minority women included in the study. Their perspectives on nurse–patient interactions occurring in hospital and later at home are highlighted. And finally, I consider the impact of health reform on these relationships. I conclude by asserting that while the patient-informants found numerous ways to support and assert themselves during their childbirth experiences, the burdens imposed by health reform on nursing staff are borne disproportionately by visible minority women. Quite possibly, this is because nurses distressed by cutbacks can ill afford the time required to address the most problematic encounters, that is, those with marginalized women. These women can hear their bodies, but can anyone but them afford to listen anymore?

Health Reform and Obstetrical Care

The Development of Obstetrical Care in Canada
Substantive changes in the treatment of women and childbirth have taken place in the past hundred and fifty years, from a view of childbirth as a natural process that could be aided by female midwives to its reframing as an illness that required the attention of, until recently, male physicians. The decline of midwifery and the expansion of biomedicine in the terrain of women's reproductive health is rooted in social and

economic changes wrought by the Industrial Revolution and Victorian ideas about separate spheres for men and women. Nineteenth-century notions that glorified motherhood for middle- and upper-class women contrasted with declining family size for this sector of the population. Allopathic (biomedical) physicians, who were anxious to delegitimize other forms of medical practice and increase their market share of healing services, successfully asserted that medical intervention was required to alleviate the illness of childbirth (Mitchenson 1991). Allopathy, associated with scientific inquiry and technological progress, appealed to these women who could afford their services, thus reducing the demand for midwives who had long served as birthing experts (Mitchenson 1991, Wertz and Wertz 1977). In addition, legislation that banned midwives from accepting remuneration for their services, effectively reduced the number of women who would continue the practice (Mitchenson 1991).

By the turn of the twentieth century, midwifery practice was relegated to the ranks of the poor and recent immigrant populations, further reducing its credibility (Ehrenreich and English 1979), while biomedical physicians offered technologically advanced inducements such as Twilight Sleep, rendering childbirth painless (Wertz and Wertz 1977). It was not until the 1930s that hospitals became the pre-eminent site of childbirth in Canada (Mitchenson 1991), and while in hospital, women and their infants were separated and cared for independently. The current practice of combined (mother and infant) care is meant to expedite the bonding of mother and child and encourage familial support for nurturing the mother–infant dyad. It owes its origins, however, as much to economic considerations as to the philosophic ones that focus on patient choice and mother–infant bonding (Phillips 1989).[3]

While coping with changes in hospital obstetric care in the past decade, nurses were also confronted with a new demographic reality, one that saw an increasingly culturally diverse clientele who demanded a new form of understanding. While the field of transcultural nursing originated in the 1950s and 1960s (see Brink 1976, Leininger 1991), the application of cross-cultural education in nursing has been variable (Carpio and Majumdar 1991). Several approaches can be found including: 1) integrating ideas about culture into the entire curriculum; 2) creating specific learning opportunities that focus on specific cultural differences; 3) encouraging students to take courses such as anthropology; and 4) instructing a core course in cultural diversity (Carpio and Majumdar 1991, McGee 1992). Some of the approaches are criticized on the basis that diversity issues are lost in the curriculum, that elective courses are the choice of only a sector of the student population, that culture is presented as static and that culture is often de-contextualized, or lacking in socioeconomic and political considerations (Carpio and

Majumdar 1991, Jackson 1993, Nance 1995). Combining communication skills, self-awareness and exploration of one's own values is often seen as an approach that can best contribute to greater cross-cultural awareness (Carpio and Majumdar 1991, McGee 1992, Nance 1995).

Nurses and Childbirth

The impact of health reform on obstetrical nursing care has been dramatic, as the findings outlined in the following section attest. Changes to obstetrical care in the 1980s already had begun to increase nursing responsibilities; however, health reform in the 1990s intensified these effects. The loss of staff due to budget cuts greatly increased the workload of surviving staff, who were compelled to train nurses from other departments, who in turn had replaced less senior obstetrical nurses. Time constraints necessarily decreased patient contact. Moreover, nurses felt uncomfortable enforcing early discharge policies with which they disagreed. Overall, health reform contributed to a decline in the morale of nursing staff and increased their anxiety regarding job security and the diminishing quality of patient care.

The age and experience of the nurses included in this study reflect the seniority of the cohort that has survived staff layoffs. The nurses, all female, ranged in age from forty to fifty-two and possessed between sixteen and thirty-one years' experience in the field. Four were university-educated and the remainder had obtained nursing diplomas. Four were foreign-born; one of these women was a native English speaker while the three others were fluent in English as a second language. Two had received nurse-midwife training; however, they chose to work in postpartum care rather than labour and delivery as they recognized that the incongruence between their roles as nurses and their training as midwives would be frustrating.

The nurses included in this study have been witness to major changes in the area of labour, delivery and postnatal care in North America since the 1980s and the current practice of combined care. While dyadic care that treats mother and infant as a bonded unit may be beneficial to the patients and be regarded as highly rewarding for the nursing staff, it effectively doubles the number of patients under a nurse's care. Coupled with changes in hospital policy that enforce postpartum discharge within thirty-six hours after birth, the increase in workload is significant. Ellen, a nurse with twenty-eight years experience exclaimed,

> I find it horrendous that these girls are leaving in 24 hours. You can't teach them anything in that time at all, you can't even talk to them anymore. We used to have five patients to last us three days or five days, that kind of thing. So if I was on a five day

stretch, I had the three same patients for that time. Now I have five patients today, I may send three of them home, get three new ones. Tomorrow, I send another five home and get five new ones.... In those same three days now I look after twenty patients. That's frustrating!

The demanding work burden has diminished the nurses' most satisfying aspect to their work–having patient contact. Instructing new mothers in breastfeeding, bathing the newborns, responding to queries and contributing to the good health of mothers and their babies have been fundamental to nurses' on-going commitment to remain in the nursing profession; however, many feel that these duties are continually being compromised. Kate said,

I mean, the most time you get to spend with a patient like that is when you are giving them a bath and that's the only time you really, really touch them and somebody in that situation really needs human contact, or I think they do, and as a nurse, you don't, you don't have time to do that and its not, its not part of your schedule. There is no where, you know, when they do that classification thing....[4] There's no where that says the man is dying, needs to hold your hand. You know, like, there's no spot for that and yet that really is as important as the rest of the stuff that you can do. But you don't get to do it, you don't.

Cost-saving measures carried out in the name of health reform have resulted in massive staff layoffs, subsequent job insecurity and increased responsibility for "survivors." Changes in policies and procedures have led to shortages in supplies, problems with patients' meals and an increase in paperwork. All of this has contributed to an overall sense of frustration and heightened levels of anxiety and stress among nursing staff. Furthermore, trust in one's colleagues—deemed by the nurses to be essential to patient care—has diminished because downsizing meant that senior nursing staff from other departments filled the positions of those with less overall tenure, but often with greater experience in obstetrics. As a result, experienced obstetric staff felt an increased responsibility to ensure that items have not been overlooked.

The reduction in patient contact has also been a major issue for nurses who have felt that although care may be adequate, it has declined in quality over the past five to ten years. The policy of early discharge has been of particular concern, primarily since problems with breastfeeding, postpartum depression or infant distress may not manifest themselves until several days following delivery. Although public health nurses provide follow-up within twenty-four hours after discharge, some nurses were not confident that a brief visit could uncover more subtle problems involving the mother or newborn, especially since they know public health nurses have heavy workloads as well. Furthermore, while some of these community-based programs, such as various hotline services and home visits from public health nurses, are highly popular, they do not always serve the entire community. In one survey of such a program, one third of the respondents, most of whom were newcomers to Canada, were dissatisfied with program changes and had hoped to stay in hospital longer (see Bubel and Spitzer 1996).

Working with ethnic minority patients was cited as both the most satisfying and most frustrating aspect of working as obstetric nurses. Interaction with women from disparate cultural backgrounds was viewed as an important and enriching experience; however, communication barriers were significant and were exacerbated by health reform measures as Roxanne explains,

> I think that if I have a patient who is East Indian or if a nurse has a patient who is East Indian, who doesn't have a good understanding of the language, I find that nurses will just avoid dealing with them. And in relation to the cuts, if the people were in the hospital longer, there's a greater chance of them to have an interpreter available or at least get those avenues checked out.

Early discharge regulations have intensified the work of nursing staff who must instruct new mothers in basic health promotion strategies, including breastfeeding, in addition to evaluating the health status of mother and infant. Patients with whom they have difficulty communicating require more time and may, from the nurses' own admissions, be overlooked in favour of easier and quicker interactions.

In addition, the brevity of a patient's hospital stay renders the services of off-site professional interpreters unrealistic as they must be contracted earlier than is often possible. As a result, nurses may improvise communication techniques, employing hand gestures or word lists that they have obtained personally. Often, friends, family members or hospital staff are asked to provide interpretation, raising ethical questions about confidentiality and concerns about the accuracy of the communication. Multilingual staff were perceived as a significant asset; however, they were often called upon by staff in other departments to provide language assistance, adding to already significant workloads tasks that are generally unrecognized and unrewarded by hospital administration.

Attitudes about Pregnancy and Childbirth

Women from the three ethnic minority groups who participated in this study approached their encounters with nurses and the hospital system with disparate histories, values and support mechanisms. While all of the women identified themselves as culturally distinct from Euro-Canadian society and its institutions (including hospitals), some respondents, most notably the First Nations and Vietnamese-Canadian women, were economically-disadvantaged as well. Thus the intersections of class and culture, as well as the individual characteristics of personality and age, contributed to each particular birthing narrative.

Keeping in mind both individual and intra-group variation, I now provide a brief overview of culturally-specific circumstances, attitudes and expectations of the birthing process for each of the three ethnic minority groups. Following that, I present some experiences of hospital treatment received by women from each of the groups.

First Nations

First Nations populations in Canada are primarily young and experience higher rates of infant and perinatal mortality than the population at large (Frideres 1988, Waldram et al. 1995). Poor health status is in part a function of experiences of trauma, including the impact of residential schooling and disruption of familial and generational ties, both the purposeful and untoward destruction of traditional social structures, substandard living conditions, poor education and high unemployment (Waldram et al. 1995). Furthermore, urban migration has destabilized the extended family and contributed to a concentration of female-led households in metropolitan areas (Kastes 1993). Family support may still be substantial, especially as many urban First Nations peoples maintain ties to family and friends in rural communities, which allows for an expansive social support network and flexibility in residential choice (Garteig 1995, Social Services 1984).

Health is conceived as a balance that encompasses physical, emotional, spiritual and social wellbeing, as well as a person's relationship to the environment and community. This contrasts with the Western scientific notion of health that is more narrowly focused and is based on binary dichotomies of good and evil or sick and healthy (Clayton 1990, Frideres 1988, Garteig 1995, Hagey 1989, Waldram et al. 1995). These understandings are reflected in the contemporary beliefs and behaviours of many First Nations peoples, both rural and urban. In her study of urban First Nations women, Garteig observed, "How you live your life summarizes the themes that emerged in women's talk about health meaning" (1995: 140).

Traditions regarding pregnancy, childbirth and postnatal care are as diverse as the First Nations themselves. In some regions, such as northern Alberta, traditional birth attendants would assist in labour, delivery and postpartum care, but were generally uninvolved in pregnancy (Neander 1988). Following birth, women were traditionally encouraged to rest and remain under the care of family members. Amongst the Blackfoot, for instance, women would stay with their mothers for a thirty-day rest period (Hungry Wolf 1982). Information about prenatal care may be provided by a mother, sister-in-law or mother-in-law and may not be offered until a woman's first pregnancy is established (Hungry Wolf 1982, Neander 1988). Women may be encouraged to moderate their behaviour by avoiding strenuous activity, resting but not sleeping too much and monitoring their thoughts and comments to ensure their emotional state has a positive impact on the infants (Hungry Wolf 1982, Neander 1988). Cecilia, a twenty-year-old Nisga'a woman commented,

> my mom always told me that how you are during your pregnancy that's how your baby is going to be.... The baby still feels things like, after, if you have emotional attachment after the baby is born, like if I got upset the baby would be upset and like, if I got into an argument with somebody, the baby would be affected by it.

Most women seek advice on pregnancy from informal sources. Distrust of institutions, shyness with strangers, lack of privacy and a lack of transportation were often cited as reasons First Nations women do not often partake in institutionalized prenatal classes (Liu et al. 1994, Robinson 1990). Materials and information presented in classes may be visually inappropriate or offensive. In the United States, over 40 percent of First Nations women under twenty years of age begin childbearing, as opposed to just over 23 percent of the general population (Liu et al. 1994). Fear of judgment by health professionals also affects information-seeking behaviour during pregnancy. Thus, while eschewing most prenatal classes, women sought information independently and obtained regular physical examinations.

Vietnamese-Canadian
Canada has become home to over sixty thousand Vietnamese since the late 1970s (Neuwirth 1987). Blending values of Buddhism, Confucianism and Taoism, Vietnamese society places a strong emphasis on family, the maintenance of roles within the household and filial piety (Rutledge 1992). Immigration has disrupted traditional household patterns, often leaving women to take on new economic and decision-making roles and

increasing role strain (Williams 1990). Settling in Canada, Vietnamese migrants contend with the stress of adaptation to a new society, downward social mobility and lack of recognition of work experience and credentials (Beiser 1990, Beiser et al. 1994, Neuwirth 1987).

> Here its cold and quiet: I miss the crowds. In Vietnam, after supper, people go for walks and talk with neighbours, here people are isolated in their families. I miss the language; in Vietnam, I can express myself easier. I know where to go. I walk to go buy milk and I can go by myself, just go, I don't need anybody to help me, to drive or to translate.

Pregnancy is considered to be a highly desirable state and requires attention to self-care and the maintenance of balance. Women may consume tonics to strengthen the mother and ease delivery (Dinh et al. 1990); they avoid foods that are too salty or sour and they are encouraged toward moderate behaviour (Mattson 1995). While the French introduced biomedicine to Vietnam in the nineteenth century, its adherents were clustered in urban areas where physician-assisted hospital birth is common. In rural areas, midwives continue to attend births (Dinh et al. 1990). Childbirth is still considered a natural process which is also the purview of women, making some uncomfortable with males attending at delivery (Immigrant Women of Saskatchewan 1993, Mattson 1995). In Vietnam, a woman might return to her mother's home for her first baby's delivery. In Canada, women relied on friends, female relatives and what they recalled from their mothers' advice to guide their behaviour during their pregnancies. Canadian physicians were seen as forthcoming with information; however, the sheer volume of pamphlets and other reading materials was seen as overwhelming and difficult to prioritize.

Indo-Canadian

The category of Indo-Canadian discloses a diversity of cultures that stretch across the globe. South Asian immigration to Canada is a relatively recent phenomenon; however, in the past few decades migration has increased from the Indian sub-continent and South Asian communities in Africa and the Pacific. As is the case with many international and internal migrants, South Asian families are often fractured, producing shifts in gender and household relations (Kurian 1989). Traditionally, pregnancy is considered a normal, healthy state and although women in some places may be given more attention and familial protection, they do not curtail their activities (Bhaskaran 1993, Kanhere 1989, Woollett and Dosanjih-Mattwala 1990). Prohibitions for pregnant women are few, except for heavy lifting and certain food avoidances that vary individually and culturally within the category of Indo-Canadian. According to the principles of Ayurveda (classical Indian medicine), pregnancy is a hot state that needs to be balanced by the consumption of cold foods (Bhaskaran 1993, Woollett and Dosanjih-Mattwala 1990). In addition, a woman's outlook is believed to affect the fetus. For example, a miscarriage can be attributed to a woman's negative thoughts; therefore, she can be held responsible should one occur (Bhaskaran 1993).

In India, a woman may return to her parents' home to deliver her first child and she will give birth with the assistance of traditional birth attendants called dais or, in some areas, dhorunis—the one who catches the newborn (Chatterjee 1989, Islam 1989). This practice of returning to the parents' home may differ according to socioeconomic status. In Gujarat, Kanhere (1989) found that lower-class women remained in their husbands' homes during pregnancy and for postnatal care, while upper-class women returned to their family home in late pregnancy. Childbirth is conceived as polluting; dais, therefore, have little status as they perform tasks that are culturally defined as defiling, such as handling the placenta (Chatterjee 1989, Jeffery and Jeffery 1993). Intense pain is believed to hasten delivery and crying out in labour is common (Jeffery and Jeffery 1993, Morse 1989). Ranjit told us,

> I had a home delivery, because in hospitals it wasn't done. In Delhi. The lady [the people like doulas—interpreter] called dais. She came, I had the baby delivered through her and she came for fifteen days after the delivery and she would massage me every day with oil and comb my hair and give the baby a bath, so I was very well taken care of.

Childbirth is generally considered a woman's matter, although research in the United Kingdom found that many Anglo-Indian husbands did accompany their wives at hospital delivery unless they were caring for other children (Assanand et al. 1990, Woollett et al. 1995). In Canada, Bhaskaran (1993) reported Indo-Canadian women refrained from participating in prenatal classes because of embarrassment, language barriers and a sense that women should not have that particular knowledge about the body or the childbirth process. A study conducted in Edmonton confirmed that Sikh husbands are less likely than counterparts from other cultural communities to attend prenatal classes or assist in the postpartum period (Nankpi 1994). Woollett et al. (1995) found that many South Asian women strongly supported biomedical practice, but they experienced conflicts in values over issues of self and infant care. For example, they were hoping to rest, while the hospitals were eager for the women to quickly take responsibility for themselves and their offspring. After birth, women anticipate a forty-day postpartum rest period. This tradition may be difficult to maintain in Canada, particularly without familial support. If a woman does not comply with this lie-in period, it is believed she will likely suffer from arthritis or other illnesses. New mothers are to be kept warm and remain with the baby most of the time. Hot foods such as ginger are recommended as are hot baths and massages. Visitors are welcome to bring gifts, but widows, women who have lost children and people in mourning are prohibited. Excessive compliments are not appropriate for fear of bringing the evil eye that may result in illness (Nankpi 1994).

Minority Women and Nursing Staff

Most of the nursing staff who were interviewed had exposure to materials designed to enhance cultural sensitivity in patient care. Often the approach is to provide the nurse with a brief overview of the cultural rules with which patients from cultural and religious minorities are presumed to abide. The nurse's relationship with a minority patient is meant to be facilitated by demonstrating her knowledge of these guidelines. The enculturation process, however, is complex, flexible and seldom reduced to assertions in a guidebook. Cultural values and behaviours change temporally, geographically and individually; a fact that proved at minimum confusing to nursing staff when minority patients did not respond in the manner suggested in the handbooks. These efforts, though well-intentioned, served to underscore one of the major difficulties with intercultural relations, that is, the temptation to produce generalizations about the Other, reducing non-dominant individuals to a uniform caricature. It is within this context that women with different expectations and varying degrees of facility with English, available support and attitudes towards institutions approached their hospital birthing experiences.

Now, I present some experiences of hospital treatment from the perspective of women from each of the ethnic minority groups.

First Nations
The average age of the First Nations mothers in this study was twenty. From the mothers' perspectives, their relative youth factored into the treatment they received in hospital. Four of the five were married or living common-law; one woman lived with relatives. Four of the women had not completed high school and one had graduated from college. The hospital birthing experience for these women appeared to vary slightly with each additional birth. First-time mothers seemed to approach the

institution with great trepidation and were reassured with the appearance of their support persons, primarily family and friends. All of the women, however, felt keenly that at some time, their treatment or that received by their relatives and friends was affected by their cultural identity. Conflict arose over hospital policy regarding visitors in the delivery room and afterward. As welcoming a new baby and comforting the mother is the purview of the extended family and community members, several women reported having large numbers of visitors. In several cases, nurses informed family members that they were to leave, despite assurances from other staff that the extended family and friends were welcome. Several women noted that their messages from friends and family were not conveyed. One woman requested her placenta be kept for ceremonial purposes, but it was disposed of after her request was made. Women repeatedly expressed that they felt accused of contravening policies when they had not been informed of the rules.

Although in some instances, women felt that nurses were overworked due to the cutbacks, evidence of overt and more subtle racist incidences punctuated these women's stories. Carey, a twenty-year-old mother of one, and Mariah, aged fifteen, shared these examples:

> She [a nurse] kept leaving the room. She'd [say] 'dirty Indians. And my mom would go swearing at her in the hallway, not helping much.... There was one doctor, he's a male doctor, he was kind of rude. He said, Well, you should have an AIDS test done. I said, okay, then he said, because most Black people and Native people have the AIDS virus ... he was, like, sort of made me feel like I had AIDS or something, and I was pretty upset over that.

Some women noted that being both young when their first child was born and Aboriginal placed them in a vulnerable position with the staff and representatives from government agencies. Other stories indicate that women not only experienced, but observed differential treatment between First Nations and non-First Nations patients. For example, Pascale, an experienced mother of two, noted,

> just as I was leaving the desk, there was a Native girl walked in ... but she didn't get like, like I noticed right away, like she wasn't cared for as much as I was ... like those nurses remember me after four ... but I noticed that she didn't get quite as much attention and she was kind of put off.

Some of the women expressed confusion and dismay over the communication problems that arose repeatedly. Women were admonished if they did not know they could pick up their infants from the nursery or if they brought visitors to see their infants in the neonatal intensive care unit. Even walking the halls by themselves was sufficient to raise comments. At times, these admonitions seemed to be grounded in racist assumptions; for instance, a First Nations woman leaving her infant with another while she made a phone call felt that the strength of the rebuke she received was tainted with the notion that she was likely to abandon her infant. Women also expressed the need to be informed of their options and be heard in their rights to make choices. For example, Pascale's attempt to give birth in the squatting position had been thwarted with her first two births. "With my third baby, that's when I told them right away. I kept going I want to squat this time. I want to squat. I made sure the nurses knew. I kept saying it repeatedly." Not all of the experiences were negative and indeed numerous staff, including kitchen and janitorial personnel, were regarded fondly for their support and kindness. Cecilia recalled giving birth to her second child:

> She [the nurse] took care of me, she was worried about my needs, like if I wanted a drink or anything like that, and she explained what she was doing. She was always checking on me and giving me options. She did lots, like ... she wasn't grouchy because there are so many people around.

Some women remarked that they were eager to leave the hospital; however, others commented that they would have preferred a longer stay in order to recuperate.

The women's experience varied with the public health nurse visits following delivery. Women generally welcomed the support and the opportunity to ask questions; they generally expressed a desire for an increase in these programs along with an expansion of parent-aid programs. However, in one instance, the mother felt as though she was treated disdainfully by one of the visitors. Furthermore, while some women appreciated the efforts of the health visitor, they were still reticent to breastfeed in front of strangers. Some women sought other useful resources for support in childcare and breastfeeding. One woman explains how her call to a twenty-four-hour hot-line gave her the support she needed to continue breastfeeding:

> I called at five o'clock in the morning and said ... I'm getting a cab and ... getting a bottle. This kid's going on a bottle because I was so nettled and cracked and finally that woman did everything I could run by her on the phone, like step by step and positioning, that was it. It was my positioning.

Vietnamese-Canadian

All of the Vietnamese-Canadian women were married and ranged in age from thirty to thirty-eight. They immigrated to Canada between 1987 and 1994. While three were university graduates, all were working either as homemakers or in low-wage occupations, thus enduring a slide in both socioeconomic and professional status. When asked about their hospital experiences, the participants appeared somewhat ambivalent.

Questions regarding their treatment by staff often centred on the attitudes of the nurses with whom they came into contact. While many Vietnamese-Canadian women were able to listen to their bodies they had different experiences communicating their needs to their caregivers. Some women were able to talk with nurses in Vietnamese and Chinese and this was comforting to them. However, for many women language was perceived as a serious problem and communication with nursing staff and physicians led to frustration and misunderstandings. Although in some cases, women had the assistance of interpreters if necessary, often they depended on family members to interpret for them. In these circum- stances, the women may have been isolated and potentially exhausted; as Vien mentioned, "I felt as though I lost my English in the middle of the night when she was in pain." The misunderstandings that arose from the failed attempts at communication were treated with humour in the course of our interviews, but were upsetting at the time. For example, Vien was given a catheter that caused her increasing pain during the night, yet every time she pressed the button to summon a nurse, she failed to muster enough English to explain her predicament. Finally, the nurse, understanding that the woman was tired and upset, thought that she must have wanted her baby taken back to the nursery and promptly removed him. Vien spent the remainder of the night with the growing discomfort of the catheter, longing for the comfort of her baby.

Communication difficulties were not always linguistic, but profes- sional. Women complained that physicians did not explain procedures or their possible side-effects. Even physicians who spoke Vietnamese and Chinese appeared not to listen to or understand certain women's re- sponses or questions. In some instances, class divisions clearly inter- ceded in willingness and ability to communicate. Yet, from an external perspective shared linguistic competency is all that is relevant.

Linguistic barriers appeared less important to these new mothers when nurses inquired about their wellbeing, demonstrated any kindnesses, spoke to them gently and were tactile. The attitudes of some nursing staff were perceived less kindly. Several women also reported having their requests for painkillers or formula denied, delayed or ignored by staff. Three of the five women reported being yelled at by nurses. One woman, who had undergone a caesarean section, and one, who had a large episiotomy, were admonished by some nurses for their inability to walk unaccompanied. Another woman who, adhering to custom, refused to wash her hair, was reprimanded by the nurse. Trinh, a thirty-eight-year-old mother of one has limited English skills; in hospital, she was hesitant to cause any conflict.

> In Vietnam, my mother said we should not take showers after childbirth, just a sponge bath. Here they said take a shower and I obeyed them. Also, on the weekend there were different nurses and one person covering two rooms. I waited for an hour for a nurse.

Care in the hospital was less than anticipated for some women. Melissa had a private room in the hospital, yet she relied occasionally on adjunct staff to help her during her stay. Later, she was discharged from the hospital without an examination, one that may have revealed an infection, and when she picked up her infant, she found him to be soiled and dirty. Melissa and others who waited a long time for nurses to answer their calls attributed the problems with nurses to labour shortages or cutbacks. Several women felt that the nurses who ill-treated them, themselves members of a visible minority, were lazy and unwilling to fulfill their duties. Still others attributed their treatment to their visible minority status. Melissa believes that her pain was not taken seriously because she is Vietnamese: "I think the nurses think you are a liar, that Vietnamese are mean."

The home visit nurses from public health nurses were welcomed for their advice, assistance with breastfeeding, for calming their fears and validating their experience. However, women also felt that more visits were needed and would have preferred getting acquainted with someone prior to delivery. In one case, a friend and her children provided an enormous amount of postnatal support and care, cooking, cleaning, taking care of the baby and the mother while she was in severe pain. This level of support was extremely helpful and, in the participant's view, necessary as her pain was so intense she had succumbed to suicidal ideation. One woman sums it up: "There's too much pressure about the family, about the baby, about how to care for the family, worries about whether there was going to be enough milk, so you get even more tense."

Indo-Canadian
Six Indo-Canadian women, from India, Trinidad and Fiji, participated in this study. Four interviews were conducted in English, one in Hindi and three in a combination of English and Punjabi. Three of the women had graduated university or college, two had completed high school and one

had finished grade ten. With a single exception, all of the women were from urban areas. Their ages ranged from twenty-four to forty; each was married and had two children.

Overall, women reported general satisfaction with their hospital experiences although each reported discomforting incidences. The support of the nursing staff was cited by a number of women as helping create a positive evaluation of their birthing experience.

> Yeah, when I have pains and stuff like that, all the nurses come and they hold me like this, one black nurse. She was there once when I was really having strong pains and she came in and hugged me, right, she was massaging my back, and that was really nice, right.

Occasionally, women felt singled out for ill-treatment because of their visible minority status. Maya, a young mother from Fiji, described how one staff member berated her for apparently not walking enough following a caesarean section.

> But I always go to washroom, right. I didn't bother any nurse to come and help me, right. But the way she said it, it really hurt because I always have pain and I do it myself, right. I know they are busy, too.

Maya's friend gave birth at the same hospital some months later. She had no problem, she remarked, but was determined to get up and walk as soon as possible to avoid any unpleasant situations such as her friend experienced.

Language barriers also proved to be a problem in hospital. Ranjit's English was limited and she recounts her efforts to order food. The nurse tried to assist her by reading the menu; however, dishes such as quiche were wholly unfamiliar. At last, she uttered a food word that was familiar—cheese. "A little cheese," she said, "when what I wanted was a mountain of dhal and roti!" Throughout her delivery, however, Ranjit had been in the presence of staff who could speak with her:

> I was really scared of hospitals, but then when I went in and saw two nurses from my own country, Punjab, I was very happy. They were asking me and they were chatting and they were very nice to me.... I didn't have the urge to run away from that place and I always get that when I'm feeling uncomfortable.

Even women who spoke fluent English noted that the intensity of the childbirth experience altered their language choice and they reverted to their mother tongue. In the event of a crisis, as Michelle who introduced this essay underwent, there is no staff available to inform family members who may not speak English about the situation. Michelle's sister Celeste provided her perspective and offered some advice:

> And for the health professionals as well, they were so much engrossed, they were running around trying to save her life rather than explaining. So if there were someone with communication skills calming them down, telling them, okay, she's in the operating room, they're working on her and we'll have to wait. You go sit with the rest of the family and we'll come to talk to you.

Some women mentioned that nursing and obstetrical staff appeared to be in a hurry, creating the perception that their own care could suffer from the effects of the staff's inattention. These concerns were amplified when they were kept waiting for assistance or treatment; they were provided treatment, such as injections, against their wishes; they were informed that side effects might develop without adequate or sufficient counselling or reassurance.

The apparent lack of assistance—nursing, obstetrical, institutional—was attributed to cutbacks in staff. While nursing staff are not responsible for the condition of rooms or the quality and availability of food services, they offer the most visible contact in hospital and often bear the brunt of patient dissatisfaction. Furthermore, attempting to resolve problems in non-nursing matters creates an additional burden on nursing staff. Tara, a forty-year-old mother of two, complained of changes in the health care system and its impact on patient comfort: "The room was filthy, no one came to change the mattress pad or the sheets ... the maternity ward was packed. If I had to do it again, I wouldn't; it was too nasty."

Women generally felt that they were discharged too soon, that they needed time to rest, and for those who had had troublesome deliveries, that they were worried about their or their families' ability to handle complications.

> He says like you are going home today, you're okay. And I said, do you think? I can't even stand by myself. He said, that's okay, you'll be fine. Well about me, I don't think so because they should keep a few more days instead of ... it's really hard to keep track of everything. Hospitals, like the nurses, they know better than you do at home. The first thing you should stay a couple of days because you've had a hemorrhage.

Women's perception of public health nurse visits ranged from out-standing to disinterested. Two women felt that the information they provided was a duplication of what they received in the hospital and from their physician. One woman mentioned that she was pleased with the visit; however, as she was responsible for hosting and providing refreshments for the nurse as well as any other visitors, visits in general were burdensome. Tara emphasized that the public health nurse brought her peace of mind: "The home nurse was really good, too... I talked to her a lot and she told me all kinds of things about being a first time mother like about the importance of sleep, how to freeze food and organize."

Birthing under Health Reform: Resistance and Advocacy

Clearly not all of the areas of tension between minority women and nurses can be attributed to health reform; yet they are all contextualized by the changes in the past several years in obstetrical and postnatal care. Communication problems feature prominently in the narratives of both patients and nurses. Cries for assistance punctuate women's stories; requests for physical assistance, pain relief and the right to enact cultural practices or personal preferences go without recognition. Nurses, pressed to care for an increased number of patients, admit to avoiding patients whom they believe to be more problematic. Some revealed they occasion-ally avoided visible minority patients who offered no linguistic barriers simply because of their assumptions about their abilities to communicate in English. These patterns of avoidance are undoubtedly recognized by patients, who perceive this behaviour as differential treatment or racism. The time constraints imposed upon nurse–patient interactions thus help reinforce preconceived notions of dominant-minority relations, creating further distrust and potential hostility.

Some nursing staff indicated that they attempt to share their limited time with all of their patients. Unfortunately, providing patients with brief, but equal interactions amounts to a disservice to minority patients and underscores one of the major flaws in hospital policies and proce-dures, that is, equating equal with equitable treatment. Equal treatment may be possible among a homogeneous population that has access to a functional support network and is familiar with the values, policies and procedures that proscribe the hospital environment. Many of the minor-ity women in this study were marginalized linguistically, economically and culturally; yet there is no time available to provide equitable treat-ment that would involve familiarization with hospital culture; inquiry instead of presumption about patients' abilities, their families and sup-port networks; and answering queries. Equitable treatment of minority women and their babies requires, above all, time.

Under current health reform practices, there is no time for answering questions and no time to listen to the bodies of women like Michelle.

> Like, take every delivery and every birth and every woman and child as an individual.... I'm a different person, this is a different child, it's a different labour.... Explain every single time and be more patient ... they've said it a thousand times.... I'm learning the first time, so teach me as if it was the first time.

The mothers in this study were not unaware of the pressures that the nursing staff face and many expressed the hope that they will be able to slow down to answer questions and attend to the women and to themselves.

Neither were these women helpless victims at the mercy of hospital staff and policies. In each of the participant communities, we saw that women experienced a loss of control when confronted with the institution of the hospital or other biomedical personnel through prenatal classes and physicians' visits. In all of these cases, we saw that women asserted themselves in an attempt to regain power and a modicum of control over their childbirth experiences. Winning back control over these situations often occurred in a culturally-specific manner. Moreover, different women were able to implement varying amounts of resources and were subject to different pressures due to the historical, socioeconomic and political context in which their relationships with dominant Euro-Canadian tradition were embedded. First Nations women were able to affirm their own strength through individual and collective means. Women looked to support from others as a means of gaining control of their own personal context. Support networks ranged from extended family and friends to volunteer agencies, a social worker who listens and nurses who provided comfort and attention. Moreover, women gained strength from that which was offered to others, in other words, from sharing their experiences, wisdom and comfort. Solidarity was also expressed by advocating for others, sometimes strangers. Some First Nations women chose to actively avoid contact with health care personnel. While some women were eager to leave the hospital; others deftly avoided interference by spending large amounts of time in the bath or shower. Some women fought back verbally and others stood up for those who could not stand up for themselves.

For many of these women, cultural identity provided a strong reference point for identifying appropriate behaviour that complemented or resisted the perspectives offered by biomedical personnel. For example, women focused on controlling negative emotions lest they imprint on the newborn and incorporating prayer and ritual into both their daily lives and childbirth. As these women have confronted inequalities and discrimination throughout their lives, it is not surprising that they have found ways, primarily through humour, anger and mediation, to resist degradation in their interactions with the health care system. Women also chose to sort through the advice given to them and care for themselves in a manner that suited them. Finally, women who had multiple births appeared to become increasingly assertive in exercising their options in hospital and at home.

As they came to know the ropes, they shared their expertise with others. The stories of the Vietnamese-Canadian women were imbued with a sense of determination in their struggles to care for themselves, their children, friends and family. Women spoke of caring for their newborn, though exhausted and in pain. They talked about deciding what was best for themselves during pregnancy and chose to avail themselves of options whenever possible. Women readily acknowledged the help of spouses, friends, family members and some nursing staff during their pregnancies and births. Solidarity with other women was vital to their experience; women perceived a need to share with other women who could offer and receive advice and support. Nurses who provided this kind of support were also highly valued and fondly regarded. Much of what these women could offer was validation of their own knowledge and experiences. Comfort from a variety of sources brought women a sense of control over their environment and strengthened their ability to thrive. Home, being cared for, their own language, the presence of loved ones, respect, a gentle voice or touch and someone to just talk to provided a sense of security and a foundation on which to re-shape their lives as new mothers.

Indo-Canadian women also attempted to do what is right, that is adhering to culturally prescribed and personally enacted models of behaviour. The advocacy and comfort provided by support people—family, friends and health professionals—appeared vital to the well-being of mother and child as well as family members. Ideas about support were closely linked with the cultural ideal, what a person grows to expect and aspire to as part of a cultural group.

In addition to underlying expectations about others, several themes arose regarding appropriate behaviour. Doing what is right was also related to self-care. Women often relied on their own judgment to decide what advice to follow or not, which materials to read, how to prepare themselves and how to pay attention to diet and exercise. All of these choices contributed to their pleasure in giving birth to a healthy child.

Conclusions and Implications

While the patients' narratives brought evidence of their agency and resistance, nurses' stories too reflected their efforts to act as advocates for their patients and their struggles in providing optimum care in an unsettled work environment. Nurses also spoke of their efforts to deepen their understanding of difference, moving beyond superficial recognition of beliefs to seeking learning opportunities, increasing self-awareness, improving communication skills and becoming more flexible in their approach. Some women sensed a shift in their relationships to minority patients through their analysis of nursing, gender and power.

These realizations speak directly to methods of enhancing nursing education. While it is laudable to familiarize nurses with a spectrum of cultural practices, where culture is studied in isolation, stereotypes are bound to emerge. Methods of teaching that commence with self-awareness may also help highlight cultural differences and assumptions, but as Jackson (1993) asserts, they may do little more than white-out socioeconomic difference. A more critical approach could aid nurses' understanding, not only of the lifeworlds of their patients, but their own. Such an approach encourages political-economic and gender analysis, acknowledges the cultural-constructedness of biomedical knowledge and ensures nursing students are placed in culturally and economically diverse situations.

The impact of health reform in hospital obstetrics wards places a greater burden on the services delivered to minority women. Women's cries for assistance are lost in the cacophony of increasing demands placed on nursing staff who have survived institutional downsizing. As economy of patient–nurse interaction is promoted, minority women's voices become increasingly marginalized in favour of what are perceived to be less problematic encounters. In other instances, the need for individualized attention is ignored as time is parcelled out into equal periods.

The brevity of, and sometimes dissatisfaction with nurse–patient encounters, is interpreted in the context of historical relations; power differentials between institutions, staff and patients; stereotypes of minority patients as non-compliant; and racist or differential treatment at the hands of mainstream institutions. While the situation may appear to be at an impasse, both new mothers and nurses were able to conceive of a common ground that would benefit all labouring under health reform, where most agree that the voices of the marginalized must be amplified.

A welcome addition to women's experience of pregnancy and childbirth is the use of bicultural and/or bilingual liaison workers who provide support, advocacy and interpretation (both linguistic and cultural). Greater emphasis on this would facilitate nursing care. These cultural brokers could begin working with women and their families from early pregnancy until postpartum, building on the existing support mechanisms already available to clients and ensuring that existing resources are within reach.

Thus, as downsizing and health reform have transformed hospital-based care, the need to support innovative community-based programs becomes more evident. This study and others (see Bubel and Spitzer 1996) indicate that the needs of minority women have been ill-served by the changes brought about by health reform. New programs will need to be established to ensure that all have the support, encouragement and opportunity to listen to the bodies of marginalized women.

Notes

1. All names are pseudonyms.
2. For a discussion of the broader health-related issues facing immigrant and refugee women see Guruge, Donner and Morrison in this volume.
3. Jane Cawthorne in this volume critically examines the tension between economic and ideological issues in the current struggles over maternal care in Alberta.
4. The speaker is referring to a workload measurement tool that nurses must use to calculate the amount of time allocated for completing a given set of patient care tasks. Each patient's care needs are "classified" according to a standardized set of time frames.

6

Obscuring a Crisis:
The Obstetricians' and Gynecologists' Job Action and Maternal Care in Alberta

Jane Cawthorne

Introduction

In May 1998, Alberta's obstetricians and gynecologists began a lengthy job action in which they refused to accept new patients. These specialists were hoping to highlight a growing crisis within their profession, but left pregnant women in the province feeling they were without options or advocates as they struggled to access care. Midwives were virtually shut out of this debate. Yet, involving them in reshaping health care as it relates to maternal care has the potential to expand the debate to one not just about appropriate remuneration to obstetricians and gynecologists but also about the goals of health care and health care reform. Indeed, if health care reform is truly to revolutionize the delivery of maternal services and improve conditions for women both as care recipients and care providers in Alberta, it is critical to question whether the dominant medicalized view of pregnancy and birth is the most helpful. Because obstetricians and gynecologists, mostly men, have authority in the institutional power structures around childbirth, they are able to obscure the view of other models of care. Involving the perspective of midwives in the health care debate opens up the possibility that an additional model could be validated through legislation and inclusion under health insurance.

Methodology

I consider this attempt to incorporate the voices of midwives into the debate about health care reform very preliminary. It is necessarily limited by several factors. It is issue specific, focusing on the obstetricians' and gynecologists' job action in Alberta. Furthermore, at the time of writing, there are only twenty fully registered midwives in Alberta. I contacted each of these practitioners in October 1998 (five months into the job action) by letter or telephone to request their response to several open-ended questions regarding the job action. Thirty-five percent of midwives responded. Although this response rate is low, many midwives responded on behalf of their shared practice, so their responses represent the views of more than one midwife. To ensure the credibility of these results, I also received input from two midwifery consumer advocacy groups (one in Edmonton and one in Calgary), the president of the Alberta Association of Midwives and I spoke informally with a number of midwifery consumers, advocates and students. There is consistency in their response to the job action, although there are clear divisions among both midwives and midwifery advocates regarding other issues faced by midwives in Alberta today. Although I mention many of these issues in passing, an in-depth analysis is beyond the scope of this work (see James 1997 and 1998).

Background information on the job action came from an analysis of newspaper articles in the major dailies in Edmonton and Calgary as well as from an interview with Dr. Paul Martyn, president of the Alberta Society of Obstetrics and Gynecology. Finally, I accessed the work of other health care reform analysts and information from government documents on health care and health care reform dating back to *The Rainbow Report* (Premier's Commission on Future Health for Albertans 1989), a document generally acknowledged as the blueprint of health care reform in Alberta.

The Basis for the Job Action

The need to critically examine the goals and progress of health care reform is clear. A recent poll indicates that health care reform has left 80 percent of Albertans wondering if the health system can meet their present and future needs (Provincial Health Council of Alberta 1998). Obstetricians and gynecologists attempted to express this same concern through their job action and their demand for higher fees. Members of their profession are under intense pressure to maintain service levels to Alberta women in an environment of cost restraints. Demand for obstetric services is high. In 1996, 99.12 percent of births took place in hospitals with 99.47 percent of all births attended by physicians as primary caregivers. Of a total of 38,067 births, only 152 (0.4 percent) were attended by midwives (Health Surveillance 1997). In Edmonton, where obstetric services are readily available, 84 percent of women gave birth under the care of an obstetrician in 1997. Obviously, obstetric services are a vital component of women's health care and obstetricians have an important role to play in ensuring these services are available in the future.

Obstetricians are concerned that their continued ability to meet the high demand for their services is currently compromised by changing demographics within the profession and conditions within which they practice. Forty-two percent of Alberta's practitioners are over fifty years old and a further 20 percent are over sixty years old (Alberta Society of Obstetrics and Gynecology [ASOG] n.d.). As these doctors prepare for retirement, the specialty is failing to attract new members. Government cuts in post-graduate funding, the high cost of an obstetrical practice and the spiralling cost of malpractice insurance in an increasingly litigious society are all cited by Dr. Martyn as barriers to entry. An even more significant deterrent is the promise of an unenviable lifestyle demanding on-call status, twenty-four hours a day, seven days a week.

These difficulties are compounded by what doctors characterize as insufficient remuneration. In the past three years, 20 percent of the practising obstetricians in Edmonton have left the province, all citing unsatisfactory working conditions and compensation as the reason (ASOG n.d.). Although these issues predate current health care reform initiatives, trying to get more money from a government determined to reduce the cost of health services has proven difficult. Prior to 1988, obstetric fees were supplemented through physician extra billing. When extra billing was banned, fees-per-delivery did not rise. In fact, the fee-per-delivery has gone down marginally in the last decade and is currently $277.78. This fee is the fourth lowest in Canada, with the lowest being $250 in Manitoba. The same amount is paid per delivery whether a general practitioner or an obstetrician/gynecologist attends, meaning there is no financial recognition for specialist care. General practitioners, facing the same issues as obstetricians, are opting out of performing deliveries, which in turn increases the workload for obstetricians. The obstetricians and gynecologists want the fee per delivery raised to $455, putting them on par with their highest paid colleagues, those in Nova Scotia (ASOG n.d.). In this way, they hope to retain current practitioners, attract new ones and keep a manageable workload while continuing to provide services to Alberta women.

In April 1998, the Alberta Medical Association (AMA) negotiated a three-year fee agreement with Alberta Health on behalf of all doctors. Unfortunately, this agreement left the fee concerns of obstetricians and gynecologists unrecognized. Unhappy with the deal, the Alberta Society of Obstetrics and Gynecology sought to increase their fees through direct negotiation with Alberta Health. Alberta Health refused to reopen negotiations, fearing such a move would lead to independent negotiations by a host of other professional groups within the AMA. In response, obstetricians and gynecologists announced they would no longer accept new patients as of May 15, 1998.

The impact of the job action was felt immediately. The impact was most severe in Calgary, a region experiencing high population growth and already suffering a physician shortage. The media reported that pregnant women were finding it almost impossible to locate a doctor willing to deliver their babies (Walker 1998a). Women experienced stress and frustration as they felt they were without options or advocates in the health care system. Although labour and delivery care at hospitals continued, women did not have the benefit of continuous care by one physician, meaning there was potentially poorer recognition of problems. As nurses were diverted to labour and delivery, existing problems resulting from earlier cuts to nursing staff were exacerbated. One mother complained her newborn was given formula against her wishes. Another mother waited over fifteen hours to see her newborn because no one was available to take her to the nursery (Walker 1998b).

As the dispute dragged on, threats were made that labour and delivery wards would close, leaving pregnant women even more worried about a potential lack of care. The protest finally ended on November 16, almost six months to the day since it began. The AMA and Alberta Health agreed to work together to find extra funding for obstetricians through a loophole in the agreement which allows extra aid for any specialty which does not have enough members to maintain adequate patient services (Pedersen 1998).

According to Dr. Martyn of the Alberta Society of Obstetricians and Gynecologists, for such an extremely conservative group of professionals to even consider refusing new patients indicated a level of intolerable frustration within their ranks. Having spent over a decade taking traditional paths to address their concerns, obstetricians and gynecologists finally felt they had no other option but to initiate a job action (Cawthorne 1998). Critics felt that pregnant women were being used as pawns in a struggle between Alberta Health, the AMA and the obstetricians, and they undoubtedly were. It is not as though women could put off having children until the dispute was over. But the obstetricians rightly argue that the circumstances within which they practise influence the quality of their work, and they equate their struggle to improve conditions within the profession with improving service for women. However, in this job action, improving conditions within their profession especially meant raising fees.

Whether or not lifestyle issues can be addressed with money is always debatable and with average yearly billings exceeding $200,000, it is appropriate to question how much money is enough. To be fair, this figure does not take into account the cost of operating a practice, nor does it reflect the investment of time and money that these specialists dedicate to their education and ongoing training. Assuming obstetricians get what they ask for and the fee-for-delivery is increased, there are still workload and lifestyle issues that must be addressed. Raising the fee-for-service also does nothing to solve the inherent problems in fee-for-service remuneration. Because physicians are paid a fee-for-service rather than a salary or by course-of-care, the only way for a physician to increase his or her overall income is to increase volumes, that is, perform more services with more patients. The implications for care are obvious. With the performance of more services, more tests and more interventions, the doctor receives more money. "It's not surprising that virtually every study of medical practice shows that substantial proportions of physicians' services—from drug prescriptions to major surgical procedures—were without medical justification" (Swartz 1998: 542) and exposed patients to unnecessary risk.

In the provision of health care, time spent with patients is equated with the quality of care provided. When there is a structural incentive to reducing the time spent with each patient, there is a structural incentive to reducing the quality of care. Fee-for-service "transforms care into a cost of doing business" (Swartz 1998: 543). Education, counselling and just simple listening are not financially rewarded. Although a fee increase allows for a boost to incomes without a reduction in time spent per patient, everyone, including Dr. Martyn of the Alberta Society of Obstetrics and Gynecology, understands fee-for-service as problematic. Since fee-for-service is part of the problem, raising the fee-for-service cannot be part of the solution. It just throws more money at a problem without solving it. The logic of doing this while health care costs are under scrutiny is mystifying.

The Midwives' Perspective

The most fundamental problem with this solution, however, is it fails to recognize the roles of alternate care providers. Obstetricians and gynecologists premised their action on the assumption that they are the only care providers capable of attending women in pregnancy and childbirth. Midwives disagree. Their response to the job action was unanimous. Without exception, they felt childbearing women were bearing the brunt of this action and that their needs were being ignored. None felt obstetricians should routinely attend "normal" or "low-risk" births, and therefore they had issues with the obstetricians' demands to receive more money for attending these types of deliveries. One midwife suggested the current fee-for-service is already quite high for those situations where "the doctor arrives, puts on gloves, catches and leaves." At the same time, all midwives felt that fees should be raised for high-risk deliveries and complicated situations where the doctor's expertise, time and skill are in high demand.

Midwives also perceive a crisis in maternal care in Alberta, but it is not the same crisis seen by obstetricians and gynecologists. Midwives are concerned about the current failure of the Alberta health care system to support midwifery while addressing the efficacy of different types of care. They understand the job action as an attempt to maintain the status quo. In their view, the status quo was never adequate, so maintaining it is not a priority. Maintaining the status quo means supporting the dominant medicalized view of pregnancy and birth. Midwives share a critique of medicalized childbirth with feminist scholars (Corea 1985, Goer 1995, O'Brien 1981, Overall 1993, Raymond 1993, Romalis 1981, Rothman 1989) and other advocates of safe alternative childbirth, including the World Health Organization (see Wagner 1994). Medicalized childbirth is widely understood to reflect patriarchal values, allowing men to gain control over women in reproduction. Within this paradigm, childbirth is understood as a dangerous, even pathological condition if left to the capricious whims of nature (and women). Active management in a controlled setting by doctors is now the routine way of handling birth. Interventions are common, adding to the perception of control while routinizing women's experience of childbirth for the convenience of medical practitioners. Although midwives express respect for the training and skills of obstetricians and the need for these skills in high-risk births, they are concerned that obstetricians attend many normal births as well. With monopoly control in childbirth, obstetricians and gynecologists obscure the view of other models of care. They determine how the rest of us understand and define appropriate care in childbirth.

This emphasis within obstetrics on birth as potentially dangerous is illustrated in a pamphlet distributed by obstetricians and gynecologists explaining the crisis in obstetrics. It reads,

> Let's take a minute to think about the care of a pregnant woman and her unborn baby. Here is one example: A patient has had a perfectly normal pregnancy. Suddenly, when she is in labour, she develops unforeseen problems and the pregnancy becomes "high risk." We all want the best outcome for this mother and her baby. In order to get the best outcome, the doctor looking after this patient has to be trained to deal with whatever may happen. That is why a properly qualified specialist, obstetrician-gynaecologist, always has to be on call. The risks, the time required to give the highest standard of care, and the expertise that is necessary

to provide that care are all a part of the complicated work of obstetrics. (Canadian Society of Obstetricians and Gynaecologists n.d.)

This approach plays upon the fear of the unknown to preference the kind of care an obstetrician can provide. Today, women in Alberta do not even need a referral from a general physician to access the specialist care of an obstetrician, whereas a referral is needed to access other specialists, including cardiologists and dermatologists. Obstetric care is further legitimized through health insurance, which provides third-party payment for the services of obstetricians, gynecologists and general practitioners in Alberta, but not for midwives. Not only is this choice presented as the "safe" choice, it is also state subsidized and more economically viable than midwifery, which is not state supported.

Although the frequency and efficacy of many obstetrical interventions are now questioned (Goer 1995, Wagner 1994), they receive little critical review within the profession and continue to be performed out of a belief that they provide a desirable alternative to the unknown. Many women never require obstetrical services and their entry into this system of care increases the chances they will experience a technologized birth that is unnecessary, dangerous and expensive (Enkin et al. 1989). As one midwife, Joy West-Eklund, puts it, "low-risk women do not fare well under high-risk care." By its very design, the health care system encourages the growth of an expensive industry in medical technology and creates new sources of corporate profits and professional hierarchy that are supported through state regulation and state subsidized insurance (Torrance 1998). "The fragmentation inherent in a system characterized by individualism and competition defies proper service delivery" (Swartz 1998: 543). Doing something is understood as better than doing nothing, particularly when doing something creates a new site for profitable economic activity (Waring 1988).

So, while obstetricians and gynecologists easily conflate their own interests with the interests of their patients, midwives recognize how these interests conflict within the existing health care system. Their own model of care offers a more holistic vision of pregnancy, one in which the interests of caregiver and care recipient are less likely to conflict. The midwife is both philosophically and physically "with the woman" (Rothman 1989: 170) in a partnership that helps the woman find her own way through pregnancy and childbirth. Care starts with what a woman can do for herself and is supported by the midwife who encourages informed choice, growth and awareness through education in a manner that is flexible, creative, empowering and supportive. Socioeconomic indicators of health that are largely ignored in mainstream medicine receive attention. Pregnancy, birth and breastfeeding are considered natural life processes in this model, and women are understood as healthy and capable (Goer 1995, Kitzinger 1988, Midwifery Regional Implementation Committee 1996). Women are encouraged to deliver their babies in the setting that they choose, with the caregivers and support people they wish to have near. What looks like a bleak option of "doing nothing" during a normal pregnancy and birth in a medical model is understood in a midwifery model as allowing a self-organizing, active process to unfold.

The scope of a course-of-care provided by a midwife is extensive. Care is offered throughout pregnancy and labour and extends six weeks into the postpartum period. A typical course-of-care takes forty-five hours in total and a midwife remains available to a woman twenty-four hours a day, seven days a week by pager or cell phone throughout this period, not just for labour and delivery. Visits last thirty minutes to one hour, with a visit of an hour or more initially and another longer visit scheduled at thirty-six weeks. Labour support is also continuous and extends into the hours after birth. Midwives limit themselves to forty courses-of-care per year in order to maintain their ability to spend considerable time with the women they serve (Midwifery Regional Implementation Committee 1997).

Typically, midwifery and obstetrical care are understood as mutually exclusive models of care. An extreme critic of midwifery, Dr. Keith Russell, former president of the American College of Obstetricians and Gynecologists, claims, "home birth is child abuse in its earliest form" (as cited in Wagner 1994: 5). An extreme critic of obstetrical practice, Goer characterizes it as institutionalized violence against women: "Seen in one light, obstetrics, far from serving the needs of childbearing women, could be described as a kind of sanctioned violence against them" (1995: 349). This rhetoric is decidedly not helpful to women and reveals more about the perceived threat each group poses to the other than it reveals about the worth of their respective models of care. Such extreme positions use the bodies of women in childbirth as the terrain over which a battle for professional power and legitimacy is waged. For example, although obstetricians do not favour home births, midwives recognize them as safe alternatives to hospital births when there is no expectation of complications and when medical support is immediately available should the need for it emerge. "No study of planned home births of a screened population of women with a trained attendant taking proper precautions has shown excess risks" (Goer 1995: 334). Home births are only dangerous when doctors and hospitals fail to provide back up services. "Thus, their failure converts an imaginary risk into a real one" (334). Both types of care and both types of caregivers are needed to ensure healthy outcomes for the woman. Any reform that ignores this contributes a conceptual barrier to solving the larger crisis in maternal care.

Throughout the job action, midwives did not argue against obstetric skills deserving proper reimbursement. In fact, several suggest that the low fee-for-delivery is indicative of a systemic disregard for women's health. One midwife, Susan James, sums up the underlying meaning of the job action, saying, "the message is: women are not important." What midwives do argue against is the idea that obstetric skills are best applied in a normal pregnancy and birth. They understand their practice to be life sustaining, even life enhancing, and ultimately ecologically sustainable as well since it requires little technological intervention.

> The demand by midwives to practice their profession is not an attempt by a less qualified group to engage in the practice of medicine, as it has most often been seen, but rather the claim of a more qualified group to practice midwifery. (Rothman 1989: 183)

With this point of view, they substantively shift the ground on which the obstetricians and gynecologists base their dispute and broaden the parameters of the discourse.

This point of view went largely unnoticed during the job action. When midwives were mentioned it was usually in relation to their fees, providing a standard by which the current delivery fee paid to obstetricians was understood as low. Such comparisons ignore fundamental differences in the scope of the two kinds of practice and were considered misleading by midwives. Their fees are based on course-of-care, not per intervention or per visit. Currently, fees range between $1,200 and $2,500 per course-of-care and this fee is paid directly to the midwife. If a midwife charging the current maximum fee of $2,500 were to be primary attendant during forty courses-of-care, she would earn $100,000. Like the gross income noted for obstetricians, however, this does not include expenses and the cost of running a practice. In the real world, though, no midwives are actually earning this much. Many midwives were so irked by the obstetricians' constant references to their fee per course-of-care that they were unable to muster much sympathy for them during the job action. Midwives know that their gross income is much lower than that of obstetricians, and they suffer many of the same difficult working conditions, such as being continuously accessible to the women they serve. In fact, their conditions are often more difficult. One midwife indicated she earned a gross income of $15,000 last year, but was left with only $2,500 dollars after deducting her expenses and taxes. The only reason she can continue to practise is because her husband's income can support their family. She cannot afford her registration or her malpractice insurance next year. Nor can she justify the continued absence from her own family and her responsibilities there for such a paltry sum. Compared to the income concerns of obstetricians, the plight of midwives is far more desperate.

Poor conditions within midwifery are grounded in the dominance of the medical model of practice. As a unified medical profession was forged in Canada, doctors gradually eliminated their competition by questioning the merit of midwives and other "non-medical" caregivers within the new empirical paradigm. Traditional and alternative care providers were absorbed into the medical model, often as subordinates to physicians, or, as in the case of midwives, were driven into a quasi-illegal status (Arnup et al. 1990, Torrance 1998). Choice is socially constructed and the decision to seek specialist care in pregnancy and childbirth is one that is validated in this culture. While obstetricians cite high demand for their services as the basis for its support, this high demand is understood by midwives to be the result of a lack of alternatives. Demand for physician services rose as other alternatives disappeared. Experience in other jurisdictions indicates that when a midwifery model of care is publicly validated through legislation and incorporation in health insurance, demand for these services rises.

> In Ontario, for example, demand for midwifery services exceeds capacity by 2 to 1. On average, for every woman who receives midwifery care, two are turned away. In Toronto the ratio is 5 to 1... Although demand cannot be met, approximately 3.5 percent of Ontario women needing maternity services are seeking midwives. (Midwifery Regional Implementation Committee 1996: 13)

There is reason to believe that midwifery could potentially catch on in Alberta if it were a socially and economically validated choice.

None of this is meant to suggest the interests of childbearing women and the interests of midwives are never in conflict, or that midwives themselves do not have conflicting points of view. This is inevitable when we recognize the diverse backgrounds of women and their differing needs, expectations and locations. With such a small number of midwives available to women in the province, their ability to reflect the diversity of the wider population is worth further analysis. For example, the needs of Aboriginal women in birth must receive more attention. Furthermore, eighteen of the twenty midwives in Alberta serve primarily urban populations. Access by rural women is severely limited. This presents another area of possible conflicting interests. But again, addressing these issues is unfortunately beyond the scope of this chapter.

One conflict that was raised repeatedly during this research was that of economic or financial access to midwifery. Each respondent expressed concern over their ability to provide services only to women who can afford to pay, and one recognized the somewhat ironic fact that often her clients are able to pay only because of an income provided by a male partner. Midwives recognize the inherent conflict between their philosophy of being with women, with *all* women, yet being accessible only to those who can afford their services. These issues of access, and others, not only divide women from midwives, but also divide the small community of midwives in Alberta.

Midwifery and the Goals of Alberta Health Care Reform

Recognizing these conflicts, however, does not alter the fundamental challenge midwives pose to obstetricians. This challenge is echoed within recent literature on health care reform.

> Everyone, including governments, providers and the public at large, is concerned about such issues as our capacity to fund health care services at the present level, the efficiency and effectiveness in the system, the impact of new technologies, the quality of care being provided, the way in which the system is organized and managed, and the overall impact of health care on population health status. (Angus 1998: 23)

For the most part, there is a tendency to think of health care reform only in terms of spending cuts. This is undoubtedly its primary goal in Alberta where any contribution to deficit reduction is politically welcome, no matter what its source. However, health care reform literature is not quite as blatant about its ultimate purpose and often demonstrates a renewed concern for the social goals of health care. This shift in policy has been defined as a movement towards a new focus on equitable access to health rather than a focus on equal access to health care (Mhatre and Deber 1998). This focus has demanded renewed attention to the social forces that influence health.

The initial blueprint for health care reform in Alberta, *The Rainbow Report*, sets six major directions for change, all of which are framed in the language of social goals (Premier's Commission 1989: 27–28). Although women's health care is never singled out for specific consideration, three of the six goals could be achieved in maternal care through the system wide integration of midwifery and a fourth, to be considered later, also has relevance. The first of these goals links human health to a healthy environment and calls for balanced economic development. Since midwives question birth as a site for economic development, their model of care would seem to be compatible with this goal. Midwifery is also congruent with this goal because there is an emphasis on the environment as an indicator of health. By this, I refer not only to the actual physical environment, but also the relationships within the family and the community that influence physical and emotional health during pregnancy.

A second goal suggests individuals will achieve self-reliance, autonomy and dignity when they assume more responsibility for health care decision-making. Again, this is clearly congruent with a midwifery model of care, which encourages self-care and informed decision-making.

A third goal is the most congruent with midwifery. It advocates education and the re-allocation of at least 1 percent of the Alberta Health operating budget to promotion and prevention programs. Clearly, the education component of the midwifery model of care meets this goal. Perhaps the greatest service a midwife provides is a supportive environment in which a woman can feel empowered during her pregnancy and beyond, learning about her body, while exploring some of her psychosocial responses to pregnancy in an atmosphere of trust. Ultimately, the goal of maternal care is not just assuring the health of the mother and newborn, but also to facilitate a healthy relationship in which the woman becomes a stronger, more capable mother, sure of herself and her capacity to provide care for her child.

In a follow-up document to *The Rainbow Report*, great emphasis is placed on the needs of the "consumer," by providing maximum access to care and maximum choice of caregivers (Alberta Health Planning Secretariat 1993: 12). This report also suggests that the Alberta Health Care Insurance Plan, through either the basic or supplementary plan, expand its coverage to include approved alternate care providers within the system to improve the mix and efficiency of services and to provide a range of less costly services. The report states,

> We must be prepared to reorganize the health care system to ensure that it is more responsive to the people it serves directly and to the changing and differing needs of our communities. There is a real opportunity to build new partnerships that are a creative mix of agencies and services specifically tailored to particular areas of the province. (40)

The Rainbow Report also recognizes the need to support health decisions that are most effective and least intrusive and to provide the easiest possible access to basic and specialized health services without financial or other discriminatory barriers (Premier's Commission 1989: 64). These recommendations read like a manifesto for midwifery, but midwifery is never specifically mentioned as a means through which these goals may be attained.

The Impact of Regulation

Midwifery is now a regulated profession in Alberta and practitioners are registered through Alberta Labour. The leadership of the Alberta Association of Midwives and other consumer groups support regulation because the process brings midwives out of their alegal status, offers consumers the knowledge that these practitioners have met specific standards and makes midwifery a more legitimate choice. This process would seem to indicate that midwives are making progress in undermining male dominance in the provision of health services to childbearing women while improving access to health through the provision of safe alternatives to medicalized birth. However, becoming a regulated profession is only one requirement in chiselling out legitimate space for midwives in maternal care. Even when many women were worried about receiving no care at all, as was the case during the obstetricians' and gynecologists' job action, midwifery was seldom mentioned as an alternative to women seeking care in pregnancy and childbirth. This speaks volumes about the continuing invisibility of this model of care in the consciousness of most women and in the dominant discourse about health care reform.

As well, registration has raised new issues for midwives that have yet to be resolved (James 1997 and 1998). Regulation has brought the practice of midwifery into the fold of the medical establishment. Many midwives question whether or not they can remain autonomous and true to their philosophical roots under these conditions (Benoit 1998, James 1997). Registration has increased the costs of practising and left many midwives with less time for the women they serve as they gain new administrative responsibilities. Even attending meetings regarding the implementation of regulated midwifery has been onerous on midwives because, with so few practitioners, almost all midwives have had to be involved in the process. One midwife expressed her dismay over being the only unpaid representative on these committees. Her greater concern, however, was her need to raise her fees in the coming year as a result of increasing costs associated with registration. This situation poses a moral dilemma for her and other midwives who are trying to remain as accessible as possible.

Regulation is not synonymous with integration or independent practice, and midwives are still outsiders in many important ways, clearly low in the pecking order of medical hierarchy. Collegiality between equally respected and supported service providers is widely recognized as a precondition for successful midwifery implementation models (Benoit 1998). But in Alberta, midwives remain subject to the authority of physicians. Unlike doctors, midwives are unable to order many routine tests and are also compelled to consult with physicians under certain conditions outlined in the Standards of Competency and Practice. Although there are certainly times when midwives willingly seek consultation with physicians and times when it is more appropriate for a woman to be in the care of a physician than a midwife, this particular rule means "the standards rather than informed choice discussions between a woman and her midwife will dictate when physician consultation is required. The midwife is required to initiate the consultation whether or not the woman chooses it" (James 1998: 25). This places the interests of the woman and the midwife in conflict and is a source of concern to midwives. It is also a source of concern to physicians who are not paid for consulting with midwives. None of these conditions encourage collegiality.

The single most important problem with the way midwifery has been implemented is the failure of Alberta Health to fully support this option through health insurance. In this way, the regulation of midwifery has been quite different in Alberta than in Ontario, where midwives are paid through health insurance. When Alberta Health refused to integrate midwifery services into health insurance, they suggested that any community wishing to support midwifery could do so through their Regional Health Authority. RHAs were created in response to a fourth goal of health care reform noted in *The Rainbow Report* that is relevant to midwifery. RHAs would permit local communities familiar with local needs to take on greater decision-making roles (Premier's Commission 1989: 28). Although this might have been an opportunity for midwives to highlight the benefits of their model of care and its correlatives with community health, it has not worked out this way. Critics view regionalization as an attempt to download responsibility for unpopular decisions onto regional groups, diverting responsibility for such decisions away from Alberta Health. Alberta Health continues to set regional fiscal targets, retains control over the appointment of board members and still holds the portion of the health care budget dedicated to physician payment. It is appropriate to wonder how much authority is really being handed to communities. Alberta Health dedicated $800,000 to the regions to go towards midwifery implementation, but as James (1998) points out, this is not enough to support the cost of administrative changes, let alone pay for actual midwifery services. To receive part of these funds, a region had to be willing to guarantee funding of midwifery services for three years. She goes on to say,

> If one does the mathematics, we quickly realize that this is no deal for the RHAs. They would receive enough to cover midwifery services for about three months. The remaining thirty three months plus additional costs to actually integrate midwives into their region would come entirely from existing budgets. (23)

Initially, all RHAs declined the invitation to implement midwifery. Some are now actively working with midwives on implementing their services, and it is anticipated that midwives will soon have greater privileges, but there will be no uniformity in the type of service that can be provided province-wide. Now the location of responsibility for failing to make the necessary changes to support midwives has been fractured.

The prospect of paying $2,000 out of their own pockets for care is fairly persuasive to most women and justifies the choice to seek care from providers who are "within the system." But beyond the economic barrier, the direct fee also presents a legitimacy barrier. Because midwifery has been considered a less valid option for care through much of this century, overcoming the stigma now associated with it requires full, unambiguous and enthusiastic support by Alberta Health. In deciding against insuring these services and allowing piecemeal implementation, the province failed to provide this support, leaving in place both an economic and psychological barrier to free choice. Midwives who responded to this survey all expressed varying degrees of shock at this outcome, having assumed that registration would be accompanied by inclusion in the health insurance plan.

Measuring the Value of Midwifery

So far, midwifery has been acknowledged within Alberta Health not so much for its ability to contribute to social goals, but for its ability to contain costs, and herein lies another problem. When birth outcomes are measured solely in terms of live infants and live mothers, and are concerned primarily with cost, practices that routinely leave psychological and social trauma in their wake can continue to be considered successful (Rothman 1989). In spite of the lofty social goals of health care reform outlined above, costs are still the primary consideration in the reform agenda. This may be because social goals are difficult to assess with a dollar value and therefore receive less focus than goals that are easily justified financially. What is the value of a maternal care model which empowers a woman to make her own decisions and increases her trust and faith in her body and her own ability to care for herself and her infant? What is the value of encouraging a woman's self worth as a mother and affirming her place in a strong supportive community? What is the value of a birth that takes place in peaceful surroundings, rejects unnecessary intervention and sees the infant placed immediately at the mother's breast? It is difficult to measure midwifery outcomes in dollars and cents, but surely this does not make their positive social outcomes any less desirable.

At the same time, looking to midwives to solve health issues that have their roots in social conditions puts an unfair responsibility on them. Social goals are achieved in a variety of interconnected ways, not just through health services. In Alberta, social spending continues to be cut dramatically, meaning any gains made through new health initiatives are less likely to succeed. For example, those who suggest midwifery can benefit clients who are economically disadvantaged forget that without social assistance, these women cannot afford to follow the advice given by midwives. In other words, cost savings in health services must be considered in relation to expenditures in other areas, making a straight cost-benefit analysis even more difficult.

Trying to justify midwifery based on cost is difficult because midwives recognize the interconnections between a multiplicity of factors related to health. They see the errors made when analysts compartmentalize different aspects of care for the sake of comparisons. Even the straightforward comparison of fee per course-of-care and fee-for-delivery is too simple. Since a course-of-care with a midwife begins with the first visit of pregnancy and ends six weeks postpartum, all the fees paid to physicians during this period must be included in an adequate comparison, not just the fee-for-delivery. In a normal pregnancy, the services of a midwife can replace not just the delivering physician, but also the labour and delivery nurse, neonatal care and the services of the district health nurse. All of these comparisons rest on the assumption that the current fee per course-of-care will remain fixed, which is not true. The fee per course-of-care is not set in stone and it is more likely to rise than remain stable, given the new costs associated with regulation. Also, being promoted as the *cost-effective* alternative rather than the *most effective* alternative in low-risk situations understandably frustrates some midwives. It feels like they are still second best and they worry that women will view their care as the cheap alternative to specialist care rather than the best care in low-risk situations.

Nevertheless, some work has been done to see if midwifery care actually saves money. There is reason to believe it might. The Midwifery Regional Implementation Committee (1996) noted that with fewer tests, reduced hospital stays (or no hospital stays with home births) and the performance of fewer procedures like epidural anesthesia, episiotomies and caesarean sections, health care costs can be significantly reduced when a midwife is primary caregiver during a normal pregnancy. An excellent Alberta study of a nurse-midwifery pilot project in one hospital followed a group of low-risk women who had all requested nurse-midwifery care (Harvey et al. 1996). Approximately half of the women received midwifery care while the other half received standard care from either an obstetrician or family physician. The rate of difference in surgical interventions was statistically significant. In the nurse-midwife group, 4 percent of the women delivered through cesarean while 15.1 percent delivered through cesarean in the physician group. The rate of episiotomy in the physician group was more than double that of the midwife group and almost double for the use of epidural anesthesia. "The results clearly support the effectiveness of the pilot nurse-midwifery program and suggest that more extensive participation of midwives in the Canadian health care system is an appropriate use of health care dollars" (128).

Midwifery attended pregnancies and births are reported to have healthier birth weights as well. The reason for this has not been established, but it may be because midwives help women to improve their nutrition and stop smoking (Rooney 1998). Alberta has a statistically higher incidence of low birth weight than the rest of Canada (Health Surveillance 1997). Since low birth weight is an important indicator of future health and results in the need for expensive neonatal care, Alberta Health considers reducing the incidence of low birth weight in the province a priority (1993: 92). Furthermore, midwives transfer fewer babies to neonatal intensive care. This constitutes an enormous cost saving, recently estimated at $1,500 a day at Calgary's Foothills Hospital (Walker 1998c).

Because cost comparisons are so difficult and because the fee per course-of-care is often cited without explanation, midwives find themselves in the unique position of being touted as both cost-effective and too costly. When midwifery is called "cadillac care" and women are told that specialist care is more affordable, the mind boggles at the sudden switch in logic. Women should get cadillac care, and in normal pregnancies and births this comes from midwives, and in high-risk situations this comes from obstetricians. Neither group should replace the other and no one model of care can adequately address all the needs women bring into childbirth. In the words of Sheila Harvey, another survey respondent, "Both groups need the other."

Conclusion

Going back to the job action, by asserting the need to increase their membership and maintain the status quo, obstetricians and gynecologists remain primarily focused on providing access to care, specifically their brand of care, without considering that this may not give access to health. They have failed to acknowledge the most negative results of their own model of care or the possibility that the burden of this care may be shared among other providers in a way that results in improved outcomes for a broad spectrum of women seeking maternal care. As a result, midwives, like obstetricians, are leaving the province. Some midwives are even leaving the profession. As of late 1998, there were only twenty registered midwives and another four with restricted registration. Of these, I learned of six midwives who do not expect to remain in practice next year, all citing grim financial realities and the conditions of practice as motives for their departure. The parallels between the complaints of obstetricians and the complaints of midwives are striking, but with less money, less prestige and less systemic support, midwives are surely worse off. Regulation has not enabled greater choice among caregivers or models of care for most Alberta women, nor has it improved the situation of women as caregivers beyond making their practice legal. The fact that obstetricians and midwives are moving to other jurisdictions and in the case of midwives, abandoning their profession, is probably the best indication that there is a serious crisis in maternal care.

If a midwifery model of care is congruent with so much of health care reform policy, why does the midwifery option continue to be unavailable to most Alberta women? Why are midwives leaving their profession? Why is government continuing to support the status quo in maternal care by facilitating an increase in delivery fees for physicians when the existing system is understood as problematic? The most obvious reason is that health policy follows the dictates of the dominant group, in this case physicians rather than midwives. "When midwifery and obstetrics conflict, midwifery loses because doctors have authority position in institutional power structures" (Goer 1995: 300). Although health care reform documents have paid lip service to the redistribution of power and the need to broaden the provision of services, the way reform has been operationalized has done little to change the balance of power within the system.

One standard solution suggests midwives regain responsibility for normal low-risk births and have their payment integrated into third party insurance plans while obstetricians concentrate their efforts and skills on women whose pregnancies and births are in a high-risk category. This change could address workload and lifestyle concerns for obstetricians, allowing them to do what they are trained to do, while providing midwives with a larger client base. Since obstetricians are currently experiencing a decline in numbers, it is a good time to undertake such a shift. If genuine health care were the true aim of the medical system, midwives would be fully privileged and autonomous practitioners. But, unfortunately, it's not that simple. There are not enough midwives to fill the gap, nor are many women currently willing to engage the care of a midwife. More education about the role of the midwife is needed to assist such a shift in care models.

Furthermore, if midwives are included in an insurance plan based on fee-for-service, they would be subject to all the problems inherent in this kind of payment plan. The Midwifery Regional Implementation Committee recommends remuneration be based on either payment per course-of-care or salary. It rejects fee-for-service as an option (Midwifery Regional Implementation Committee 1997: 3). Obstetricians also argue that their practices would fail under these conditions without a change in remuneration plans. While midwives gained business, obstetricians would lose business and considerable income. If, however, obstetricians were to become salaried, they could provide the necessary care to patients in high-risk categories without destroying the income base that low-risk care provides. Currently, they can only afford to dedicate the requisite time to high-risk situations because their low-risk patients, in effect, subsidize their practices. In the current fee structure, there is no way to adequately compensate obstetricians for the extensive care they provide during routine office visits throughout high-risk pregnancies and births. An alternative solution is to substantially increase fees for pregnancies and deliveries that are high-risk. This imposes a tiered fee system in maternal services. Midwives argue that this tiered system already exists because obstetricians are paid per intervention. But additional fees for interventions do nothing to support the needs of women in high-risk pregnancies for increased time and attention in the nine months prior to birth, nor do they support the needs of physicians to be properly remunerated for providing such care. Any of these solutions will likely require an increased investment in maternal services and the chances of this happening in an environment of cost restraint are slim.

The challenge facing those of us committed to improving maternal care in Alberta and elsewhere is to concentrate on what enables a positive outcome for the childbearing woman and her family as she defines it, while setting aside divisive issues of professional power and politics. The groundwork has been laid within health reform literature for achieving these goals. Ideally, women should choose between equally validated models of care that best suit their needs and have the option of altering the provision of care as new circumstances arise. Power must reside with women who determine their own needs in collaboration with health care professionals. Creating such a model necessitates "breaking the circle of medical dominance" (Rothman 1989: 184). The obstetricians' and gynecologists' job action diverts attention away from this goal and puts energy back into maintaining the status quo. Ultimately, this will not serve women because the crisis in obstetrics does not define the crisis in women's health services. Paying attention to the voices of midwives clarifies the view of a much larger problem. It allows us to reconsider the definition of appropriate care, the social goals of health care, the complexity of cost analyses, the problems in fee-for-service remuneration, the plight of women as care providers in a male dominated world and the systemic failure of the health system to fully address the needs of women in pregnancy and childbirth. When midwifery is understood as both a life enhancing and sustainable practice, systemic barriers to its full implementation can only be seen as perverse. Obstetricians and gynecologists do not have the vision to single-handedly determine what is needed within women's health care. The voices of women as caregivers and care recipients must also be heard before the health care reform will be able to adequately address their needs.

Notes

1. I would like to thank the midwives, midwifery advocates and obstetricians who spoke to me regarding this work.
2. This information was made available by the Alberta Society of Obstetrics and Gynecology in a series of press releases and internal information sheets that are undated and untitled. All future references will be noted within the text as (ASOG n.d.).
3. Doris Grinspun in this volume explores the multiple impacts on care and caring labour wrought by the shift toward the business paradigm.
4. Douglass Drozdow-St. Christian in this volume examines some responses of aging women to the structural incentives that reduce the amount and quality of time spent with a physician.
5. For discussion of the impact of regulation on health professionals in Ontario, see Lum and Williams in this volume.

7

Dissolving, Dividing, Distressing: Examining Cutbacks to Programs Responding to Sexual Violation

Si Transken

> Marnina [a SACC social worker]: It's pretty nuts, you know! How do I think budget cutbacks and restructuring have impacted [on victims of sexual violation and their social workers]? I would think that it's made it so we can't be as holistic. Perhaps, we don't provide services for as long as they're required. People are left on waiting lists for longer. People maybe aren't provided the group counselling combined with individual counselling as often or as frequently.... I think society feels the strain of them [social service cutbacks]. I think for a woman who may be in a physically, sexually, emotionally or abusive relationship in general she may be more hesitant to leave that relationship. Society isn't seen as a very supporting environment with which to run to. I think that. It just doesn't feel as safe. They're more isolated. It further isolates women and children.

Introduction

This chapter is about the two programs in Ontario that are funded to respond specifically to sexual violation, about the women who have experienced sexual violence and/or who work in the area of attending to victims of sexual violence, and about the serious effect of funding cutbacks and health care restructuring on these programs and people. Specifically, I discuss how social worker interviewees in nine sexual assault treatment (SATs) programs and nine sexual assault crisis centres (SACCs) are coping with budget cutbacks. I describe how social workers themselves are feeling more vulnerable and how they are watching their clients go through more intense periods of crisis than in the past. This chapter shows that service to victims of sexual violation is dissolving, that the Ontario government's health care reform has served to sometimes divide those who deliver service, and that service providers, clients and the larger community are all in greater distress because of these changes.

Women's episodes of body-spirit-mind crisis are responded to by our health care and social services systems with a decreasing recognition of women's whole personhood and diversity of needs. I offer a personal observation by way of example: In the months during which I considered and undertook this research, I went through many personal changes. In the last six months, much has happened to my body-spirit-mind: a common-law marriage I had been in for thirteen years concluded, I had a tubal ligation, eye surgery, recurrences of a long-harassing neck and shoulder injury and countless migraines to fight my way through. Regardless of my emotionally, spiritually and physically draining experiences I had to, as most women do, continue working full-time and part-time at paid positions. Also, I continued in my community activism and in the caring relationships in my personal life. Had it not been for the support and encouragement of women caregivers (formal and informal), these changes would have disappeared me from this project.[1] In fact, it feels like a miracle has happened in that this chapter has been written.

For good reason I link this private information about myself to the public scholarly project of producing this chapter. Our species exists with our body-spirit-mind always connected; we cause damage and distortion when we pretend otherwise (Transken 1995 and 1997). Much has been written affirming this body-spirit-mind connection, but it has been minimized or lost in Western imaginings of humanity (Carver and Ponée 1989, Charmaz and Paterniti 1999, Dua et al. 1994, Laidlaw et al. 1990, Messing et al. 1995, Ng 1 in press[2]). Non-western approaches to wellbeing often not only recognize, but celebrate the intrinsic body-spirit-mind inseparability. (Charmaz and Paterniti 1999, Ng 1997, Silvera 1994: 324, Tomm 1995: 77–114, Waterfall 1996). The fact is that during my troubling experiences of the last year, my body-spirit-mind underwent pressures and challenges. Some of these positioned me to think and feel alertly and mournfully about what was happening in the health and social services sectors. In some ways my own life echoed those of the women social workers[3] I interviewed. It is precisely this fundamental body-spirit-mind experience which Ontario government health care reforms now aim to ignore by viewing sexual violation through a medical model, rather than as an issue which requires that victimized women be empowered in order to wholly heal.

In this chapter, I outline the dramatic changes Ontario's health care services have undergone in the recent past. Social support and care services to women are being dissolved or distressed. As the interviewees I quote here describe, some women's supports are being divided and conquered; some services are becoming so burdened that the staff are distressed to the point of taking stress leaves, gradually changing professions or even quitting their employment without having other options in place. As the interviewed social workers tell us, these patterns have meaning in that more women are vulnerable to sexual predators, and that once violated, fewer women are able to fully access appropriate healing resources. Sexual violence is a prevalent experience in women's lives (Bart and Moran 1993, Blume 1990, Buchwald et al. 1993, Burstow 1992, Gil 1988, Laidlaw, et al. 1990, Maltz 1992, Roberts and Mohr 1994, Sumrall and Taylor 1992) and this has multiple and long-term mental and physical health care consequences.

In the interviews quoted in the pages to follow, social workers tell us that programs which have evolved over the decades to respond to victims' needs are being reshaped toward a medicalized and less politicized approach, and away from a grassroots and politicized feminist social justice model. A shift toward single-problem and short-term crisis therapy (or Brief Solution Focused therapy) is a central feature of this reshaping. I discuss a provincial government plan called the *Maguire Report* and show how this report's suggestions could move us more toward an American service delivery model. This would mean that women who have been violated might access some basic supports from the publicly funded programs, with any supports beyond that (more extensive individual or group counselling) paid for privately. The very fact that SAT programs are being created in hospitals and that they are hiring social workers as support staff in these programs suggests a movement to a medical model. All of the practitioners whom I interviewed expressed concerns about these trends which are constricting and damaging women's lives. Most indicators suggest that, at least for the immediate future, women will continue to face these threats to their access to services, their safety and their dignity (Demetrakopoulos et al. 1997: 76–100). We can fight to hang onto little everyday miracles or find new miracles, but the fight can be brutal.

Methodology

> Nancy [a SAT social worker]: I just think that it's very important that we have an opportunity to voice these interests and concerns. I'm really really pleased that you are doing this [research], because I don't think that enough research is done in this field and it gives me a chance to sort of say, and have somebody listen to what I *think is important* about my work and about what is important *for women* in this community. So I just want to thank

you very much for initiating this kind of work. I think it's really important, we need more of it. It substantiates kind of where we're at. If it's not studied, it doesn't seem like we exist.

These research findings are based on extensive qualitative interviews with eighteen women social workers in Ontario SATs and SACCs spread out all across the province.[4] An equal number of women was interviewed from SATs and SACCs. All interviewees chose their own pseudonyms; some minor details (of geography or exact years as a staff member in a program, for example) have been changed to protect anonymity. This chapter is further enriched by my own three years of experiences as a social worker in a SAT program; my ongoing private practice with women who have been violated; my own experiences as a survivor (of years of childhood sexual abuse) who has used a variety of healing services; and my learnings from three years in my role as an assistant professor supervising social work student's internships in women's services.

All SATs and SACCs in Ontario were faxed and/or mailed on more than one occasion a letter of introduction and an outline of proposed interview questions. These written materials were followed up within four weeks with at least one phone call initiating contact. From here appointments were scheduled for telephone interviews. This process invited considered analysis from the interviewees as each participant was able to discuss the questions with her peers and to reflect deeply on how she wanted to answer the questions. The questions they were each faxed/mailed and then asked during the phone interview were:

1. Are you familiar with SACCs and their herstory? If "yes," how do you think they might be similar or dissimilar to SATs?
2. How do you think the mission and vision of SATs connects with the mission and vision of SACCs?
3. To your knowledge, how are SATs and SACCs funded? How does the funding have meaning and consequence for the programs and for the service recipients?
4. How do you think budget cutbacks and restructuring have impacted upon service delivery in the SATs and SACCs programs?
5. Many changes have happened in regards to how social services and supports such as legal aid, welfare, unemployment insurance, subsidized housing, etcetera for women are delivered. How do you think these changes in social service and support programs have impacted upon women in regards to sexual violence?
6. If present trends continue what do you think SATs and SACCs

will be like ten years from now?

7. Are you familiar with "Brief Solution Focused Therapy?" What meaning, if any, does this therapeutic approach have for women who have accessed services from places like SATs and/or SACCs? What meaning might it have in the future?

8. Are you familiar with the Maguire Report? What meaning has it had for SATs and/or SACCs?

9. Are there any other thoughts or feelings you would like to share about the themes and questions raised in this interview?

These questions gave many social workers an opportunity to vent their frustration and to use the interview preparation and process to make more sense of the changes with which they were being forced to cope.

Representatives from about one-third of all established SATs and SACCs completed interviews. Only one person from all those approached actively refused to be interviewed for reasons I discuss later. The programs from which no interview took place did not respond to repeated messages left on their answering machines. My present belief is that many of them were just too understaffed to give an hour or two of their time to a researcher on the phone. I infer this because any of the women whom I did "catch" live (versus the telephone answering machine) repeatedly agreed to do the interview with me "next week" or "as soon as they had more time" but eventually I discontinued my pursuit of them due to my own time and resource constraints.

Defining Sexual Violation as a Health Care Issue

> Cher [a SAT social worker]: about physical injuries, I learned my biggest lesson probably with the first client I ever had when I went in and I said to the lady, "Are you hurt at all?" and the volunteer [from a SACC] who had been a volunteer for years looked at me like I had absolutely lost it and I didn't know what she was looking at me so strangely for and she looked at the client and she said to her, "She means do you have any physical injuries, are you hurt anywhere [on your body]?" My question of "are you hurt?" was probably one of the stupidest things I've ever said in my life. Her heart was broken. She had been hurt. She had been sexually assaulted by her partner and I'm saying, "Are you hurt?" So I learned a big lesson there!

The medical model was referred to by many interviewees and is a term commonly used in this line of work. Cher, the SAT social worker cited in the preceding quote, in describing a moment of "unlearning" the medical model. Armstrong, Choiniere, Feldberg and White (1994) comment on this approach by referring to it as the " 'engineering' approach to treatment and care, which views the body as a collection of parts to be fixed" (55). Later they say,

> The system is based on a model of health that sees the body as a collection of parts that can be treated separately, and illness as primarily biological. Only with such assumptions can care be divided into discrete tasks and units of time and recovery be assigned a limited period. (82)

A medical model refers to seeing only the immediately visible physical injury and efficiently attending to that. It is imagined as the opposite to a feminist social justice model because the medical model does not see the whole life of the woman before this moment when she appears in the emergency room or where she may be going when she leaves this emergency room.

Preventative care and all of the social conditions that lead to a woman being sexually violated are not part of the discussion within a medical model. Maya, a SACC social worker, describes the medical model as a,

> focus more on collection of forensic evidence, addressing health needs, and maybe narrowly focusing on just the physical types of injuries ... the medical model might ... not emphasize, emotional, maybe some limited emotional work, of course, but there's a more ... medically quantifiable, physical manifestation ... very much like a crisis intervention ... very short term.

Mary Ann, a SACC social worker, describes how even victim/survivors can come to damagingly internalize dictates of the medical model because it can seem safer. Women victim/survivors sometimes believe that being diagnosed and medicated will cure them of the damage inflicted by sexual violation.

> The medical model may condescendingly define women helpers in SACC programs [as] we're just women talking. And he'll [a psychiatrist] have given her [the victim] a diagnosis which she just holds onto for dear life. Because it's about the diagnosis, about "my illness." This is about *my illness* as opposed to, this is about the fact that my *father screwed me* every morning of my life [which is too overwhelming to face]. It's my illness. And that can be treated with drugs. We don't want to take that away from her

by any means. We try very hard to work with the system so she isn't feeling like she has to chose. That's often what she feels like she has to do.

The conceptualizing of the medical model and how sexual violation relates directly or indirectly to the medical model are central questions for any woman in this line of work.

The terms sexual assault and sexual violation benefit from a discussion also. I prefer to use the term sexual violation because it is larger, it is more inclusive, and it more effectively recognizes women's experiences. Within the meaning of sexual violation I include women who have been sexually harassed in the workplace or elsewhere, women who have been date raped, and/or women who have been violated by a member of their family. I include any woman who has had her body violated and/or who has experienced the threat of having her body violated. I also include women who have had their psychological space violated because this is a psychological and physical health hazard. All of these violations have the possible consequence of inflicting health issues (Blume 1990, Burstow 1992, Courtois 1988, Maltz 1992, Terr 1990). For example, a woman who is being criminally harassed may develop an eating disorder, a sleep disorder, or a drinking problem. A woman being sexually harassed in the workplace may become so overwhelmed and depressed that she begins using prescription and/or street-level medications in an attempt to cope.

Representatives from all SACCs and SATs would agree that sexual violation damages women and girls on many levels. There are immediate and readily obvious health care issues of acute sexual assault such as unwanted pregnancy, broken bones, cuts, bruises, internal injuries, sexually transmitted diseases and emotional shock. Sexual abuse has also been linked to drug abuse, alcohol abuse, self-mutilation, depression, suicide attempts, eating disorders, insomnia, headaches and irritable bowel syndrome (Blume 1990, Burstow 1992, Courtois 1988, Maltz 1992, Terr 1990). In some cases a woman's sexual violation has been linked to her neglect or abuse of her own children. This then creates health care issues for children. Further, when a man who has sexually abused one woman goes unreported and unpunished he may continue to abuse. Therefore, a system of effective, immediate and substantive health (and legal, political and economic) care for women and girl victims means that more of them will report their abuser and thus prevent future abuse situations. Common sense tells us that if all violators were reported and our justice system was effective (in restraining perpetrators and in giving them appropriate counselling and education), fewer women today would need to heal from violation.

Funders often attempt to deny that sexual violation is a health care issue on many levels: both short term and long term. If sexual violation were responded to as a health care issue, with more emphasis on prevention of violence and the provision of quickly available depthful counselling, more health care dollars would be saved in the long term.

Funders, in contrast to social workers like Oprah, do not always have a complex long-term analysis of the consequences of sexual violation. Funders, administrators, those advocating the medical model or a Brief Solution Focused Therapy model, segment and quantify women's lives and their pain. More than a decade ago, Campbell and Ng examined "how power relations are embedded in state funding" (1988: 41) showing how funders use money and the administrative process to monitor and control women's services. They write,

> the routine use of document-based management practices, including Program Evaluation, does more than provide accountability; the power implicit in such a management process is its capacity to authorize a particular viewpoint. Program Evaluation lends scientific authority to the particular version of truth about the program which the information system constructs. It is that the evaluator adopts a "ruling" standpoint regardless of intention. (43–44)

A case can be made that the intentions of funders and administrators involved in SAT and SACC issues are to deny or offload responsibility for women's body-spirit-mind wellbeing.

Defining and Comparing SATs and SACCs

SATs and SACCs are the two services publicly funded to respond to survivors of sexual violation. I want to clarify, through this research project, the degree to which women in these two groups were informed about each other.

Sexual Assault/Rape Crisis Centres (SACCs)
SACCs arose on Canada's social terrain in the 1970s (the first one opened in 1974) in a grassroots effort to respond to women's pain and isolation. Originally SACCs were called Rape Crisis Centres and many people still refer to them with this name. These places usually emerged on a tiny budget of community raised funding and were staffed by volunteers. Many of the volunteers are women who had been sexual violated themselves and who made helping others part of their own healing journey.

Presently, most SACCs have a core of paid staff who are from both the grassroots movement and/or from the helping professions. SACCs have always been connected to many political movements and activities. As service agencies, SACCs evolved their way into existence from many other services being sought in women's referral and resource centres. This grassroots and politicized feminist heritage means that most SACCs have a tradition of seeing their work as being profoundly connected to the work of unions, Take Back the Night organizing, International Women's Day events, Gay Pride Parades, the Pro Choice Movement, etcetera. In fact, most SACCs have retained the role of leaders of these activities in their communities. Certainly, in my own community this has been the case.

SACCs provide care for women who have been hurt in the recent or distant past. No secondary referrals are required for clients to access services. SACCs have traditionally provided as much counselling as a woman expressed an interest in receiving (i.e., there were no limits on how many therapy sessions were available to women). The formats and processes of counselling also were customized to the women victim/survivors' requests.

SACCs are largely funded by the federal government through the Solicitor General but many also receive a portion of funding from Health and Community and Social Services. Almost all SACCs participate in some type of community fundraising efforts. Their stated goals are to provide the following services to women who have been sexually violated:

> 24 hour crisis counselling over the phone; Accompaniment to the hospital and/or police station; Advocacy and referrals; Crisis follow-up face to face counselling (usually within a few days); Court support; On-going counselling; Group counselling; self-help groups; Outreach support including diversity work; Public education, resources and information libraries; As well as speakers and workshops for the public and professionals. (Aikens 1996: 2)

Throughout the years of their existence and continuing into the present, many SACCs supplement their Solicitor General money with projects (e.g., anti-racism workshops, conferences on violence, creation of educational materials and so on) funded by the Ontario Women's Directorate, the United Way and the like. Much of this supplementary money has dried up in recent years. Solicitor General money has been, according to my interviewees, reduced by 10 to 15 percent in 1996; reduced again by 4.8 percent in 1997; and again by 4.8 percent in 1998.

Not all SACCs have had their budgets cut in identical ways. Some were the only centres in their communities who responded to any women's issues. Other communities have multiple types of agencies which respond to different aspects of women's oppression. Therefore, some communities divided up the scarce resources and SACCs in these communities felt more cuts. In other communities programs continued with minimal cuts to their SACCs. According to my interviewees, all but one SACC has experienced some type of funding cutback during the last three years.

Although Jill's agency had not faced cutbacks at the time of this interview, her agency's waiting list was almost two years long.

> I'm the only worker for [a large geographic region] and so that translates into about a twenty-two month waiting list. So that's enough actually for another social worker to have her full case load right there. And then with whatever slack there is [we could] do a group. So there would be enough work certainly to have another full-time social worker on board but that's not [going to happen]. We've applied for various grants and we've been told that there's just no money there.

For many women victim/survivors, twenty-two months of time means defeat. By the time their sessions begin they may have fallen over that edge (i.e., they may have lost their job, quit school, been repeatedly abused, developed an alcohol or drug problem, attempted suicide).

Many SACC women have hostile feelings toward the medical model, which they perceive as being the dominant frame used at SATs. SACC women work with, or in resistance to, the medical model but it is always a dimension of a woman's story that they must consider.

> Bubbles [a SACC social worker]: We see ourselves as an alternative for women. [Women] have been screwed over by the medical model time and time again. The majority of women who come to our centre have a history with psychiatrists and medical practitioners that's horrifying. Around the kind of medication they've been prescribed, around the kind of treatment [women have received]. Whether it's been the shock treatment stuff. They are survivors of abuse and nobody is listening to them say that. Nobody is saying, "You know what? Maybe that [sexual abuse] is the issue to deal with!" as opposed to, "Well let's just make you feel better by killing all your brain cells [with medication]. 'Cause if you can't remember it [the abuse], then things will be better."

Sexual Assault Treatment Programs (SATS)

> Lynne [a SAT social worker]: SAT programs have a medical
> mandate first, like they take care of the health needs first …
> sexually transmitted diseases and in terms of being intact in their
> body, and also they [SATs] have a mandate to collect medical,
> legal evidence. So that's very different than SACCs where they
> have more of a mandate of providing crisis counselling, short-
> term and long-term resources, group support.

Sexual Assault Treatment Programs (SATS) are a more recent addition to the social terrain. Most came into existence within the last five years and are still in the process of defining exactly what role they can and want to fulfill within their communities. A few existed, at the time of my inter- views, as mainly a phone number in a hospital emergency ward. Women who called this number were connected to pre-existing or pre-deployed staff who had a personal mission to be of as much assistance as possible regarding sexual abuse issues (i.e., a whole program did not exist to support victims of sexual abuse).

To my knowledge SATs have always been staffed by paid profession- als (i.e., not necessarily victim/survivors or volunteers). They have arisen within a hospital context, although in some communities it was not only the health care professionals who advocated for SATs to exist. It was also the SACCs who advocated for creating SATs because, of course, SACCs recognize that some type of specialized medical support is needed for survivors of acute sexual assault. SATs provide this acute care treatment for sexual assault victims of any age and both sexes. SATs have prided themselves on becoming specialists at providing medical care for sexual assault victims who have been hurt in the recent past (usually defined as within hours or days) of the assault. I have no evidence to suggest that in this regard they are anything less than excellent. The medical dimension of care provided by SATs is provided by highly trained professionals who are continually developing their knowledge base and their technology. Consensus seems to exist among all SAT and SACC representatives regard- ing this aspect of care.

Within the last year, seven SATs have added domestic violence programs to their services. These are pilot projects for which some SATs had a funding increase in their overall budget. At the same time these SATs were assigned substantially increased workloads. SATs offer many types of care including: providing a full medical exam; preparing a forensic kit that assists victims should they decide to lay charges; assisting clients to ensure an unwanted pregnancy does not take place as a result of the assault; assessing whether the victim has been exposed to infectious diseases and attending to these if exposure has occurred; and providing public education and follow-up counselling.

Most of the staff in SATs are nurses and these nurses rather than social workers are more likely to be the program's coordinators. Caring professionals with a social work background are often the most peripheral members of the SAT teams and their area of work (counselling and public education/advocacy) is exactly the terrain that is most ambiguously situated within SATs. Katherine, a SAT social worker comments on how the medical model maintains certain tasks for staff to provide but that other tasks can quickly be eliminated when money restricts options:

> It is difficult to provide the same level or frequency of counselling or availability of counselling with the cutbacks. We've had minor cutbacks through the Ministry of Health, okay.... And what it did to us personally is all the education that we do in the community that's all [now] volunteer work.

These role dimensions of counselling and public education or advocacy from SATs is also the most ambiguously received and viewed by SACCs. I certainly encountered this sense of ambiguity about my own role as a social worker in the SAT program I worked in for three years. Many SAT social workers experience internal tension between what may be their personal level of feminist or politicized analysis and commitment to activism, and what the professional role as a social worker in a SAT program invites or allows for. Some SAT workers chose to do volunteer work to fill the gaps their program disallows them to formally participate in.

SATs are funded by the provincial government through the Ministry of Health. Initially SATs' monies were kept in a separate pool which could only be spent on SAT initiatives, staff, etcetera. Recently, most SATs have had their money pooled into their hospitals' overall budgets. This one event has enormous potential consequences. This means that a large portion of control has been lost by SAT program coordinators. Regular hospital administrators and medical personnel are now making decisions about SAT programs' wellbeing, needs, staff training budget and so on. When a hospital administrator has to make tough decisions regarding where a cutback will be made, administrators may feel that funding for heart health care, head injuries victims, or high-tech equipment is more important than the emotional wellbeing of sexually violated victims.[5]

When there has been a budget cut across the whole hospital, of course, SATs have their budget decreased regardless of whether their workload has been increasing. Almost every one of my interviewees from SATs confirmed there has been a notable decrease in the amount of resources available to them to do their work, in spite of promises to the contrary declared in a recently produced pamphlet sent out by the Ontario Women's Directorate (n.d.). Katherine, a SAT program coordinator summed it up like this, "I am running as hard as I can and so are my team members. But I do have real fears for the security and the longevity of our program."

Dis/Similarities Between SATs And SACCs

SATs and SACCs often have been and/or have felt distanced from and pitted against each other (and against some other women's services).[6] It could be said that they are similar in the potential to perceive each other as a competitor for funds, status and credibility. Tension is something they have in common. It could be said that what they should have in common is respect for each other's rightful role in survivors' journeys. Mary Ann, a SACC activist, describes recent tensions at press conferences and community committees where SAT and SACC representatives have been invited to participate. She also alludes to the imagery that I often encountered during my three years as a SAT worker, and elsewhere since then, that SAT women were "nicer" and more open to co-optation and that SACC women were "bad " or "rebels."

Oprah, who works with a SAT in a remote part of the province commented on the scarcity of resources and how that was a commonality among SATs and SACCs:

> We are so exhausted. It's the divide and conquer thing at the moment where you know, those of us, and there are *so many* of us [advocates for women's issues and survivors of oppression] that are marginalized or disenfranchized because we can't gain access to the resources that we *need* in spite of our hard work.

Identifying the specifics and particulars of this potential distance and conflict between SATs and SACCs was an intriguing aspect for me in designing this research project. I asked myself: How much do they have in common? How significant is the ideological gulf between them? My findings have been that they do have much in common. They do have some ideological disharmonies but their commonalities and their harmonies are being overshadowed by their location as competitors for government funding. The allocation of money can foster or destroy harmony.

Ideologically, SACCs are more committed to understanding sexual violation as a type of force which keeps all women feeling vulnerable. In other words SACC women do not forget that women who have never experienced any overt physical assault have still been damaged because the threat of sexual abuse and harassment has restricted their/our lives.

SACC women, especially in their roles as volunteers (as unpaid activists they cannot be dismissed or reprimanded), are more likely to see and speak out about a multitude of oppressions. SAT representatives are often quite informed about such issues on a sociological level but not all of them take the same kind of passionate ownership over the process of change. Many SAT social workers may hold equally passionate feminist sociological views and may display these perspectives when they are alone with their clients, but they are not as able to overtly display these views as activists within a SAT. Some SATs are more comfortable delegating the protest work and social activism work to other organizations. This is partially because they do not want to overlap in the task areas that everyone has agreed belong to SACC programs (and other women's advocacy and public education organizations). It does not seem to be the case that SAT program workers do not want the work to be done. Instead, SAT workers have recognized their organizational locations and limitations, and they seem to feel confident in the abilities of SACCs to do the loud and dirty work (high-risk political work) of social reform. Consequently, some SACC workers feel they are taking the risks of being punished by funders and they feel that the silence they sometimes witness SATs offering on issues is a form of collusion with oppressors.

A large portion of the perceived dissimilarities are actually myths created by misunderstandings and misinformation by government funders playing SATs and SACCs off against each other. I was well aware of these tensions between SATs and SACCs, and I was not sure how each organization would respond to my research inquiries. I tried to look for commonalities that would inspire them to share their perspectives with me. One of the shared things I first noticed was that SAT and SACC workers feel they are invisible right now. They feel the governments and funders of the day are not listening to SATs and SACCs and their concerns.

What did SAT and SACC people say were similar or dissimilar aspects of their programs? Nancy, a long-time activist in women's organizations and a SAT program social worker who is in one of the most mature SAT programs, felt SATs and SACCs had a great deal in common. She said,

> Nancy: [We have in common] that feminist analysis, *that* we really believe in and we can support that, both of us can support that on each other. We might operationalize it differently but I think that is basically there and we support each other in those endeavours either sort of in a community support basis or whatever, activities that they are holding, we support those, and they do for us. We get together and collaborate on some things.

Not all social workers share Nancy's perception that all SATs and SACCs share a common feminist vision, and not all interviewees believe that SATs and SACCs "support each other" or "collaborate." Nancy notes the disharmonies:

> There is some difference [between SATs and SACCs]. I think there is, how people perceive rape crisis centres is quite often different than how they might perceive SATs and I think that they are perceived as a very grassroots organization because they have had a lot of credibility over the last you know twenty-five or thirty years. And certainly SATs are much newer there, we operationalize our vision very differently and we have a little more structure perhaps, we have to deal with than they do. For instance we are housed in a hospital and we are sort of part of that system, unfortunately or fortunately, so we have more limitations perhaps in being more political.

This restriction of being governed by an organizational structure that is large, hierarchical, medical-centred (a few are also religiously oriented, e.g., Catholic hospitals) and usually male-dominated is one of the major differences between SATs and SACCs.

One primary aspect of the difficulty between SATs and SACCs is that of client understanding of the programs' differences. The funding is organized so that an "acute care victim" (where the term "acute care" may be defined anywhere on a continuum from "within twenty-four hours" to "within the last year") is expected to go to a SAT and have her wounds tended to and her medical needs met and then she is expected to move on to a SACC program in those communities where a SACC exists. If a woman was sexually violated a long time ago (i.e., the consequences of the "crime" are no longer seeable on her body, which is the "site of the crime"), then she is supposed to be encouraged to begin her healing journey with a SACC program. Complications may arise in process and definitions of where it is most appropriate for a woman to receive help; a woman may present in a hospital setting with an injured limb, an attempted suicide, a drug overdose, serious mental health problems (e.g., an admission for being an hallucinating street person), an eating disorder—and she may also have sexual abuse issues. This can be stressful for a SAT worker. As well, clients do not always understand funding structures and neither should they be expected to. The process of moving through this system is potentially awkward and disorienting.

Restructuring and Budget Cutbacks

On March 21, 1998 Ontario Premier Mike Harris wrote,

> Consultation has always been and always will be the hallmark of
> the Harris Government. I value the feedback I get from every
> Ontarian—men and women from all walks of life.... The difficult
> choices we have had to make for ourselves and for Ontarians
> were necessary to protect the services we all cherish: Top-quality
> health care that's there when you need it. (5)

My interviewees did not feel Harris had been listening to them! Their
definition of "top-quality health care that's there when we need it" is
dramatically different from the Harris regime's definition. To SAT and
SACC social workers the definition of "health" involves a much more
holistic array of services including food, shelter, psychological support
services, physical protection services and options regarding medical
care.

Questions in my survey about funding generated an enormous
amount of dialogue around the despair that social workers and their
clients are confronting right now. Budget cutbacks in a variety of programs (welfare, legal aid, subsidized housing, training allowances,
childcare, student loans and so on) impacted upon women's experiences
of assault. The vast majority of victims of sexual violation (81 percent) are
hurt by someone they know, such as their father, their husband, their
boss, their neighbour, their teacher, a classmate, or an extended kin
member (Canadian Panel on Violence against Women 1993: 9). When a
sexual violation happens and the woman wants to protect herself from
further abuse it may mean, for example, that she has to leave her home,
quit her job, move into another neighbourhood or drop out of school. As
social support programs are being cut, women have fewer options
available to them to effectively restructure and resettle their lives. Further, the justice system has also been under increasing demands with
scarce resources. If women decide to lay charges, sometimes there is a
two-year turnaround time between the day of the violation and the final
day in court. This means that women's lives are held up in the air, in fear,
in confusion and in despair as they wait for their perpetrator to be
removed from the community or punished in some way. Many women
feel stuck and can't move forward in their healing process until the
court's activities have concluded.

Changes in Ontario's response to sexual violation issues could be
thought of as having happened in at least four ways. The first is for staff
themselves. The second type of change could be thought of as the wider

community's lessened tolerance for the neediness of oppressed or vulnerable populations. The third change could be thought of as resulting from the first two. Staff have constricted emotional and material resources to give. The wider community's mean-spiritedness and the climate of scarcity impacts upon how many women are sexually violated. The wider community's messages impact upon victims' belief in their entitlement to reach out for supports. Women have found there is less available when they do reach out, and the intensity of neediness that they exhibit when they do finally reach out is higher. The fourth change in Ontario's response to sexual violation is related to the changes for social workers, clients and the wider community. This change is the movement toward Brief Solution Focused (BSF) therapy for the care of women who have been sexually violated. Now I look at each of these changes in turn.

Changes for Staff and their Experiences of Themselves
Social workers in these programs are feeling defeated, overwhelmed, under-regarded, disrespected and fearful for their own futures. Many of them are seeing more clients and clients with startlingly high levels of needs. Some of these social workers have had their programs restructured so they are trying to cope with lots of changes. Some have had their co-workers laid off and this can invoke grief and a sense of guilt. Many have had their hours cut. Some social workers now have two or three part-time jobs, and this changes how they experience themselves as caregivers. Cher describes the meaning for her of having two part-time jobs and of only being able to offer BSF therapy to clients.

> No matter what your role [within the client's healing process] ... they can't do a good job looking after the patients or clients in the way they were educated to do. So I find that probably a lot of people are taking that home and it's stressful knowing that you didn't complete what you wanted to do with the client ... and you don't get to see the end result, sometimes, because of the fragmentation. You don't get to see the end result. You don't get to see the outcome for the client.

It sometimes feels like a miracle that women continue doing the kind of work that we do in these organizations. Their/our compassion and stamina are testaments to the potential of the human body-spirit-mind.

Changes in the Larger Community
The cuts in all kinds of services have generated a climate of competition and fear. People are feeling protective of their own turf, their own jobs, their own little lives. Many people may want to think, "Well, sexual

assault will never happen to me so why should I worry about that issue?" They may feel inclined to fall back to a position of victim-blaming or denial of the frequency and seriousness of sexual violation.

"Cognitive dissonance" is a term social workers might use to describe this phenomenon. Cognitive dissonance is "an uncomfortable psychological state in which the individual experiences two incompatible beliefs or cognitions. Cognitive dissonance theory holds that the individual is motivated by the attendant discomfort to act in such a manner to reduce the dissonance" (Chaplin 1975: 94). If we blame the victim for her own abuse then we do not experience cognitive dissonance when we say to her, "Solve your own problems—you made these problems for yourself. Leave me alone!" If we recognize that any of us could be sexually violated at any time and there is no perfect way to keep ourselves safe, then we know we are morally obligated to help someone who has been hurt. If we recognize that we owe vulnerable people support, but that this support is not being provided, this causes cognitive dissonance. So by imagining that sexual violation rarely happens and that when it does the person brought it onto themselves and thus they themselves should heal the damage done, we are freed from responsibility.

Given that I did not ask about the ethnocultural identities or special needs of the eighteen social workers I interviewed (or about clients who might be defined as having additional oppressions to contend with) and I did not ask any questions that specifically explored the meaning of cutbacks for multiply disadvantaged women, I feel disqualified to speak extensively to this question. I do know that, in many programs, success has not been achieved at securing the resources for translation, sign language, affirmative action hiring practices, staff development regarding the needs of statistically smaller populations and so on. The needs of ethnocultural minority women, immigrant women, First Nations women and disabled women are often disregarded in this restructuring of priorities. This is not news; multiply disadvantaged women are frequently disregarded in how social services and health care are delivered (Kavanagh and Kennedy 1992, Masuda and Ridington 1992, Sehdev 1987, Stimpson and Best 1991, Tudiver 1994: 96, Waxler-Morrison et al. 1990).

Some interviewees did comment on how these harsh attitudes arising in our communities more intensely impact upon multiply vulnerable women. Scarcity of resources often breeds competition. Unfortunately, in small agencies, when there are limited amounts of time and money, often the needs of the statistically few can become overlooked while the needs of the many are crisis managed.

Changes for Clients because of Cutbacks

Clients are surely being affected by the exhaustion that some SAT and SACC workers are feeling. Clients also are being left to struggle alone through some very tough situations and decisions. Many social workers describe their clients' hard situations:

> Oprah: I'm certainly seeing more women in acute homeless situations, as a result of perhaps a sexual assault that's made following up on certain things or decision-making perhaps difficult without those other supports. I certainly see women making choices about their children and I'm not sure they would be making them if they weren't forced to do that by those budget cuts. Getting the children over to the partners that they don't feel safe about doing, putting children in care that they really don't want to be putting in care [Children's Aid Society or foster care] but they don't feel that they are able to cope.

In the near future it is even possible that people going to hospitals without their health care card on them will be refused service ("No card, no care" 1998). Is it possible that women arriving at the hospital to be cared for after they been violated (but who have no obvious physical injury) will be told to go home and get their health card? Tragically, women may feel so disentitled that they do not even reach out for help. They may give up on themselves. These women who do not contact a helping agency or the police may create the inaccurate impression that services are no longer required.

> Faith: The reality is that there are more barriers than open doors, that just serves to reinforce that hopelessness and powerlessness. I know that there have been less reports [of sexual abuse] the police have even said so. They [the police] had this huge, pat-themselves-on-the-shoulder day, when you know so many less reports regarding sexual assault. No doubt! I believe that some of that has to do with the fact that women don't or can't access legal aid as easily as they used to be able to. Five years ago and even then it was hard enough to access services [like welfare, housing, etc.] and we should have been looking at increasing legal aid support services and the opposite has happened. So with these barriers posing tremendous amounts of stress and hopelessness in women who are trying to heal their lives, they often feel even more overwhelmed. And this serves to paralyze their process [of reaching out for help]. How can they stop themselves from

feeling hopeless and powerless when things around them seem to be shutting down?

The formally constructed statistical profiles of what exists in women's lives and the *truths* of women's lives may be different. Within hospitals, social service agencies and other helping contexts many women are having to wait longer periods of time for supportive counselling. One SACC, for example, has had waiting lists of between eighteen and twenty-two months. These waiting periods between first contact and access to individual counselling have remained this high in this one agency for the last five years. The waiting periods tend to be higher for adult clients who are survivors of childhood sexual abuse or survivors who are not in their "acute" phase of healing.

Brief Solution Focused (BSF) Therapy

A fourth change (and in my opinion, a dangerous one) that is related to the previous three changes (changes for social workers, clients, the wider community) is that Brief Solution Focused (BSF) approaches to therapy are becoming more popular (some people have referred to this approach as "drive-through McTherapy"). In contrast to the opinion of one SAT worker who actively refused to be interviewed, I believe (as did the eighteen women who consented to be interviewed) that the therapeutic approaches advocated and practised in an organization are unavoidably linked to funding realities. To my clinical social worker's ear the one refusing interviewee's voice suggested she felt fear. My sense of what motivated her refusal to be interviewed was that she might have been afraid for her agency's wellbeing and/or for her own promotion possibilities or employment. She said she felt that restructuring and cutbacks in services were unrelated to therapeutic approaches to the care of women victims/survivors.

In my opinion BSF is the perfect ideology to rationalize budget cuts. BSF and downsizing are profoundly related to each other. Here, Mary Ann, an experienced SACC worker explicitly states the connection:

> The meaning for me is that most of the funding that both our services [SACCs and SATs] have had is for crisis services so we've had to institute approaches like BSF therapy because we can't have clients stay in our programs indefinitely. And rape crisis centres have had way more flexibility in the kinds of programs that we offer in that there is group and that we have done some long-term [counselling]. The Solicitor General doesn't know the difference between "crisis" and "long-term." Many women's centres are using their dollars to do long-term as well. We get our

centre's special funding for the long-term [counselling that we do] from Community and Social Services and Health and everybody always asks me how we got it. I'm not really sure how we did it but we did it.

Mary Ann sees the potential for resistance to BSF approaches only in that her primary funder has not realized how other funders and programs are now impelling women to accept less than they deserve.

BSF cannot be fully described here (but please read: Cade and O'Hanlon 1993, Epstein 1992, Furman and Ahola 1992, Guldner 1995, Miller et al. 1996, O'Hanlon and O'Hanlon 1991, Weiner-Davis 1995), but because this therapeutic approach minimizes the significance of the past and because it has no sociological or political analysis, it can be seen as the opposite to a feminist anti-racist approach (which examines herstorical and structural causes for women's oppression and contextualizes women's lives). Evelyn Wolf,[7] a social worker in a SACC program in my community told me this about BSF,

> Many First Nations women experience their pain as spread through their whole lives. It is not just the pain of sexual assault. They may have learned to contain that pain but it is the grief of their whole lives and their whole context that they want to talk about. They struggle with all of that.

BSF, when applied in its pure form, only allows for the one issue to be discussed for one hour, once a week, for ten or twelve weeks. Another First Nations woman who teaches in a university social work program, Barb Waterfall,[8] does not support BSF. She said, "Do you honestly believe that BSF therapy is going to undo five hundred years of damage!"

Mental health care providers in many SATs and even some SACCs have been moving (and are being pushed) more and more towards a BSF approach to counselling. BSF is time-limited, single-problem focused, does not recognize the meaning of historic/herstoric factors and can be seen to have a neoconservative agenda. With a BSF approach, women are being abandoned without the healing care they deserve—and potentially they are blamed when they cannot "succeed" and complete their recovery by the conclusion of their budgeted sessions. Further, social workers may feel blamed also when they cannot, in the system's view, cure their clients in the allocated ten or twelve sessions.

Each emotional wound a woman experiences may link to the other wounds in her life. The wellbeing of her body links to the wellbeing of her spirit and her realization of her full intellectual capacities. Each woman is more than the sum total of her body, spirit and mind parts. As I described at the beginning of this chapter, my own healing journey continues. Many healing circles, groups and more than 250 hours of individual therapy over twenty years have forwarded me but not necessarily solidly healed up every wound and weakness. Cutting a woman off from therapeutic support when she still feels she needs this kind of body-spirit-mind care may not only insult her but it may be experienced by her as yet another act of aggression, violation and/or abandonment. Some of the techniques or ideas within BSF are appropriate with some women for a time. My belief in women victims/survivors' common sense suggests that women will not attend therapy sessions unless they are benefitting from them. Social workers, also, would not encourage therapeutic relationships if the women clients were feeling strong and focused.

The Maguire Report[9]

> Susan [a SAT worker]: Nobody really knew what the implications of the Maguire Report would be. I think people got nervous and scared and put their heads together and got mad about it.... People aren't talking to each other, and may not be talking to each other even more, or talking to each other less because there's some threat to their programs. The split is settled back into place again. People aren't talking to each other ... something that was being thrown about [within the Maguire Report] was the amalgamation of SATs and SACCs. That [recommendation] has not resulted in very positive relationships, you know, between the two groups. So if there was some initial putting our heads together, and there was, absolutely [some putting of heads together] I think that's kind of died down a lot. People are back in their own corners and very much protecting their own territory.

The Maguire Report could be thought of as wanting to create a one-stop shopping centre approach to women's services. It could be thought of as wanting to create a monoculture—only one growing life-form on the terrain—and we know how vulnerable to one type of predator a monoculture is. When the Maguire Report was released in 1996, I co-organized a local protest to demand that its recommendations not be implemented. Many other individuals and communities also organized protests and wrote long reports back to the provincial government (Aikens 1996, Family Service Centre of Ottawa-Carleton 1997, Ottawa-Carleton Community Coalition 1997, London Sexual Assault Centre 1997). Much material was produced by women activists and social workers challenging the Maguire Report (Aikens 1996, Family Service

Centre of Ottawa-Carleton 1997, London Sexual Assault Centre 1997).

Certainly the SAT and SACC workers (with one exception) shared my own deep concerns. Note the concerns and anger about the Maguire Report that Mary Ann, a SACC social worker expresses:

> Totally [the Report suggested that feminist/women social service providers have no knowledge or expertise] all the way through the Maguire Report they kept quoting women and it's [the quotes are] from a twisted [perspective] and that's what angered me. There are abused women that used services generally that, and they [the report's authors] twisted their words and the same they were talking about all the victim assistance and witness assistance services [which are varied and complex]. There's this sexist assumption that autonomous women's groups are a bunch of financial idiots and we can't manage. We're under far more scrutiny than any other service or other services. I could go on about that for hours.

If this monoculture or one-stop shopping mall of services were created within a hospital context (and it most likely would be within a hospital context), then it could be controlled by a well-defined pre-existing administration which has a certain worldview. These new monoculture/malls would have little control or ability to resist. Presently SAT coordinators themselves have little control. They have marginal control within the walls of their small offices: but decisions about how large those offices will be, who will work there, how long they will work there, what they will be able to say when they interact with the wider community and so on is controlled by someone above and outside of the SAT programs. Even the advisory boards, which are supposed to give guidance to SAT programs and advocate for their rights within hospitals, are relatively powerless.

Some SATs have had their workers' hours cut and some have taken hours of SAT time and "farmed out" their social workers to other programs. SAT program activists clearly do not want to receive funding at the expense of other women's services funding. At the same time, most of these SAT program workers realize that the present climate disallows the government to expand funding in both directions. Therefore, it follows that the expansion of one stream of programs will probably mean an eventual downsizing of the other.

Another aspect of the Maguire report that insulted SAT and SACC specialists was that the government was suggesting we are not deeply informed, effective, creative, dynamic workers. They suggested we have historically had too many resources at our disposal and we were too casual with how we invested these human and material resources. On the contrary, we have always been devoted to doing the best job possible for our clients. We have always been running these organizations on a shoe string. We have always been doing more with less—in fact *we have always been doing more and more and more with less!*

Another insult to our integrity as professionals and caring activists that the Maguire report suggested was that we deliberately create dependency situations. The report inferred that we create "make work" relationships with our clients and that they (the funders) would like to come and teach us how to be more effective in our role as healers of women who have been abused and victimized.

The Maguire Report inspired some practitioners to work more closely together, at least for a short time. Largely, we were united in our disenchantment and rage. The implementation of aspects of the Maguire report still lurks on the horizon. The Maguire Report moves us closer to an American system of care that offers minimal choices for those using public services and more depthful resources and supports for those who can afford to pay for private-practice counselling (and legal advice, housing and so on).

The Future of SATs and SACCs and Care for Women

Tragically, many of the women I interviewed feel that the future will not unfold in the ways they would prefer. Some SAT and SACC workers do seem to be on the edge of admitting defeat. Workers in both SATs and SACCs feel worn down, and they feel that inevitably and eventually there will be a one-stop shopping mall version of services and it will be housed within a hospital context.

SACCs have been around for years and the feminist movement has been around for decades, so we have accumulated a lot of experience and wisdom about how to do resistance. This whole situation is not new. We have been here before.

> Maya: It's important that we not just see ourselves as victims within these organizations. That we not just feel that we're all just a product of budget cutbacks and that's all we will ever be. I think that would be our biggest mistake, if we sat back and said, not necessarily passively, but not that it doesn't actually alter our organization, it does. Realistically it does [if we have less resources]. To be conscious of how it does, to be strategic at the same time and say: "what are we going to do about this?" Are we going to just be victims to cutbacks? If these organizations like

SACC … could start within the climate that it started. It was a time of upheaval the seventies where everything was being questioned. If it could be established in the first place, when nothing existed before it, then we still have something worth fighting for now. We still have to celebrate what we have left and work from there. So I think that's one strategy that is really important.

As Maya says, we can chose to celebrate what we still have left. We have our feminist knowledge; we have all of these SAT and SACC programs still doing the best they can; and we have the possibility for resistance. SAT and SACC workers could unite more effectively if they / we came together and focused on commonalities rather than on differences. Some of our programs have been dissolving, some of us have felt divided (within our own agencies and networks, and across agencies and networks) and all of this is distressing. At the same time we do have access to information, an empowering ideology, potential support from and for each other, and we have been through more struggles with less resources in the past. There is nothing that neoconservative regimes can tell us about surviving that we don't already know. They may tempt us to consider surrender. Then we remember our visions and land on our feet again ready for the next challenge. Eighteen women social workers in SATs and SACCs still have offices, programs, phones to answer, work to do. They, and many more like them, have not admitted defeat. Their doors are still open and they are still providing services for women. Largely as a result of support from women like these SAT and SACC workers, I am still here. I have a computer set up in my new home. Today I have excellent health. I have written this chapter. None of us have admitted defeat. In spite of government efforts to dissolve our programs, divide us from each other (and from our visions)—in spite of the distress encountered in my professional and personal life I try not to give up on the possibility of minor daily miracles.

The patterns of vulnerable women being expected to aggressively seek out and pay for their own nurturance and healing are expanding. The few services that do remain are often delivered only to those most in crisis and delivered conditionally. These trends towards care services being provided more rapidly and extensively for those who can afford to pay for them are intensifying. Healing from sexual violation is always a process involving the whole body-spirit-mind. I am still a work-in-progress. I am not uncommon in the rhythm or pacing of my healing journey. I am not a failure. I am not an "unmotivated" client or a "resistant" client. Neither am I someone who is becoming "dependent." The following poem is disturbing but truthful. Writing this chapter dredged up pain.

My Life Now Whole?

I repulse from this admission.
so much effort-full purging's
been done to full-fill the opposite
& yet he exists there on the sludgy edge
of a dream, a thought,
a name, a place,
or a sentence I want to speak.
he remains a vague vulture-presence;
half my blood line & bone structure
are from him & more than half my scars.
as I pirate & acheologize
my whole life for treasures he swoops.
his talons puncture through a muscle or vein
of who I am / becoming;
as I experiment & alchemize
for possibilities he preys
& his beak sinks into a joint or organ
of who I am / becoming.
I don't talk about these assaults
from the shadow-sticky
past unjustly often
it seems I am knowing
his existence continues
in my present & DNA;
I did not ask for this hurt.
25 years later
250 therapy hours later,
a Ph.D., an ideology
& multiple revolutions later
an unblinking instant of eye contact
with a blue-eyed blond-haired stranger,
in a mall, for example,
can return me to under
his horrible touch.

Notes

1. I particularly want to thank Ginette Demers (my research assistant); Tina Lacoste, Yolanda Coppolina, Marnina Gonick, Morgan Gardner, Melanie Robitaille, Sandra Edwards (my sisters / comrades / friends); Irma Howe (my therapist); Paulette Dahl, Carol Trepanier and Sally Power (from the creative

writing circle); Robert Kominar (an intellectual supporter and peer) and with rivers of affection, Diana Gustafson (my patient Goddess of Editing).

2. I especially want to thank Dr. Roxana Ng for the extensive work she has done in this area and for the depth of effort she made to bring me forward in my understandings of health and illness and my own body. She taught a variety of courses that linked with this theme (the multiple layerings and connections between body-spirit-mind) and I was fortunate enough to be a student in her classes from 1992 to 1996.

3. Throughout this chapter I use the term "social worker" to identify the professional backgrounds of the women interviewed but some of the women may define themselves as counsellors or nurses who have training in social work. The term "social worker" is about to become a very specific label to be used only by those who are licensed to practice. The letter of introduction and question format that were sent to all of the SAT and SACC programs specifically requested that I interview social workers in these programs. I did not specifically ask the formal academic qualifications of each interviewee. Some women did communicate specifics but to identify those specifics here would breech their confidentiality so I have been deliberately vague. I am a certified social worker myself and I teach in a university level social work program.

4. I thank Laurentian University's Research Funds for contributing to the transcription costs for these interviews. I thank Latisha Dionne, Anne Biggar and Cathy Jewel for their transcription and research work.

5. Doris Grinspun in this volume examines the shift from the carative-curative paradigm to the business paradigm.

6. Lum and Williams in this volume examine how government legislation and health system restructuring is exacerbating tensions among care provider groups.

7. Evelyn Wolf has been a social worker in our Sexual Assault Crisis Centre in Sudbury for five years. I thank her for sharing her insights with me on this topic and others on many other occasions.

8. Barb Waterfall took up this topic extensively in her workshop titled, "Culture Appropriate Service Responses and Native Human Services" at the Native Women and Disabilities Conference held on May 20, 1999, at the Holiday Inn in Sudbury, Ontario. Her thoughtful exploration of First Nations women's needs made vividly clear that budget cutbacks are having a substantively destructive impact on many First Nations women's lives.

9. This report is commonly referred to among activists and social workers in this field as the Maguire Report but the document itself has no authorship on it.

8

The New Wageless Worker: Volunteering and Market-Guided Health Care Reform

Elizabeth Esteves

Introduction

The recent process of health care reform in Canada has received increasing scholarly attention. Within a hospital context, studies have focused on the impact of these reforms on the paid providers of health care services and/or their recipients and families (Armstrong et al. 1993, Armstrong et al. 1997). Similar attention has not been given to the impact of reform on hospital volunteers whose unpaid health care services historically have been provided predominantly by women.

This chapter considers the impact of health care reform on the caring work of such volunteers. I argue that hospital volunteer work is fundamentally linked to market guided health care reform and that this changes the social relations constituting volunteer work. Volunteers, many of whom are women, are being transformed into wageless workers with less control over their caring work. I demonstrate that market-driven health care reform has transformed all work, paid and volunteer, in a process which limits caring and instead emphasizes task-based work. Also, it appears that younger volunteers are beginning to dominate volunteer membership, as they are perceived to be able to perform more task-based, unpaid labour. Older women, those with the greatest volunteer experience, once brought to hospitals the caring component traditionally centred in volunteer activity. But today they are less valued for this contribution and as a consequence, many have resigned.

This examination of organized hospital volunteer activity in the existing context of health care reform is based on my research in progress at a major metropolitan hospital in Ontario. Given the lack of research on hospital volunteer work and the incomplete nature of research at the time of writing, the intent here is not to present conclusions but rather to illuminate key issues and illustrate them with data gathered from participant observation during one year's anthropological fieldwork. This examination presents realities encountered in fieldwork. By situating such realities in the historical and contemporary contexts in which they are embedded, I begin to explore some of the social relations which serve to govern volunteer work.

At the time my fieldwork began, January 1998, people who volunteered at City Hospital[1] did so within a structured volunteer department and/or auxiliary organization, which were products of a particular social and historical process that originated at the turn of the century. This process was tied to the history of the hospital and ultimately to the historical development of health care in Canada. The activities performed by these volunteers are part of an historical tradition of allocating certain work to individuals specifically organized for its performance. They provide an example of the historically gendered allocation of volunteer work, of certain types of caring labour, to women. This delegation of responsibility to volunteers accords with a wider social valorization of voluntary participation. Unfortunately, the social and cultural construction of volunteering in Canada, in national and regional contexts, has received very minimal scholarly attention.

Scholarly study of the voluntary sector has tended to focus on volunteering on a macro level. Increasingly sophisticated statistical surveys have measured the magnitude of the nation's voluntary sector, of which *The National Survey of Giving, Volunteering and Participation* (NSGVP), a large-scale survey even by international standards, is the most recent example. According to the NSGVP, 31.4 percent of the population aged fifteen and over volunteered for a non-profit organization in the period November 1, 1996 to October 31, 1997 (Statistics Canada 1997a). This figure, representing 7.5 million Canadians, is indicative of the widespread participation of Canadians in voluntary organizations. These statistical surveys are useful in the data they yield regarding the scope and scale of voluntary participation, but they are limited in their examination of transformations within the voluntary sector.

Some theoretically oriented literature examines the historical and contemporary relationship between voluntary and state sectors. Of particular relevance to this discussion are the works of Mishra, Laws and Harding (1988), Rekart (1993) and Valverde (1995). Their investigations, which consider specific contexts of voluntary participation within the voluntary sector, yield data which large-scale surveys are unable to provide. Each examines the complex relationship between the voluntary non-profit sector and the state in the provision of social services.

Mishra et al. (1988) investigated privatization as part of Ontario's social policy under a Conservative government' in power until 1985. These scholars argued that conservative ideology played a significant role in the complex process of the privatization of social services. The

Ontario Progressive Conservative party (re-elected to power at the time of this writing) continues to assert an ideological commitment to privatization. The contemporary effects of privatization were also the focus of Rekart's (1993) work. Her examination of the privatization of social service delivery in British Columbia demonstrated the increased dependency of voluntary organizations on the state and illuminated the relationship between the voluntary sector and the state in a contemporary context. Valverde's historical examination of a mixed economy of social service delivery challenged the opposition of state and civil realms and pointed instead to a "complex web of relationships linking the two supposedly separate realms" (1995: 34).

Collectively, these works provide the theoretical framework for my examination of volunteering at City General Hospital. This chapter demonstrates the inter-connectivity of the voluntary sector and the state sector, and the ways that volunteer services in one hospital context are being transformed by health care restructuring.

My exploration of the work of hospital volunteers in one Canadian hospital proceeds in three sections. The first section presents the historical development of volunteer work at City General Hospital. This serves to introduce volunteering in this location and to stress that contemporary volunteering is a product of a specific historical process. The second section explores the transformation of volunteering in light of current health care reform. It details changes in volunteering at both organizational and performance levels. In the third section, I argue that market-driven reform initiatives are transforming volunteering and constructing volunteers as wageless workers. I begin with a brief description of the methodology.

Methodology

The data presented here are the result of ethnographic research in a major metropolitan hospital in Ontario initiated in January 1998. Primary data were gathered both from participant observation and archival research. In addition to observing volunteers as they carried out their volunteering and engaging in informal discussion with volunteers, I conducted interviews and attended meetings relating to volunteering both inside and outside the hospital. Forty semi-structured interviews with volunteers were completed at the time of writing. Non-volunteer hospital staff were also interviewed.

In order to discover the history of organized volunteering, I researched, with the permission of the Auxiliary, the loosely organized material contained in the archives of the Auxiliary of City General

Hospital. These archives consisted mainly of the minutes of the committee meetings of the hospital's volunteer organization, dating from 1911. Early records consisted of minute books while later material was organized yearly into binders. Each binder also included reports of other official meetings, such as annual meetings. During the time I began researching the archives until the time of this writing, the archives, which had been the private domain of the Auxiliary, became the property of City Hospital and are now being processed by the hospital.

The historical examination in the first section of this chapter draws extensively on archival data and every effort is made to fully cite the sources. These data, while providing some information on the organization's structure and activity, focus on the activities of the organization's executive body. The greater visibility of the leadership body in archival material and the difficulties this generates is acknowledged by historians of women's organizations (Prentice 1985). In order to address the limitations of archival material, I also draw on the experiences of volunteers. During the course of research, I interviewed women with a considerable history of volunteer work at City General Hospital. Through these various practices undertaken in ethnographic research, I was able to conduct in-depth analysis of volunteering in this local context. Drawing on these various resources, I examine the transformations in volunteering at City General Hospital.

The Historical Development of Organized Volunteer Participation

Organized volunteering at City General Hospital began as a semi-autonomous association of white, middle-class, Protestant women founded in 1911 and developed over time into the contemporary context of volunteer participation directly and exclusively controlled by the hospital's Volunteer Department. In this section I show how volunteering at City General Hospital not only responded to, but was a part of, connected processes that involved the transformation of gender relations and the rise of the welfare state.

Gender and Volunteering

Volunteering is largely the work of women, both in terms of its symbolic construction and material performance; therefore an analysis of gender relations in the development of volunteering at City General Hospital is of key importance. City General Hospital's volunteer organization began in 1911 with fourteen volunteers and for over fifty years was exclusively composed of women. While membership expanded to include men in the mid-1960s, volunteer activity continues to be predominantly performed by women. While white, middle-class women founded and dominated most of the history of organized volunteer work at City General Hospital, this, too, has changed in recent years.

The formation of the Ladies Committee in 1911 was typical of urban[2] pre-welfare-state responses to poverty in Ontario. In one of the few examinations of the history of Canadian women's association activity, Brandt (1985) notes the formation in the 1880s and 1890s of organizations devoted to addressing Canadian social problems resulting from industrialization and urbanization. Typically, these associations were formed by a membership of English Protestant middle-class women. Although Auxiliary archives do not provide explicit data on the membership of the Ladies' Committee, it is, however, possible to infer that the founding members of the Committee were white, Protestant and drawn from the upper and middle classes. This homogeneous group of women raised funds through garden parties and teas and were able to secure the presence of prominent political figures such as the lieutenant governor at their annual meetings. Thus, the work of social reform performed by the volunteer association at City General Hospital was linked with women of a particular class, age and race.

The work of social reform undertaken by the Ladies' Committee was also linked with changing female gender roles and grounded in the essentialist notions of femininity of the first wave of feminism in Canada. By engaging in the public work of social welfare these women confronted the state. As advocates of health care reform, for example, they wrote letters to municipal officials, usually petitioning the mayor directly (Minutes of the Regular Monthly Meeting, March 6, 1913, City Hospital Auxiliary Archives). Additional historical sources point to the participation of members of the Committee in the women's movement. Roberts notes that they were central figures in "the first self-conscious generation of women activists in Canadian history" (1979: 45). The committee's approach to social welfare was consistent with the ideology, namely maternal feminism, that governed the activities of many women reformers at the time. Kealey defines maternal feminism as,

> The conviction that women's special role as mother gives her the duty and the right to participate in the public sphere. It is not her position as wife that qualifies her for the task of reform, but the special nurturing qualities which are common to all women. (1979: 7–8)

In 1917, the hospital's superintendent thanked the "ladies who, through their nurturing efforts, support" social service endeavours (Annual Meeting, Social Service Department, City General Hospital, January 9, 1917, City Hospital Auxiliary Archives). The social reform work of women challenged traditional notions of the proper sphere of engage- ment for the upper- and middle-class woman (Roberts 1979: 19) while retaining and building upon the essentialist notions of women's activities as caring and nurturing. The gender link between women and volunteer work continued throughout the history of organized volunteering at City General Hospital, yet in a process that responded to women's changing roles.

The most significant transformation in gender relations to affect voluntary participation occurred following the second wave of feminism with the entry of increasing numbers of middle-class women into the workforce. Jill, eighty years old at the time I interviewed her, had volunteered at City General Hospital for forty-eight years. She quit her work as a hospital lab technician and began volunteering after her marriage to a City General Hospital doctor. Jill explained her decision saying, "Socially it was the thing to do. Women didn't work in those days, they were expected to volunteer, to do something." Jill's decision to cease paid employment upon marriage and begin volunteering was typical of women who began their volunteering at City General Hospital between 1950 and 1970.

Increases in women's labour force participation transformed the nature of women's volunteering and volunteer membership at City General Hospital. Student volunteers began to account for an increasing portion of volunteers with the inception of a female youth volunteer program in the 1960s. Falling membership became a significant concern, as evidenced by the many Auxiliary membership drives during the 1970s and 1980s. Men were recruited in the 1970s and male membership was recognized by the renaming of the volunteer organization in 1977. This change is marked in this discussion by the fictitious title Auxiliary of City General Hospital, which replaces Women's Auxiliary of City General Hospital. Older individuals also began to account for an increasing number of volunteers, specifically in the Auxiliary. Membership diversi- fied in terms of race, religion and class as well. The reasons for these various aspects of diversification are complex, elusive and worthy of further exploration. I limit the discussion here to the gender-related transformations.

Phillips and Phillips point to a revolution in married women's labour force participation, especially with respect to women in their mid- twenties (1983: 37). Armstrong and Armstrong (1984: Table 20) note that in 1941 less than 5 percent of married women participated in the labour market while in 1981 this figure had risen to more than 50 percent. The career volunteer also vanished. When women married, they were not leaving the paid sector to join the voluntary sector. My fieldwork reveals that by the 1990s women were becoming volunteers in response to retirement, joining the organization after their labour force participation. In addition to these gender-related transformations, volunteering at City General Hospital was also influenced by the development of the welfare state.

Volunteering and the State

When the Ladies' Committee formed, the Advisory Board of the City General Hospital appointed the committee as "voluntary helpers" for a social service nurse (City General Hospital Minutes of Medical Advisory Board 1910–1911, Cases from Social Service Department, October 11, 1911, City Hospital Auxiliary Archives). In addition to raising money for the salary of a social service nurse, the committee members also organized and provided relief to the needy by visiting patients in the hospital wards and in patients' homes. At its origin, the work of this committee had two dimensions: financial responsibility for a social service nurse and the practical work of patient care. Through the course of its history its contribution, both financial and practical, in the form of voluntary patient care work, increased and diversified in scope.

This organization of fourteen women volunteers played a key role in funding and administering what would gradually become a hospital department devoted to social services. The Social Service Department was composed of the superintendent of the hospital, nurses and volunteers. In 1921, the Social Service Department reorganized and the volunteer association was renamed. The Ladies' Committee became the Social Service Association. It was composed of "active" members, who assisted with the work of the Department, and "sustaining" members, who supported the Association financially. This separation of membership into active and sustaining members continued throughout history. The objectives of the Social Services Department and its Association were outlined in the department constitution:

> To assist the medical profession in all branches of preventive medicine by cooperation in the Hospital, the Out-Patients Department and in the homes of the patients. To endeavour to effect family rehabilitation and to cooperate with all charitable organizations engaged in similar work by interpreting the medical viewpoint, physical, mental and moral that will enable them to deal intelligently with the social problems of the families. (Constitution of the Social Service Department of the City General Hospital. City Hospital Auxiliary Archives)

City General Hospital's voluntary social service organization was a characteristic outgrowth of a particular type of pre-welfare-state initiative to address the needs of the poor in Canada. Approaches to poverty varied regionally across Canada. In their historical examination of the beginnings of the welfare state in Canada, Moscovitch and Dover (1987) outlined three organized practices toward social welfare in pre-confederation Canada. In the Maritimes, relief was guided by English poor laws. In Quebec, welfare organizations were primarily church run. Ontario, which did not adopt so-called "poor laws," evolved a system of poor relief, which linked private and public sectors. In this mixed economy of social services, voluntary charitable organizations played a key role.

The evolution of Ontario's mixed economy of social service delivery can be traced to the ideal of an independent civil society. Valverde's (1995) analysis of the development of government funding and the inspection of charities in Ontario illustrates that the emergence of a mixed economy system is related to a prominent ideal in the development of Ontario. Valverde explains how the mythical "image of a self-sufficient civil society of hardy pioneers and charitable philanthropists" (1995: 43) existed alongside a system of private and public cooperation in social welfare. This construction continues throughout Ontario's history. City General Hospital's voluntary organization reflected the partnership between public and private sectors in addressing social welfare in Ontario.

The development of organized volunteering at City General Hospital was also related to the state's evolving approach to social welfare. Originating as a self-financed association directing and funding social service programs, this association gradually began to expand its activities and to receive public funding, channelled through the hospital. In the 1930s and 1940s, it held a prominent role in managing social programs and developing social services. By the 1950s, its social service role had diminished and City General Hospital's organization of volunteers decided to expand the scope of their activities to address the needs of patients in other hospital departments

Moscovitch and Dover (1987) trace the development of the welfare state and identify three periods: "Reluctant Welfarism 1891–1940"; "The Establishment of a Welfare State 1941–1974"; and "The Appearance of Fiscal Crisis 1974–78." The transformation in volunteering at City General Hospital may be understood using these periods while attentive to the mixed economy nature of social service delivery in Ontario.

The formation of Canada marked increased state involvement in social welfare, but the period of 1891–1940 was one of reluctant government spending on social welfare. In the early years of this period, Moscovitch and Dover note that the establishment of a wide range of political and social movements characterized by social ferment resulted in only minor changes in state social expenditure (1987: 20). They insist that relief was largely a private undertaking achieved through "so-called scientific philanthropy and the more systematic organization of charity" (20). Volunteer organizations dedicated to social relief, such as the self-financed Ladies' Committee of 1911, played a key role during this period of limited state spending in social welfare. By the 1920s the Social Service Association had joined with local charity organizations, depending on them, not the state, to finance their increasing social service efforts. Moscovitch and Dover argue that even though state involvement in social welfare expanded during the period, the state was devoted to strengthening Canadian capitalism (25) and social expenditure remained relatively insignificant until the 1930s. The depression of the 1930s forced the expansion of social expenditures, establishing the principle of major state involvement in welfare (38).

The period referred to by Moscovitch and Dover (1987) as the "Establishment of a Welfare State 1941–1974" was characterized by a marked change in the state's response to social welfare. The expansion in state expenditure led gradually to a substantial number of social reform programs. Social expenditures, for example, on social welfare, health and education, grew from 4 percent of the Gross National Product in 1946 to 15 percent by the mid-1970s. The state's new approach to social welfare is evident in the area of health. The *Hospital Insurance and Diagnostic Services Act* in 1958 put in place national legislation to cover the cost of hospital care for all Canadians. Hospital insurance was followed by comprehensive and universal health insurance with the establishment in 1966 of the federal and provincial *Medical Care Insurance Act*. These developments transformed Canadian health care. They reshaped the role of hospitals as major components in the delivery of health care and in so doing affected related volunteer organizations.

During this period, City General Hospital's volunteer organization assumed a new role in social welfare provision as it entered into a partnership with the hospital and the Welfare Council. This new status involved establishing and improving social service provision and developing student training in social services (Report to the Finance Committee, The Social Service Association of the City General Hospital, January 19, 1953, City Hospital Auxiliary Archives). Gradually, the hospital assumed some of the financial burdens of the Association. In the 1940s, it began to pay the salaries of some of the Social Service Department workers. In 1949, the hospital took advantage of increased state funding to apply for federal health funds for the Social Service Department. Demands for provisioning social service work soon outstripped the Association's possibilities. In 1953, the hospital assumed complete responsibility both administratively and financially for its social services endeavours (Annual Meeting, The Social Service Association of the City General Hospital, January 26, 1954, Report of the President, p. 3, City Hospital Auxiliary Archives).

This organization of volunteers entered into another phase in its existence. Relieved of its social service responsibilities, the Association directed its fundraising efforts and patient care work to a variety of hospital departments and patient needs. This shift was marked by a name change in 1955 as the Social Service Association became the more expansive Women's Auxiliary of City General Hospital. In 1956, 323 of the Auxiliary's 416 members actively volunteered their time in the hospital, with the remaining inactive members supporting the work of the Auxiliary financially (Annual Meeting, The Woman's Auxiliary of the City General Hospital, January 31, 1956. City Hospital Auxiliary Archives). These auxillians visited patients and served as clinical aids, interpreters, receptionists, hairdressers and librarians. They also organized sewing committees and seasonal festivities, such as Christmas parties. Volunteers also administered gift shops which served as key sources of funding. Within a decade, the scope of voluntary effort in the hospital increased substantially. Just as the hospital assumed the responsibilities of the Association's social service work, in time, it would assume the increasing volunteer work organized and performed by auxillians.

In 1967, City General Hospital administrators created the Department of Volunteers, which together with the Auxiliary, administered the activities of volunteers. The hospital-appointed Director of Volunteers worked with the Auxiliary to provide, facilitate and extend patient care delivered in the hospital by volunteers. The partnership into which the hospital and the Auxiliary entered was ill-defined. The distribution of powers and responsibilities was unclear; yet this partnership in volunteering was successful for twenty years. In the intervening years the Auxiliary expanded its activities in response to the challenges posed by the next stage of the development of the welfare state.

Moscovitch and Dover (1987) identify the years 1974–1978 as a period of fiscal crisis marked by cuts in state funding of social services. These cuts affected the hospital's delivery of health care. The Auxiliary responded by strengthening its volunteer services and fundraising efforts. First mention of the effects of hospital budget cuts was made in documents of the Auxiliary's January 14, 1975, Executive Committee Meeting. The minutes of this meeting note the hospital's request to the Auxiliary for volunteers to fill positions left vacant by staff cuts. In the March 9, 1976, Executive Committee Meeting, Auxiliary leadership considered supplying facial tissue in patient rooms because it was no longer provided by the hospital due to budget cuts.

The Auxiliary's fundraising efforts expanded throughout the 1980s in an attempt to address the hospital's increased requests for funding. These requests amounted to hundreds of thousands of dollars in one fiscal year (Minutes of the Executive Committee Meeting, Auxiliary of the City General Hospital, May 31 1983, City Hospital Auxiliary Archives). The Auxiliary was not able to undertake such major fundraising efforts. Its Long Range Planning Committee recommended on April 20, 1985, that large-scale funding projects should be left to the hospital's Foundation (an association dedicated exclusively to hospital fundraising). While the Auxiliary continued to raise modest amounts of funds for the hospital, it decided to focus its efforts on the practical work of patient care.

The history of organized volunteer participation reveals various transformations in volunteering with respect to gender and the state. Originally, the exclusive preserve of White English, upper- and middle-class women, volunteer membership responded to wider developments in gender relations. Material changes in the volunteer work accompanied the diversification in membership composition. Volunteer activity also responded to the changing role of the hospital in the development of Canadian health care. Organized volunteer participation continues to undergo transformations in response to contemporary health care reform.

Contemporary Changes in Organized Volunteer Participation

The most fundamental changes in the organization of volunteering in the hospital occurred in the 1990s, especially in 1998. During the course of my research, the City General Hospital Auxiliary experienced a merger and then a dissolution. The hospital's Volunteer Department became the only structure organizing and controlling all aspects of volunteering within the hospital. This subsection describes the contemporary organization of volunteering.

At the onset of my research, City General Hospital volunteers included both Volunteer Department volunteers and Auxiliary volunteers. As of January 1998, total membership of the Auxiliary of City General Hospital was 529 (City Hospital Auxiliary 1998a: 22). Based on my observations, women continued to dominate as volunteers. The composition of volunteer membership was also significantly marked by age. The majority of volunteers were largely either student volunteers in their late teens and twenties or retired volunteers aged fifty-five years and over, with older volunteers dominating the Auxiliary membership.

At the onset of 1998, two auxiliary organizations existed at two of the three hospital sites and were in the process of merging. City General and

City Western Hospitals, two of the three hospital sites composing City Hospital, each contained auxiliaries which were very similar. They shared a comparable process of historical development and were alike in their organization, composition and functioning. Efforts to merge the auxiliaries began with the merging of the two hospital sites but these efforts were resisted by auxiliary members. Interviews with auxiliary leaders in both of the organizations revealed that the merger was resisted because a newly merged organization would put an end to the distinctiveness that each auxiliary organization was felt to have held. Ultimately, auxiliary leadership decided to accept the hospital's requested merger plans, and the hospital agreed to delay the merger until the auxiliary of the Western Hospital site celebrated its one hundredth anniversary. By the spring of 1998 the unified City Hospital Auxiliary came into being. In general, auxillians that I interviewed were satisfied with the process of the merger and they held a positive outlook on the organization's future. Both the existence of the unified auxiliary and the positive outlook were, however, short lived.

By the fall of 1998, the City Hospital Auxiliary had ceased to exist. Within months of its unification the Auxiliary began a process of dissolution. Its president resigned in response to changes in the reporting structure of the Auxiliary and as a result of increased difficulties in dealings with hospital administration. The Volunteer Department assumed an increasingly active role in Auxiliary affairs, unprecedented in the history of its relationship with the Auxiliary. As conditions deteriorated both parties came into increasing conflict. Speaking on behalf of the Auxiliary, a leader within the organization explained after the dissolution, "We didn't like the interference in Auxiliary affairs, but we hoped that we could work something out."

As mentioned earlier, the archival material indicates that the distribution of powers between the Auxiliary and the Volunteer Department was not well defined. The Auxiliary had always enjoyed autonomy even though it was ultimately subject to the authority of the hospital's executive leadership. In the course of the history of organized volunteering at this hospital, the reporting structure of this semi-autonomous association had changed very minimally. In 1988, the Auxiliary reported to the hospital's president through his vice-president or the vice-president of nursing (City Hospital Auxiliary, Administrative Organizational Chart, revised March 1988, City Hospital Auxiliary Archives). In City General Hospital's Organizational Chart (1998a), the Auxiliary had become a division of Human Resources. While the Volunteer Department was listed as a separate division, also within Human Resources, the Auxiliary's activities became increasingly controlled by the Volunteer Department's administrator.

With the dissolution of the Auxiliary, the Volunteer Department became the only body controlling and developing volunteer programs in the hospital. The dissolution resulted in the departure of many auxillians. The Volunteer Department assumed some Auxiliary administered and staffed programs, such as the patient library. Auxiliary fundraising projects were discontinued with the exception of the lottery program. Between 1997 and 1999 the hospital's Volunteer Department grew considerably. At the time of this writing the Volunteer Department at City Hospital, a branch of Human Resources, is administered by a volunteer director aided by a senior secretary. Three site managers, each assisted by a secretary, report to the volunteer director. Two years prior, when City Hospital was composed of two, not three hospital sites, combined administrative staff totalled three individuals. The organization of volunteering has changed considerably at City General Hospital since the inception of the Ladies' Committee. The contemporary changes I outlined occurred within a particular climate characterized by health care reform, which is the focus of the next section.

Volunteering and Health Care Reform

This section focuses on the way in which market-driven health care reform is transforming volunteering alongside and in connection to the way in which it reshapes the work of paid hospital health care staff. Drawing on the work of scholars who have explored the impact of health care reform on paid health care work, this section begins with an outline of the context of health care reform. The reforms identified by these scholars are then considered in relation to the organization and performance of volunteering at City General Hospital at the time of my research.

A neoconservative agenda has resulted in market-driven health care reform. Armstrong and Armstrong argue that "the North American Free Trade Agreement has further consolidated the conservative agenda, based as it is on the understanding that free market principles will apply in all aspects of society" (1994a: 31). The running of health care like a business has become increasingly dominant within the health care sector.[3] The result is a significant impact on volunteering, given the relationship identified by Mishra et al. (1988), Rekart (1993) and Valverde (1995) between the volunteer sector and the state in providing social services.

Hospitals, as key components in the delivery of health care, have experienced the impact of the market on a variety of levels. Armstrong and Armstrong argue, "The pressure to cut costs, combined with the pervasive business philosophy, has been a major factor in the transformation of health care delivery" (1994a: 36). A privileging of market management within hospitals has occurred with a resulting increase in the power of management.

> The threat of transfer to private management firms, combined with significantly reduced budgets and a new ideology of efficiency defined in money terms, encouraged pubic sector managers to follow the practices developed for profit-making systems. Private and public, these managers have sought to rationalize the system, intensify labour, and increase control over workers. (36)

In Ontario, hospital mergers and closures have been a significant dimension of health care restructuring. Armstrong and Armstrong note that "like big business, hospital's and other health care services have been merging as a means of reducing costs and increasing control" (1994a: 36). City Hospital is a prime example of hospital merging practices. City Hospital is a composite of three geographically separate hospital sites. In addition, it has incorporated some of the services of a hospital forced to close under provincial directives. This mega hospital provides the new context in which volunteering occurs, a context characterized by a tightening of administrative control. These mergers have facilitated the application of corporate sector techniques aimed at rationalizing production and intensifying labour (38).

In her examination of the impact of reforms on nursing work, Armstrong et al. write, "Cutbacks have meant an intensification of labour, a reduction in jobs and a disciplining of workers" (1993: 40). The development of management techniques such as task-based formulas are also noted as part of an attempt by administrators of large urban hospital's to control workers (43). Cutbacks have increased the demands placed on nursing work, resulting in work which is more carefully monitored, with an emphasis on measurable tasks (45). Market management and the resulting mergers and reorganizations in paid health care labour have also had an effect on the organization and practice of volunteering. For instance, health care reforms have allowed City Hospital to increase its control over volunteering.

Mergers have been a technique used by hospital administrators to increase control over sectors within the hospital. Armstrong and Armstrong write, "In addition to negotiating mergers and combinations outside their institutions, health care managers have also been rationalizing and merging sectors within their institution" (1994a: 38). The merger of the auxiliaries in 1998 was connected to the hospital's response to legislated hospital reform initiatives which related to the tightening of control, financing, cost reduction and revenue generation. The merger represented the first step of the hospital's attempt to gain full control of volunteering and resulted in the loss of one of the two auxiliary seats on the hospital's Board of Trustees. While the seat continues to be associated with volunteering, it is now held through the hospital's Department of Volunteers, and is thus under hospital control.

In the creation of one auxiliary organization, the hospital was able to focus its attempt to control auxiliary activities by dealing with one single auxiliary governing body. Increased interference by hospital administrators in Auxiliary affairs and changes in the Auxiliary's reporting structure resulted in its dissolution. A senior member of the Auxiliary's leadership body recounted the repeated attempts by the Auxiliary to reach a compromise with the hospital and stated, "We could never get through. It had to be [name of the volunteer director's] way or [name of the hospital president's] way or the highway."

The demise of the Auxiliary also allowed the hospital to control the Auxiliary's principle revenue generating source, the gift shop. Two of the three hospital sites contained gift shops that sold a variety of merchandise, such as flowers, greeting cards and personal care products, to patients, visitors and hospital staff. Since their inception, the Auxiliary had maintained complete responsibility for administering and operating the shops, although revenues raised in the shops were turned over to the hospital. In 1998, the City General Hospital gift shop reported a profit of $135,000, more than half of the Auxiliary's $233,059 contribution to the hospital for that year (City Hospital 1998a: 14). Despite these profits, hospital administrators felt that the shops were not run efficiently and attempted to increase their control over the running of the shops. Even prior to the official dissolution of the Auxiliary, the administration hired consultants to increase the gift shops' profitability. The new gift shops will take their place alongside the many profit ventures, such as the coffee shop and pharmacies, dominating the entrances at the three hospital sites. These provide a physical document of the impact of the market in the hospital.

The assumption by the Volunteer Department of complete responsibility for volunteering within the hospital resulted in a concentration of power in the hands of hospital administrators. Prior to its demise the Auxiliary's organizational structure allowed for a distribution of power among volunteers. Auxiliary-elected volunteers led the organization and its development of programs and services. In accordance with the City Hospital Auxiliary Constitution, the Auxiliary was governed by an executive committee composed of officers, the immediate past president, the elected coordinators of services and four members-at-large (1998b: article III, section 2). Executive officers and members-at-large were elected annually by auxiliary members (article III, section 3), providing them a degree of power in the administration of volunteering. The Volunteer Department, in contrast, is part of the rigid bureaucratic structure characteristic of mega hospitals.

With volunteering organized exclusively within the hospital's Volunteer Department, administrators have increased their control over volunteer membership. As Armstrong and Armstrong (1994a) show, health care reform resulted in a corporate sector approach to delivering care in hospitals. This is evident in the recruitment of new volunteers. A prospective volunteer is given a seven-page application package, consisting of two reference check forms, in which applicants are asked to be evaluated on their reliability, flexibility and communicative, interpersonal and time management skills. Volunteers are also provided with an eighteen-page handbook outlining the guiding principles of the hospital and of the Volunteer Department (City Hospital, n.d.). This material informs volunteers of what is expected of them. It also provides an indication of the extent of control the hospital exerts over them. For example, the "Volunteer Code of Ethics" specifically forbids a volunteer to "speak on behalf of the organization or mention any affiliation with the hospital to the press or other public groups (unless written approval has been given by the Department of Public Affairs)" (5).

In addition to the transformation of the organizational structure and membership composition of volunteering in the hospital, the activities performed by volunteers also have been effected by health care reform. As Armstrong et al. (1993) found with nursing work, volunteers are experiencing in health care reform an intensification of certain aspects of their contribution and a minimization of others. Concerns have been raised by volunteers about their ability to provide care in a context in which they are called upon to perform an ever increasing number of task-based activities. A volunteer in one of the surgical waiting rooms noted how her volunteering had changed over time. "We used to be able to sit with distressed families, to get them coffee and to talk. We don't have time for that anymore. It's rush, rush, rush." She went on to outline the various tasks that were expected of her, tasks whose completion resulted in very little time for her to provide care. These findings are similar to those reported among paid health care workers. Armstrong et al. said of nursing work, "with the emphasis on measurable and visible tasks, there is little room for the caring work" (1993: 45).

Such an intensification of certain components of volunteers' activities is related in part to the relationship between paid and unpaid work in the hospital. Volunteers are assuming more work as a result of reductions in paid hospital staff and the loss of volunteers following the demise of the Auxiliary. In response to cuts in paid hospital staff, volunteers are assuming activities not previously undertaken. For example, volunteers comment on having to clean their work areas, previously maintained by paid housekeeping staff. Volunteers are also providing support services in various hospital departments. In the hospital's endoscopy unit, volunteer assistance is provided by three individuals, and many of their activities are essential to the unit's functioning. Rita, one of the endoscopy unit's paid hospital staff, explained how these volunteers assisted her by preparing patients for their medical procedures and by compiling the unit's statistical information.

Volunteers are aiding the work of paid hospital staff, yet their role is not exclusively one of support to paid labour. In some instances volunteers are completely assuming work previously undertaken by paid hospital staff. At City Hospital, General Division, the entire department of information desk workers was laid off, and volunteers were called upon to provide information services. Within the hospital, volunteers are prohibited from replacing unionized staff, but the jobs of non-unionized staff are not similarly protected.

This issue of labour replacement has been problematic for volunteers, not to mention the paid staff they replace. While all volunteers stressed the value of their contribution in providing essential services, opinion varies among volunteers about assuming previously paid jobs. Some volunteers shared the hospital management's labour cutting goals. They viewed their activities as free labour and thus cost saving for the hospital. Anne, who had volunteered at City Hospital, for one year, constructed her volunteer activity as free labour for the hospital.

> The job that I'm doing now is the office work of the hospital. It is not extras. It is something that has to be done. But I see nothing wrong with it. If the cutbacks can improve other areas in the hospital that's fine.

Many volunteers, in contrast, expressed considerable distress at the prospect of serving as labour replacement. Janet, a volunteer at City General Hospital for fifteen years, said that she had often felt that she was "taking away someone's job." Later, she added, "but who would do the job, it would just go undone." Viewing volunteering as labour replacement has significant implications that are the focus of the next section.

The Volunteer as a Wageless Worker

Volunteering is in a certain manner undergoing a process of commodification. It is not a process in which the activities of volunteers are gradually coming to be remunerated monetarily and thus commodified, but one in which volunteer activity is constructed as if it were commodified labour, governed by the market sphere of exchange. Volunteering as the giving of time captures relations which are located within the sphere of gift exchange. Mauss[4] (1925/1990) delineated the opposition between gift and market spheres, pointing to a dichotomy between free gift and economic self-interest as a particular creation of western society. Parry (1986: 458) further stresses Mauss's contention that relations occurring within the market sphere are opposed to those in the gift sphere, as each are governed by contrasting ideologies. The result is market exchanges which are defined as obligated and based on self-interest, and gift exchanges premised on notions of freedom and disinterest. The existence of two opposed and separate spheres of exchange is a key Western construction which illuminates the relations which compose volunteering. With the increased market influence on volunteering, the opposition between gift and market spheres has been blurred, challenging key conceptual boundaries. In this final section I will demonstrate the breakdown of this dichotomy by detailing how market principles have increasingly dominated the practice, evaluation and valuation of volunteer activity in a process in which the volunteer is becoming the hospital's wageless worker.

The administrative relocation of the Volunteer Department under Human Resources rendered volunteers *de facto* workers. Volunteer activity is treated as if it were interchangeable with wage labour. It is this perspective that has allowed administrators to find solutions to budget cuts by replacing paid hospital staff with volunteers. Volunteer labour has been used to assist, and in some instances, completely replace the work of paid hospital staff.

Market principles are evident in the construction of volunteer labour as paid labour. The handbook, which is given to new volunteers by the hospital's Volunteer Department is a good example (City Hospital, n.d.). In the handbook, volunteers are referred to as if they were paid workers. The language used to discuss volunteering is the same as that which is used in commodified work. Additionally, it reflects the material changes underway in volunteer activity. It has become mandatory for all volunteers to sign in and out at the "completion of their shift" (15). Volunteers intending to take a "vacation" or "leave of absence" are required to provide a two-week notice in writing to the Volunteer Department (15). Shaping volunteering as work has been a mechanism by which hospital administrators have been able to increase their control over volunteers and their activities.

Market principles like productivity and efficiency guided hospital administration in their evaluation of volunteer participation. The ideal volunteer was a younger and more efficient individual, active in, or seeking entry into, the workforce. Older individuals who were no longer in the paid workforce were less welcomed by the Volunteer Department. Many elderly volunteers sensed the hospital's unwelcoming stance toward them as tensions escalated between the hospital administration and the Auxiliary. Through official and information meetings, volunteers learned that age would become an important factor in the evaluation of their performance. During an Auxiliary Executive Committee Meeting, the Volunteer Director informed the Committee members that "experienced" volunteers would be matched up with "less experienced" volunteers, namely students, in an effort to facilitate their work. Volunteers understood that the value of their contribution was been questioned because their age rendered them less efficient. Not surprisingly, when the Auxiliary, composed largely of older members, later dissolved, many auxillians ceased volunteering.

With the escalation of tensions between the hospital and the Auxiliary, the hospital's attitude toward the older volunteer was more directly stated. I was told on various occasions by auxillians that a senior member of the Volunteer Department referred to older auxiliary volunteers as "geriatric retreads." One Auxiliary member commented on the change in attitude of hospital management towards volunteers,

> The trend now with volunteers as far as I can see—what they want is they want capable staff that aren't paid.... You are supposed to come in and do a job for four hours. And this job matters and is enough for you. And the fact that you can't perhaps run up and down the passages as many times as the teenager means that you can't do the job, so go away.

Although precise statistics on the age of volunteers were not available to me, it appeared to me that younger volunteers have begun to dominate volunteer membership, and they represent an overwhelming majority of new applicants.

The construction of the volunteer as a wageless worker is further evident in the hospital's valuation of volunteering. Volunteers are not valued because their work brings to the hospital a caring dimension, rather they are valued because they provide unpaid labour. The contribution of volunteers is quantified and it is measured monetarily. The City Hospital *Staff Newsletter* (1998b) profiled a seventy-year-old retired orderly who volunteered at City Hospital, providing volunteer labour four days a week, seven hours a day, in the hospital's hemodialysis unit. The efforts of this volunteer were praised because they "save the hospital more than $100,000 a year" (2). Hospital administrators are primarily concerned with the hours of labour delivered by volunteers. The Volunteer Department was unable to provide precise information on the total numbers of individuals volunteering in the hospital. Monthly totals of the number of hours volunteered at the hospital were, however, available. The Volunteer Department's market-driven concern with an abstracted labour contribution of volunteers, measured in time, results in a depersonalization of volunteer effort. It contributes to reshaping volunteers as wageless workers.

Care by volunteers has suffered with the loss of the Auxiliary and it also continues to be weakened within the hospital's Volunteer Department. The approach to volunteers as wageless workers minimizes the caring component traditionally central in volunteer activity. It is not that commodified labour is, in and of itself, an anathema to care. Care is a component in both paid and unpaid hospital work. The danger of health care reform is that it is transforming all work in the hospital, both paid and unpaid, in a process which limits care. The reduced delivery of care is a product of the intensification of volunteer activity and its refashioning as task-based work. The impact of minimizing the care in volunteer work is greatly significant. Care serves not only to describe the type of activities that volunteers, like paid hospital workers, deliver; it is also fundamental in the non-market relations governing volunteering. Volunteer work is being transformed on many levels of which its material practice is but one.[5]

Volunteering is not work in the sense of commodified labour. However, the activities of volunteers do constitute a non-wage form of labour, which is valuable in the hospital setting. Within anthropology, arguments have been made for broadening definitions of work to include non-wage forms of work, in order to more fully comprehend work which contributes to the maintenance of major social institutions (Wadel 1979: 368). Within sociology, feminists who have specifically examined caring work have also stressed the need to view such work as involving not only psychological elements but also as constituting labour (Graham 1983). Volunteering, while not commodified labour, is a form of labour. The transformation of volunteering underway has resulted in a contradictory relationship between volunteer activity and commodified labour, between giving and market exchanges. Health care reform has resulted in a fashioning of volunteer activity as wage work. This examination has attempted to uncover this change in volunteering which has the potential to remain obscured by the very opposition of volunteer work and market work.

Transformations in volunteering have had an impact on those individuals who deliver care and on the delivery of care. Volunteers have increasingly assumed work that was previously undertaken by paid staff. Changes in paid health care work have lead to an intensification of the work performed by volunteers. Volunteers are assuming more work in an organizational structure which limits their ability to determine the performance of work dominated by market principles in its practice, evaluation and valuation. Their work is increasingly task-based and under the control of the hospital's bureaucratic structure. Market-driven health care reform has resulted in the decreased ability of volunteers to deliver care. Many auxillians, women with the greatest volunteering experience, have resigned. Their resignation has resulted in a loss of the skills they have acquired over time. A member of the Auxiliary who had been volunteering for seven years noted in the beginning of 1998 the contribution of the older volunteer,

> These women are amazing. They come in, sometimes it takes them the whole day. They live a way out. They take buses. They come in the cold and they do their four hours…. They don't take off for being sick, and if it is very bad weather they are bound to come in. They are amazing. But they are old. So they are slow. I'm not sure the hospital wants this. They want people who are younger and smarter and faster and you can see why, because their focus is that this is a job.

Implications for Future Research

With its focus on hospital volunteers, this chapter addresses a neglected dimension of health care reform scholarship. I argue that market guided health care reform is transforming the volunteer into a wageless worker and reorganizing volunteer participation. Volunteering currently unfolds within a context of reform characterized by market-driven management practices designed to cut costs through mergers and the reorganization of labour. These reforms have resulted in volunteer work which is performed under greater hospital administrative control. In order to put these contemporary changes into context, I took an historical look at this localized practice of volunteering, outlining the development of organized volunteer participation at City General Hospital with respect to gender and the state. The unpaid health care services provided predominantly by women have undergone transformations in relation to the state's evolving approach to health care. Further research is required to explore this historical process of change in its social, political and economic contexts.

While the structure and composition of organized volunteer effort at City General Hospital has changed over time, individuals have always contributed their time to the hospital. The contribution of these individuals and the way their work is constructed must be examined within the wider social context in which it is embedded. In a mixed economy of social service delivery, exploring the part played by volunteers in Canadian health care is vital. Various avenues of research are open given the relatively unexamined role of volunteers in Canadian society.

The long-term impact of contemporary transformations in the social relations that govern volunteering still needs to be explored. How will a market approach to volunteering alter not only the practices of volunteers but also the meaning structures which govern the symbolic construction of volunteering? What are the consequences of the dominance of the market in giving with respect to our key cultural dichotomy of gift and market exchange? In addition, future research needs to examine the implications of the changes identified in this discussion, not only on the construction of volunteering but also on the delivery of care. For example, who will provide services previously performed by women volunteers with a long history of volunteer participation? My investigation, together with the analysis of these and other questions, will contribute to a greater understanding of this female dominated domain of unpaid work and in so doing will unravel the complexity of one aspect of voluntary participation in Canadian society.

Notes

1. The names of hospitals, organizations and people used in this discussion are pseudonyms. City Hospital refers to the corporation formed of the merger of City General Hospital with two other area hospitals. This chapter focuses on the history of volunteering at one location, that is, City General Hospital.
2. These organizations was more common in urban contexts than in smaller communities where "women played little or no role in poor relief" (Marks 1995: 80).
3. Doris Grinspun in this volume critically examines the shift in Canadian hospital management from the carative-curative paradigm to the business paradigm.
4. Mauss is most remembered, not for his delineation of the dichotomy of gift and market spheres in the West, but rather for his elaboration of obligated and interested giving in non-market societies where a system of reciprocity played a key role in the maintenance of social relationships. Parry (1986) contends that the implications of Mauss's theoretical perspective on exchange has largely been overlooked in the West.
5. For the purpose of this examination, the intersection of caring and volunteering is discussed on the level of care as a material activity performed by volunteers, as the actual delivery of care through voluntary participation. This narrowing of focus does not imply that the material work of volunteers can be separated from other aspects which combined constitute volunteer-

ing as a whole. By virtue of giving their time freely, volunteering is performed in non-market relationships structured by care. Researchers have
argued that the commercial relationships prevailing in the market are
contradictory to the relations governing the health care system, relations
which are based on care (Armstrong et al. 1997). White (1997) also identified
the problems with treating paid health care work as a commodity.

9

Home Care Before and after Reform: A Comparative Analysis of Two Texts-in-Action[1]

Diana L. Gustafson

Health care as business has become a widely accepted social fact.[2] As a nurse and a clinical educator with over twenty years experience in the health sector, I wondered how this so-called fact had come to displace the more traditional goals and practices of health care workers who coordinate home care services for the ill, injured, elderly and disabled in Ontario communities. This chapter explores one way in which government goals of cost-containment and efficiency have penetrated the actual work processes performed by people working in home care agencies. This means looking at *what* these work processes consist of and *how* various health care workers enact these processes. Specifically, I compare two administrative procedures: one used in an Ontario home care agency in the early 1990s, prior to the major restructuring of community services; and the other used in a community care access centre (CCAC) in the late 1990s, after restructuring. This analysis illustrates how the process of coordinating home care services has been reconstituted so that health care workers (predominantly women) come to act in business-oriented ways that may not be consistent with their knowledge and perspective and that contribute to the downloading of caring labour onto other women, usually unpaid family members.

My interest in this issue was sparked by the case of a young woman pregnant with her second child who suffered needlessly because cost outcomes outweighed health outcomes in the management of her care. Bev,[3] a thirty-year-old White woman living in a middle-class suburban neighbourhood required dozens of sutures to close a gaping leg laceration sustained in a car accident. After a few hours in the hospital emergency department she was sent home with a bulky pressure dressing on her leg, a pair of crutches and verbal instructions for assessing and caring for the wound. No one told her that she might be eligible for home care services.

Bev managed as best she could, considering she was new to her neighbourhood, had no friends or family in the local area to whom she could turn for support and her husband was on assignment out of the country. Twice she returned to a walk-in clinic as she was concerned about the condition of her wound and was experiencing pain so severe she was unable to bear weight on her affected leg. Following her second visit, she was hospitalized—her leg red and swollen to twice its size, her wound burst open and draining pus, her pregnancy at risk. After three days in hospital, she was sent home, this time with a referral for home care services.

The visiting nurse called on her daily, listened to the fetal heart rate and showed Bev how to change her medicated dressing four times a day. Bev received no other services such as light housekeeping or meal preparation that would have lightened the burden of caring for herself, her pregnancy, her young daughter and her home. After four days, the nurse determined that Bev could manage her own care and discontinued home care services. Two days later, Bev was back in the hospital with a blood infection that threatened her life and that of her unborn child.

This case stands in stark contrast to the government's vision of a more accessible, client-focused, community-based health care system (Ontario Ministry of Health [OMOH] 1994, Working Group on Health Care Services Utilization 1994). Shorter hospital stays, faster patient turnover and community-based care, which in Bev's case was too little too late, contributed to this woman's extended and complicated recovery with all the attendant financial and human costs. Equally troubling to me were the actions and inactions of health practitioners working in the hospital, the walk-in clinic and the home care agency. Decisions made by these workers, traditionally regarded as patient advocates and caring practitioners, seemed focused less on quality patient care and more on the bottom line. How has this come about? How does the government's business orientation come to penetrate the everyday activities of health practitioners like those involved in Bev's case? How do interests in the fiscal health of the state merge with and displace interests in the health of the individual and family? These are the questions I address in the following pages.

Institutional ethnography offers the framework for examining these questions. The assumptions guiding this method of social inquiry are introduced in the first section. The second section provides a detailed description of two sets of administrative processes in place at two different historical moments in Ontario's home care history. Comparing the actual sequencing of bureaucratic practices illustrates how home care workers have become unwitting and, perhaps, unwilling agents of a government agenda that puts cost outcomes above health outcomes.

Institutional Ethnography: A Method of Social Inquiry

To engage in this comparative textual analysis, I turned to a method of social inquiry called institutional ethnography. Institutional ethnography examines the ways that everyday activities and social relations are coordinated and linked to the exercise of power both at and beyond the local setting in which they occur (Smith 1987: 92). The "relations of ruling" (Smith 1987: 3) or the extralocal forms of control that regulate local activities are what we might refer to as bureaucracy or management or administration (Smith 1990b: 6). These organizational controls are neither an "abstraction" (Grahame 1998) nor are they readily recognized as concrete by individuals engaged in their daily work. Instead these ruling practices may be experienced by women and men as "bureaucratic red tape," those nonsensical or pointless operations that workers perform that seem disconnected from the knowledge and experience they bring to their jobs.

To examine the disjuncture I experienced in reviewing Bev's case, I focus on one type of document and the work activities and social relations linked to that document. The document is an intake record used by health workers to initiate the process of linking individuals who need home cares services with community agencies who deliver those services. When completed, the intake record becomes the source of data about the patient or client[4] and her or his health care needs.

My analysis, however, does not treat the intake record as an independent document whose meaning is located solely in the words and tick boxes printed on the page. Instead I view the intake record as a single component in a complex set of documentary practices that mobilizes the activities of health workers in an actual social and historical location. This is the first of four assumptions underpinning institutional ethnography as a method of inquiry. The term "text-in-action" captures the real-time movement of documents from one worker to the next as well as the concrete nature of bureaucratic activities enacted by real people in the movement of data along a communication route. Furthermore, as Dorothy Smith notes,

> In taking up a text as a constituent of a social relation, we are constrained not only to understand it as a moment in a sequence, but also to recognize that the interpretive practices which activate it are embedded in a relational process. Textual practices are operative in the work of accomplishing the social relations in which texts occur. (1990b: 125)

Included in this citation is the second assumption. No single person completes all activities related to the text. Nor does any single worker take an individual case from its inception to its conclusion. Therefore, rather than focusing on the work of a single health worker I attend to the way social relations are organized by and in relation to the intake record as it passes from one individual to the next at several concrete sites. Ellen Pence refers to these concrete moments as "processing interchanges" (1996: 60). At each processing interchange the document is received, then interpreted, modified or acted upon before being passed along to the next interchange. According to Pence, "It is the construction of these processing interchanges coupled with a highly specialized division of labour that accomplishes much of the ideological work of the institution" (1996: 60).

Third, the actual activities: what data is entered into text and the sequencing of each processing interchange, when and to whom data is communicated, is institutionally organized by the text itself and by other bureaucratic practices internal and external to the organization. For example, legislation (texts external to community agencies) and administrative policies and procedures (internal to these agencies) regulate and standardize the kinds of information that are collected, communicated, interpreted and acted upon as the intake record is passed from one worker to the next. Therefore, this set of bureaucratic activities is only understandable in the larger context of the health care system in which the community-based agency is embedded.

Fourth, bureaucratic activities generate texts that constitute the institutional record of what is and what happened—a documented account of reality. This "textual reality" (Smith 1990b: 79) represents objective knowledge or "facticity" (79). The power of institutional facticity lies both in its concreteness as text and in the relations of ruling that give authority to documented accounts over oral histories. Thus, the intake record and the work process it organizes produce objectified knowledge about an individual person needing home care. That textual reality comes to represent and be disconnected from the subjective knowledge and experience of the individual needing home care services. Furthermore, the institutional facts of the case disqualify or displace the subjective knowledge and experience of the individuals enacting the work processes.

Comparing Two Texts-in-Action

In this section I compare two texts-in-action: the Home Care Program Medical Referral form and the CCAC Client Assessment form. At both historical moments these intake records and the sequence of activities health care workers performed in relation to these texts regulate who receives home care services, what kinds of services are delivered and for how long. This discussion illustrates: 1) how these texts and the work processes they organize changed with home care restructuring; and 2) how the work of CCAC staff is restructured and standardized in ways that accomplish the functional work (the coordination of home care services) and the ideological work (accountability for cost containment and efficiency) of the health care system in which the agencies are embedded.

Home Care Program Medical Referral Form—Before Reform

Prior to restructuring, two government-funded agencies, each with offices in regional health departments across Ontario, coordinated the delivery of insurable health care services provided in their respective communities.[5] One of these, the Home Care Program, assisted an individual to return home from hospital, or remain in their home, with the support of appropriate health care services. For example, this agency coordinated services so that an elderly widow could convalesce at home after hip replacement surgery. The other, the Placement Program, served the needs of persons who required more support than could be provided under the Home Care Program guidelines but who did not require the type of acute care services provided by hospitals. For example, this agency assisted individuals in accessing a suitable level of care in community facilities such as a nursing homes, homes for the aged and daycare programs for seniors. Later I discuss the restructuring of these two programs.

The Home Care Program Medical Referral form was an intake record used during the early 1990s at one Ontario Regional Health Department. In separate interviews with four workers who had used the document, together withmy own experience of using this document, I mapped the details of the process: who completed various parts of the document, the kinds of information included and the sequence of individuals who handled the text as it moved along the case route.

To illustrate this process, I present here a typical, uncomplicated scenario. This is the fictitious case of Ruth, an elderly white woman who broke her hip falling on an icy sidewalk. Previously in good health, she recovered well following surgery to repair her fracture. On the eighth post-operative day, her physician performed a standard clinical assessment strategy that considered all aspects of Ruth's past and current physical and mental health. The assessment indicated Ruth was ready for discharge home with support.

The process began when the physician completed a Home Care Program Medical Referral form. Legislation (texts external to the local setting) restricted this authority to physicians. In most instances, an individual with a health problem consulted first with a general practitioner (in keeping with legislated funding arrangements). The family doctor frequently had an established relationship with the patient, knew her or his medical history and managed the bulk of patient-physician interactions. Consequently, the family doctor was usually in the best position to provide follow-up treatment and continuity of care between acute care episodes.

The doctor obtained the intake record from the receptionist on the patient care unit. The specimen text is a single-page with "Home Care Program Medical Referral" printed across the top. A rectangular space in the upper right hand corner of the page was used for imprinting the patient's vital statistics. Six data fields at the top and bottom of the form were for fixed responses. These included tick boxes for indicating the patient's prognosis (i.e., improve, remain stable, deteriorate), whether the diagnosis is known by the patient and the patient's family (yes/no) and the type of home care services requested (e.g., nursing, physiotherapy, homemaking and so on). There were also lines and spaces for dates and signatures of various text readers. Four free-text fields took up most of the page. These fields are entitled, "Diagnosis," "History," "Medications," and "Specific Orders." Medical knowledge and practical experience guided the kinds of data about a patient's medical history that a physician entered into each field. The free-text design allowed a doctor more latitude than fixed-response fields in using that knowledge and experience to create an account of a patient's health status. This, in turn, allowed more subjective data about the patient's needs and treatment goals to enter into communication.

The doctor was the first text reader and this was the first processing interchange along the case route. In Ruth's case, the physician ticked most of the fixed fields including Prognosis: *improve*; and Services Requested: *physiotherapy*. Additionally the doctor added information about the patient's health status to all free-text fields. Typical documentation may have looked like this:

> *Diagnosis:* Previously healthy active 76 year old woman; Lives alone since death of husband six months ago. Presenting problem: fractured left femur; eight days post-op hip replacement; uneventful recovery.
> *History:* none significant.
> *Medications:* Tylenol #2 q4-6h prn for pain.
> *Specific orders:* physio consult

After dating and signing the intake record in the space provided, the doctor left the document on the patient's chart for the next text reader. In that way, the patient's health needs were made concrete in text and constituted as a Home Care case.

While it was the physician who made the referral, all members of the multidisciplinary team (nurse, home care case manager and physiotherapist, for example) were responsible for identifying patients who might require home care services upon discharge. Four formal communication channels were used for sharing information. Routinely, team members communicated details about a patient's progress and discharge planning by writing in the patient's chart, adding to the patient's care plan, and sharing verbally with other team members during shift changes. Team rounds was a fourth communication channel. This multidisciplinary team met regularly to share patient information, identify patient care problems and plan patient care, including discharge plans.

In this fictitious case, all members of Ruth's care team evaluated her progress toward recovery and discharge home. The surgeon or family physician, Ruth and a member of her family may have attended weekly team rounds to discuss discharge plans and the need for home care services. While any team member may have facilitated the referral process, communicating with the physician was often undertaken by the nurse in charge of a patient's care, the nurse manager, or the home care case manager.

The second processing interchange occurred when the unit receptionist, the second text reader, found the intake record in the patient's chart. The receptionist used an addressograph to stamp the right upper corner of the document with the patient's vital statistics including name, age, address, date of birth, hospital identification number and admission date. Then the receptionist phoned the home care case manager, giving her the patient's name, diagnosis, hospital room number and expected date of discharge. In the space provided in the left upper corner of the document, the receptionist added her initials and the name of the home care case manager with whom she spoke.

This apparently simple act of recording the fact of a conversation illustrates how extralocal forms of control penetrate the actual activities performed by a health care worker. Adding to the text was a real-time moment in a bureaucratic sequence. The unit receptionist knew that Home Care Program procedures (texts external to the hospital setting) allowed the case manager twenty-four hours notice to organize patient services. The unit receptionist responded to these ruling practices by making the phone call in a timely fashion and certified that act by filling in the appropriate field on the intake record. Her actions established communication between the hospital staff and Home Care Program staff. Thus, acting upon and adding to the document were organized by the text, linked to the exercise of power both at and beyond the local setting, and operative in accomplishing the social relations between other health care workers.

The same can be said of the actions of the third text reader, the home care case manager. A registered nurse, the case manager operated from an office in the hospital and was a liaison between the hospital and the Home Care Program who employed her. The third processing interchange began when she picked up the text from the patient care unit, read and interpreted it. In Ruth's case, the physician ordered a physiotherapy consultation. One benefit of such a broadly articulated order was the way it allowed the case manager more flexibility in planning services to meet the full range of a patient's needs. However, responding to a broadly articulated order was more time consuming and labour intensive. A narrow and specific order such as "physiotherapist to teach crutch walking" might have been less time consuming but it also left less room for interpretation and limited the degree to which a case manager could apply her professional expertise to meeting the specific needs of a client.

The case manager reviewed the patient's chart and care plan to familiarize herself with Ruth and her medical history. From these internal hospital documents created by Ruth's caregivers, the case manager learned about Ruth's health care needs and her level of physical and mental functioning. In addition to this textual account of Ruth's health status, the case manager consulted in person with Ruth and her hospital caregivers. Whenever possible, the case manager met with a family member and made a home visit for additional information about Ruth's needs for convalescing at home. Based on her interpretation of these data, the case manager added her recommendations for home care services to the "Specific orders" field at the bottom of the intake record. The home care case manager's notation may have looked like this:

> *Goals for treatment:* Return to self-care and optimum level of mobility. *Treatment plan:* Physiotherapist to assess safety in ambulating and making transfers from bed to chair. Teach crutch walking and stair climbing. Supply crutches, wheelchair, elevated toilet seat. Health care aide daily for assistance bathing and dressing. Homemaker for laundry and light housekeeping twice weekly. Meals-on-Wheels five days / week.

Then she dated and signed in the space provided at the bottom of the intake record. Because the doctor in this fictitious case ordered a professional service (physiotherapy), Ruth was entitled to receive the nonprofessional services (homemaker) she needed to convalesce at home. In cases where the doctor did not order a professional service,[6] patients had to assume the costs of retaining any nonprofessional service.

The fourth processing interchange in the documentary process occurred when the hospital-based case manager communicated details of the referral to her agency-based colleague. The intake record organized the telephone conversation between the case managers. Documented details about Ruth's health constituted the institutional facts of her case. The agency-based home care case manager listened to and interpreted these data and created her own notes about Ruth's health and the specific orders for her care.

Following this conversation, the hospital-based case manager sent the intake record by inter-agency mail to the Home Care Program office. This worker's action was a concerted response to the instructions printed in a small box in the upper left corner of the intake record. These instructions stipulated that the intake record be submitted to the agency office within five days of initiating a referral. Upon reaching the Home Care office, the intake record became the first document in Ruth's permanent patient file.

The agency-based case manager did not wait to receive the intake record. Instead she acted upon the text she created during the conversation with her hospital-based colleague. This meant phoning the coordinator of a community agency with whom the Home Care Program had a government contract. During this phone conversation with the coordinator, the case manager communicated Ruth's health needs, type of care required and goals for treatment. Later, she mailed a copy of the intake record to the agency.

During this fifth processing interchange, between the home care case manager and the coordinator of the community agency, the coordinator created her own text by completing her agency's administrative documents. As in previous processing interchanges, the newly created text constituted the institutional facts of a case as created and sent by one worker and received and interpreted by the next. That document and a copy of the intake record became part of the permanent patient file of that provider agency. Acting upon her interpretation of the facts of Ruth's case, the coordinator scheduled a physiotherapist, a home care aide and a homemaker to begin home visits.

The sixth processing interchange in the sequence occurred when the health care provider (in Ruth's case, the physiotherapist) reviewed the text passed on to her by the agency coordinator. In preparation for meeting Ruth for the first time, the physiotherapist interpreted the data and created her own documentation including information about Ruth's diagnosis, health status and preliminary treatment plan.

The patient-caregiver interaction that took place in the patient's home was the seventh processing interchange. Here again, the actions of the caregiver were organized by the data written on the intake record beginning with the physician and added to by the various text readers along the communication route. In this example, the physiotherapist assessed Ruth's general health and mobility in planning day-to-day caregiving activities aimed at meeting the goals for treatment (return to self-care and optimum mobility). With each visit, the physiotherapist documented both her own and Ruth's assessment of her progress toward meeting the treatment goals. These notes remained in Ruth's home for all caregivers assigned to her case to consult and add to with each visit.

When the goals for treatment as written on the intake record were met, the caregiver documented her findings and discussed them with her team leader (the eighth processing interchange). The texts created by the various caregivers became part of the permanent patient file stored at the agency. When services were terminated, the agency coordinator notified the Home Care Program case manager. This was the ninth and final processing interchange. Closing the patient file terminated the communication.

To summarize the process in place prior to reform, an individual with a health need hooked into agencies that provided home care services when a physician initiated an intake form. The text was a single component in a complex documentary process that was itself organized by other texts such as provincial legislation, professional standards and Home Care Program policy and procedures. The predominantly free-text design of the document allowed health practitioners to use their knowledge and experience in shaping the kinds of patient information that entered into the process. Also important to note is the way the patient's subjective assessment and experience of health entered into the process at several points leading up to and during the bureaucratic process. As a result the patient's health needs remained at the centre of the communication and decision-making. Each text reader acting in relation to the text was accomplishing both the functional and ideological work of the Home Care Program. That is to say, the sequencing of the activities as well as the activities they enacted, centred around coordinating the delivery of appropriate home care services to the individual.

Client Assessment Form—After Reform
In the mid-1990s, the Home Care and Placement Programs were replaced by forty-three community care access centres. Each CCAC is governed by a local community board and this is expected to improve the program's responsiveness to local needs. Home care restructuring was part of the Ontario government's vision of a more cost-efficient, client-focused, community-based health care system. One goal was to eliminate unnecessary costs associated with the duplication of administrative processes, services and resources. This involved reducing the total number of the staff positions, reorganizing the physical plants and restructuring work processes. In this section, I examine the work process organized by a CCAC intake record.

Obtaining a current CCAC intake record and mapping the work process proved difficult. My phone calls to one CCAC were never returned. My requests for interviews at a second CCAC were declined. Secrecy and suspicion marked my interviews with staff at a third CCAC and, on at least one occasion, I was given misinformation. None of the three CCACs I contacted were willing to give me a copy of the intake document they used or let me observe the intake process. The specimen text I describe here came from an informant who would not name her CCAC contact or the region where the form was used. I was told that the CCAC contact feared reprisals if she were found disseminating agency documents. The contact used liquid paper to erase the agency logo on the form and I received a photocopy of that altered form. Furthermore, my informant asked that I conceal her identity as it may allow readers of this chapter to trace the identity of her CCAC contact.

In this section, I map the bureaucratic process used in one CCAC region after home care reform in Ontario. As before, each processing interchange is numbered sequentially with the corresponding number appearing on the process sequencing map. Although details about what text readers do with and in relation to the text may vary from region to region, two contacts who reviewed the map confirmed that the process I describe here is the same in the CCACs where they work.

Since the restructuring of home care services, anyone—a family member, a concerned neighbour, a nurse, a physician, or the individual in need of care—may initiate a home care referral by calling their local CCAC. A caller to the CCAC may be greeted by the receptionist who screens incoming calls. The receptionist transfers the call to the CCAC worker assigned to information and referral. In some agencies a caller may not have this first human contact but may be greeted by an electronic call-answer system. If the caller is able to follow the instructions and input the appropriate digits, she or he is connected to an intake worker or their messaging system. The first processing interchange occurs when the intake worker[7] initiates the CCAC Client Assessment form. This text standardizes the caller's interaction with the CCAC intake worker who fills in the form.

The specimen text is two pages long. While the first page consists entirely of fixed response fields, the second page has both fixed response and free-text fields. Like the earlier text, there are fields on the first page for the client's vital statistics. Now, there are also spaces for other data not collected prior to reform, including the client's social insurance number, the physician's billing number and the expected dates of discharge from hospital and from home care services. Like the earlier text, there is a field for services requested. Now, there are eleven rather than eight tick boxes as well as spaces for the names of therapists. Information about the client's diagnosis is no longer a large free-text field but is limited to three spaces: one for each of the primary and secondary diagnoses, and another for the name and date of any surgical procedure. Also previously a free-text field, treatment goal is now a set of ten tick boxes each associated with a code number. These include: "assess level of care required," "teach treatment protocol," "reintegration into community," "adjustment to altered functional status," "return to total care by parents," and "return to total self-care." Another fixed-response field lists support services including drugs, dressings, equipment, diagnostic/lab services, transportation and oxygen, each associated with a code number and a space for the name of the supplier.

In the right upper corner of the first page is a field entitled "Admission Status," with four tick boxes: "Admitted," "Service Delay," "Not Admitted," and "Transferred in." Another new field entitled, "Reasons for Non-Admission" has eleven tick boxes each associated with a code number. Three of these are "no OHIP coverage," "needs can be met as an outpatient," and "condition inappropriate." Other tick boxes in this section indicate that an applicant can be denied home care services if their condition is not expected to improve, if the applicant's home is "not suitable" (however that might be construed), or if the family is not available to participate in care.

One-third of the second page is devoted to fixed response fields. Various aspects of a client's physical and functional status are listed, each with a tick box for either "independent" or "dependent." There are three choices for describing a client's mental status: "lucid," "forgetfulness," and "confusion." Data about the client's mobility and place of residence are similarly condensed. The remainder of the second page is divided among six free-text fields for present health and social history, past history, medications, treatment orders, goal and plan. This allows space for some subjective data to enter the process.

The intake worker collects and documents as much health and non-health related data as the caller is able to provide. If a physician initiates the referral, the intake worker ticks the "yes" response in the "medical referral" field. When a potential client or other individual initiates the referral she ticks the "no" response. According to one CCAC director, the majority of referrals in her region still come from the family physician. All physician referrals are forwarded to the CCAC district case manager, who handles referrals for a specific geographical territory. If the intake worker determines that a referral made by another individual also merits further consideration, she passes it along.

At this second processing interchange, the district case manager reviews, interprets, adds to and acts upon the form. For example, the case manager checks the field indicating whether or not a client gave consent for treatment. In cases where the client did not initiate the referral, the case manager must, in accordance with provincial legislation, obtain consent. She does this when she arranges to meet and assess the potential client either in the home or the hospital. If the client did not initiate the referral, this may be the first time the client's subjective experience enters into the process. But it is not the client's subjective experience of her health that determines how this exchange plays out. Nor is it the case manager's knowledge and experience that organizes the interaction. Again, the text regulates the engagement and the kinds of health and non-health related information that are collected and entered into the decision-making process.

One field is entitled "Client lives with" and another "Next of kin/ Support." These fields include tick boxes and spaces for recording the name, age, relationship and phone number of persons who may participate in the client's care. Collecting these data reflects 1998 guidelines requiring that individuals first exhaust the support of friends and family before turning to publicly funded support (Aronson 1999). The same goes for exhausting other sources of private coverage. A field called, "Financial Information" has tick boxes for indicating the type of subsidy, if any, whether or not the client is employed, the kind of private coverage, if any, the names of other agencies involved, such as Department of Veteran's Affairs, public health nurse and so on. Many of these fields are linked to codes that the case manager uses in determining if and what kinds of services the client is eligible to receive and for how long.

If, based on the available data, the client is deemed eligible to receive services, the district case manager calls one of the service provider agencies with whom the CCAC has contracts. During this third processing interchange, the case manager communicates to the agency coordinator the documented facts of the case including the estimated date of discharge from care. This date is based on another text that defines the standard course of care for a specific diagnosis. The case manager follows up with a faxed copy of the intake record. Upon receipt of the text, the coordinator interprets and acts upon the text by scheduling an appropriate caregiver. According to two women employed by service provider agencies, the "appropriate" caregiver is the one able to provide the necessary care (as stipulated on the intake record) at the least cost to the agency.

The fourth processing interchange occurs when the assigned caregiver receives her assignment, refers to the patient file and creates her own text based on the documentation provided. Then she goes into the client's home. Her interaction with the client and the term of engagement are regulated by the documented facts of the case. Each visit is expected to take a given length of time based on workload measurement standards.

So, for example, performing a complex wound care may be expected to take twenty minutes while teaching a client or family member to care for the wound may take the same time. The number of visits in a course of a client's care is also regulated by the text. According to one case manager, continuing visits past the targeted date of discharge written on the intake record must be carefully documented and justified. She went on to say that a caregiver will routinely involve the client and family in caregiving activities to maximize the benefit of her visit and encourage a return to independence.

Lindsay Wizowski (1994) found that many nurses support client and family participation in care as being of both medical and moral benefit to the individual and the family. One home care case manager disagreed, saying, "Get in, teach and get out. That's what we do." In her experience, the emphasis on teaching the family how to manage the client's care has more to do with meeting standardized targets for discharge than providing client-centred care. This was true in Bev's case. Despite Bev's history of being unable to adequately care for herself and her leg wound, the visiting nurse spent most of her time teaching Bev how to change her own dressing. When that goal was met, Bev was discharged from home care services.

To summarize the process in place since restructuring, anyone may contact their local CCAC to initiate a referral for home care services. The process of considering a client request for services begins when a Client Assessment form is initiated. While the form devotes roughly the same amount of space to information about the client's health needs as the earlier Medical Referral form, an equivalent amount of space is devoted to collecting non-health related data about family/kin support and insurance coverage. The predominance of fixed-response fields over free-text fields standardizes much of the data collected. Coding procedures linked to other texts regulate eligibility for services and the course of care. This means that the knowledge and experience of those health professionals who enact the process are no longer central to decision-making. Furthermore, the client's health needs are evaluated in terms of the short-term fiscal considerations of the agencies in which the texts are used.

Work Processes: The Penetration of the Fiscal Imperative

Moving health care "closer to home" (Armstrong 1994: 95) was part of an overall health care reform strategy initiated in Ontario in the early 1990s.[8] Three years into the reform process, a community health framework was still in the early stages of development. The promised infusion of dollars

into the community had not materialized. Despite the provincial government's promise that public health and community services would have
more money at their disposal, the operating budgets for some community-based services declined (Ontario Council of Hospital Unions/Cana-
dian Union of Public Employees [OCHU/CUPE] 1995). This problem was
further complicated as restructuring in the hospital sector[9] increased the
numbers of ill and injured persons discharged into the community
(Armstrong 1994, Neysmith 1998). The resulting gap in community
resources encouraged growth and competition among service provider
agencies (Armstrong 1995).

Provincial funding to CCACs increased slowly in the latter part of the
1990s. However, these modest infusions did little to keep pace with the
increasing demand for services (Aronson 1999, Neysmith 1998). CCACs
are faced with the challenge of operating a more accessible service, over
longer hours, more efficiently and more cost effectively to a growing
population that is sicker and in need of more and more complex care.

Herein lies the conundrum. Hospital restructuring increased the
demand for home care services. The demand was further increased by
legislation that redefined an insurable service as any service that can
reasonably be provided in the home that supports an (eligible) client
remaining in the home. Government funding to CCACs lags far behind the
growing demand. Service provider agencies who compete successfully
for their share of the home care dollar often do so on the backs of the
women they employ.[10] Still there remains a gap between the demand for
insurable services and the available funding to meet that demand. The
result is a fiscal imperative to ration resources.

Women, more than men, and some groups of women more than
others are disadvantaged by this rationing of resources. Studies of health
care recipients show that transferring care from the hospital to the home
is negatively impacting on aging women (Aronson 1999, McDaniel and
Gee 1993),[11] immigrant and refugee women,[12] Aboriginal women[13] and
poor women (Morris et al. 1999). Reforms are also impacting on women
who assume the care of an ill, disabled or elderly relative (Abel 1995,
Canadian Study of Health and Aging 1994, Keating et al. 1994, Neysmith
1998, Watkinson 1999). This is especially onerous for women who must
reconcile paid employment with unpaid caregiving responsibilities.
Working poor women, especially those tied to an hourly wage are more
severely penalized financially for taking time off than are women in
salaried employment. Poorer women who assume family caregiving
responsibilities tend to be more burdened because there is generally less
money to pay for complementary health care services or respite care
(Abel 1995). Reforms are also impacting on paid home care providers
working for service provider agencies. Some are nurses displaced from

hospitals; many are poor women and women of colour working as health care aides. Their labour is characterized by lower wages and poor job security (Morris et al. 1999, Neysmith and Aronson 1997).

Comparing texts-in-action illustrates how this fiscal imperative penetrates the work processes of women who must decide which individuals and their families benefit from the timely delivery of limited resources and which individuals and families must wait, or pay for private services, or (mis)manage their own care.

In this section I discuss two sets of conclusions drawn from the comparison of work processes in place before and after reform. Collectively these conclusions illustrate how the new intake record, as a constituent of social relations among health care workers, accomplishes both the functional work of the CCAC and the ideological goals of the restructured health care system in which it is embedded. More specifically, these conclusions offer some insight into how administrative processes mobilize the everyday activities of home care workers (predominantly women) in ways that contribute to the downloading of care.

Changes in the Referral Process: Power, Knowledge and the Business Discourse

Prior to restructuring, only the physician could initiate a home care referral. Since restructuring, any person may initiate a referral. Widening the portal of entry to services is not without merit. This change advances the right of individuals to be advocates for their own care or that of a family member. Furthermore, the change is consistent with other legislation, such as the *Regulated Health Professions Act* that recognizes the competence of all health professionals to negotiate care options with a client.[14] In principle, this means any health worker may make a direct referral on behalf of a client without speaking through the voice and authority of the physician.

In practice, however, physicians continue to initiate most of the referrals. Several factors contribute to this outcome. A wider portal of entry assumes that the individual or other concerned person is knowledgeable about home care services and how to access them. As Bev's story suggests, this may not be the case. When asked why so few referrals are initiated by a potential client or family member, one CCAC director explained that the public is "uneducated about the change." She said that CCAC efforts to heighten public awareness through information drives and community consultation have not significantly changed the pattern of referral. While this may be so, my frustrated efforts to learn more about CCACs and their work processes suggest that greater public awareness may not be a priority. My other difficulties contacting staff and gathering texts and information from three CCACs are strongly suggestive of a dynamic of consolidating and concealing authority that is systemic rather than agency specific (Gustafson 1998a).

On at least one occasion that I can substantiate, I was given misinformation by a CCAC director. When I asked how a worker determined who received home care services I was told that anyone with a valid OHIP card is eligible to receive home care services. As I later discovered, the CCAC intake record lists eleven conditions for denying services. Even without this evidence, the director's claim does not make sense in a light of the pressure to be fiscally responsible, to reduce waste and to monitor abuse and misuse of services. Only with persistent questioning did the director admit that CCAC workers use eligibility criteria when reviewing requests for homemaking services. The criteria, she said, reflected a "common sense" notion of who and under what circumstances a client was considered eligible for this non-professional service. The director's use of this term had an eerie ring in the Conservative days of Mike Harris's "common sense revolution." Recalling that Bev did not receive any homemaking services during her convalescence suggests that a worker's common sense does not drive decision-making in Harris' Ontario.

I argue, therefore, that rationing information is consistent with the campaign to ration resources. A public ill-informed about how to access home care services is more likely to assume responsibility for their own care, like Bev, or in the case of more privileged women, to seek out and pay for services. An ill-informed public is less likely to consume products and services.

If knowledge about how the system works is not available to me who can claim status as a health care insider, it is at least as inaccessible to individuals needing home care services. Potential clients, the very people represented in the institutional texts I examine here, cannot become better informed about restructured services if accurate information about how the intake forms organize outcomes is considered ineligible for discussion.

It appears there is a tension between widening the portal of entry for home care services and rationing the consumer's knowledge about how to access those services. Three flawed assumptions sustain this tension. First, inherent in a business-driven system is the notion that the consumer has the responsibility to be as well informed about a service and the alternatives as the provider of those services. Yet, little in the history of our physician-driven, patient-dependent system has prepared care recipients to assume the role of informed consumer and owners of their own health. In addition, funding arrangements that reward acute care treatment (Armstrong and Armstrong 1994a) rather than long-term health promotion, encourage interactions between care recipients and care providers that are discontinuous and unpredictable rather than regular and planned. Take Bev, for example. Her interactions with the system were urgent and not conducive to thoughtful or considered decision-making. Her inexperience with the system made her less able to negotiate decision-making in a knowledgeable way or do so during a time of stress.

Second, introducing a mechanism of self-referral assumes that an individual in need feels entitled to receive home care services. This assumption is also flawed. Jane Aronson (1999) found that many women living with chronic conditions and disabilities did not ask for help because they feared they could not demonstrate sufficient need. In a climate of fiscal constraint, some women *feel* disentitled to receive home care services. This was true of Bev. Because the doctors and nurses did not discuss the option of home care services, she believed she *ought* be able to manage on her own. Their professional expertise disqualified her own experience of need.

Third, empowering other health care workers to initiate the process assumes they have sufficient time and opportunity to assess an individual's need for home care and make a referral. In Bev's case, the physicians and staff in the emergency department and the walk-in clinic had neither. They focused on caring for her wound, not on caring for her. Recall that it was only after her fourth contact with health care practitioners— following her first hospitalization—that home care services were initiated. This is not an indictment against individual practitioners. Rather it illustrates how staffing cuts, shorter patient stays and faster patient turnover (all business-driven outcomes) severely restrict the time and opportunity available for caregivers to provide comprehensive, client-focused care. This leads me to a review of changes in the ways social relations are organized among health care providers, and between the health care worker and the client.

Changes in Social Relations:
Subordinating Subjectivity and Experience

Prior to restructuring home care services, the physician initiated the referral and was the first person to contribute data to the intake record. Other health professionals who cared for and assessed the patient's needs supported the initiation of a referral and contributed relevant data. Granted there were power inequities in the relationship between the patient and the physician and other health care professionals. And an unequal relationship impacts on the nature and scope of communication and the kinds of information shared. Still, the patient's health-related data constituted the facts of the case, and the bureaucratic practices that organized decision-making were grounded in medical discourse. New administrative practices reorganize the client-worker interaction in four ways that are consistent with the shift toward the business paradigm.

First, the new CCAC Client Assessment form is completed by a health professional who does not know the client. The physician, client or other concerned individual supplies the information to the intake worker who initiates the intake record. Getting the physician's approval for specific home care services is very different from having the patient and her doctor working together, sharing responsibility for health care outcomes.

The need to obtain physician approval raises another issue not readily apparent to those who enact the current work process. According to one CCAC director, the presence of the medical referral field reminds text readers to consider the need for physician approval for care. Virtually every scenario I proposed (except those involving homemaking services) was construed as one requiring a physician's approval. The director claimed that obtaining physician consent ensures there are no medical contraindications that put the client at risk for receiving a home care service. This means that a potential client or non-medical health practitioner may not, in practice, be able to initiate care independent of a physician's expressed consent for treatment. So while, anyone may, in principle, be able to initiate a referral, the text reasserts the role of the physician as the guardian of home care dollars in a restructured, business-driven system.

I turn now to the way the format of the text regulates the actual conversations between workers and between the worker and the client. Fixed-response fields require brief, discrete responses. Because it takes less time to collect data and construct text for nominal-type fields, this portion of the form can be completed with rapid-fire questioning. The format of the new text creates a tension between the way client and the intake worker *may* wish to communicate and the way the intake worker *must* sequence the interaction in order to complete the form and her interaction in a timely, efficient manner. As a result, the actual process of constructing a client's case becomes disconnected from the caring discourse that once guided the worker-client relations.

Second, the text regulates the kinds of data that the intake worker gathers to construct an account of the client's need. The process reconstitutes a real person with health care needs into a paper image shaped by both medical and business knowledges. The client's health care needs do not frame communication as they did in the earlier process. The actual conversation between client and health care worker must produce details about the client's health needs and the client's sources of financial and family/kin support. Before services can be arranged, these data must be gathered for review and interpretation against eligibility criteria shaped by legislation and budgetary constraints. These data can then be used to justify transferring the burden of care from the agency to the family and from paid workers to unpaid family members. As others have noted, transferring the labour and costs of care to other groups and individuals is the same as reducing the demand (Angus 1994, Evans 1998, Glazer 1993).

Take, for example, the issue of eligibility for services. Some of the criteria listed suggest a *more* acute need for home care services rather than reasons for denying services. Services can be denied to a client whose condition is not expected to improve. Is this not the case for the elderly infirm, the chronically ill, or the disabled? Services can be denied to a client whose family was not available to participate in care. Is this not the case for many single or elderly women and single parents? I submit that each of these reasons for non-admission are conditions which would extend or increase the cost of providing insurable home care services. More expensive, more labour intensive and long-term services drive up CCAC operating costs. Denying home care services to clients who need these services shifts the work and the cost of care from the government to the private sector, from paid workers to unpaid family members, or worse yet, as Jane Aronson (1999) said, from someone to no one. In this way, the text's design and coding procedures accomplish the business goals of the health care system by requiring the worker to collect data that she must then use to disqualify clients who require more costly support. A similar trend was reported by researchers from George Washington University who studied twenty-eight home care agencies in nine American states (California Healthline 1999). They found that two-thirds of those agencies, in response to reduced funding for insurable services, were taking steps to reduce the proportion of very sick Medicare patients they served.

Third, the format of the new intake record text standardizes the client data that enter into the sequence of communication. Much of the information offered by the client is interpreted by the worker and that interpretation squeezed into an appropriate field. Women who have limited experience with the health care system, who do not speak French or English fluently or who are not savvy advocates for their own health will have difficulty offering the kinds of data that constitute the eligible client (New and Watson 1983: 61). Client data that does not fit into a text field may be excluded, and as a consequence, rendered unavailable for interpretation or further action by subsequent readers. Only client data that is entered into text is available for coding and consideration. Completing a text made up of both free-text and standardized data allows health workers to more quickly determine if and for how long a client will receive a given service. Regulating and standardizing the data that enter into the work process is evidence of the way business discourse competes with medical discourse as the central organizer of client data. Health care workers who enact the new textual process produce an institutional account of the client's needs and resources. These objectified facts are used by the workers to make decisions about who receives home care services and for how long. The worker's subjective knowledge is no longer central to decision-making. Similarly, the client's subjective experience is subordinated to a bureaucratic process designed to ration home care resources.

Conclusion

In multiple ways, the new administrative practices are linked to the exercise of power both at and beyond the local site, and are operative in accomplishing the social relations between workers, and between the worker and the client. Dorothy Smith says, "Power is always the mobilization of people's concerted activities" (1990b: 80). This chapter explores one way that government goals of cost-containment and efficiency penetrate the everyday activities of people working in home care agencies. Comparing the actual work processes performed at two moments in Ontario's home care history reveals how health care workers (predominantly women) have come to act in business-oriented ways that accomplish the functional work and the ideological goals of a restructured home care system. Their concerted activities result in the delivery of limited resources to some clients, the offloading of some labour and costs to private agencies and government subsidized programs, and the downloading of caring labour onto other, unpaid women. It is under these conditions that women are implicated in and affected by the merging of the fiscal health of the state with the health care needs of the individual and family.

Notes

1. My thanks to Dorothy E. Smith and Si Transken for their comments on earlier drafts of this manuscript.
2. See Doris Grinspun in this volume for a discussion of this point.
3. This woman's name and identifying details of her story have been altered to protect her anonymity.
4. While *patient* is the term still used by lay persons and many health workers in everyday communication, the term *client* is used with increasing regularity in Ontario Ministry of Health documents, professional standards of practice and health professional educational curricula. The shift in terminology from patient to client reflects the shift away from traditional discourse of health care delivery toward the discourse of business wherein a client is

constructed as a service recipient rather than as a care recipient.

5. Home care and long-term programs across Canada underwent changes similar to those affecting Ontario during the 1990s. The nature and process of those changes, however, varied from province to province. As Sheila Neysmith (1998) notes, this is because there is no federal legislation comparable to the *Canada Health Act* that organizes these programs or their budgets. Instead budgets for community-based programs usually reside with the provincial ministries of health "where they must jostle for resources alongside the powerful interests that represent acute care" (Neysmith 1998: 235).

6. At this time, professional services were defined as those provided by a nurse, physiotherapist, speech-language pathologist, nutritionist, occupational therapist, social worker or laboratory technician.

7. The intake worker is usually a nurse although other health professionals such as a social worker, occupational therapist or physiotherapist may be trained to perform this job.

8. Other Canadian provinces also proposed similar strategies for shifting the responsibilities and costs of caregiving into community-based programs, into the home (Angus 1992, Neysmith 1998) and, consequently, onto the shoulders of women.

9. Hospital restructuring took the form of shorter patient stays, increases in same-day surgery, higher patient turnover, displacement of hundreds of professional and nonprofessional staff and cuts to programs and services. These initiatives had multiple and varying effects on women as caregivers and care recipients (Grayson 1993, Gregor 1995, Gustafson 1996 and 1998b, OMOH 1993 and 1994, OCHU/CUPE 1995).

10. Nurses displaced by hospital downsizing and eager to work for economic survival accept part-time jobs with no benefits in community-based agencies where they make considerably lower wages than their hospital colleagues (Gustafson 1996). Paying lower wages to qualified personnel allows service provider agencies to submit lower bids, win government contracts with CCACs and sustain their own viability.

11. See also Douglass Drozdow-St. Christian in this volume.

12. See also Denise Spitzer and Guruge, Donner and Morrison in this volume.

13. See also Denise Spitzer and Simpson and Porte in this volume.

14. For a discussion of the multiple and contradictory effects of the RHPA on professional practice in Ontario, see Lum and Williams in this volume.

10

"And Then There Were None": An Experience in Building an Integrated Health Service among the Chippewas of Georgina Island[1]

Patricia E. Simpson and Sheila Porte

June 29, 1998—The front page of the weekly edition of the *Georgina Advocate* laying open at the checkout at the Foodland store on Baseline Road in mainland Georgina, boasts an "[h]istoric self-government agreement..." between Indian Affairs and the Chippewas of Georgina Island.[2] Outside, a six-month-old announcement of the October 1997 local performance of Agatha Christie's "Ten Little Indians"[3] remains lettered on the glass-encased notice board. The board is a stone's throw from Sutton District High School, where courses in the Ojibwa language and Native Studies are held up as signifiers of the community's collective tolerance of difference. Yet, Chippewa students at the school are required to relocate from their homes on the Georgina Island reserve to the mainland each fall because it is too dangerous to cross the lake on a regular basis during the school year, what with the variability of water and ice conditions through the channel and a car barge known to catch fire mid-crossing. "Death by misadventure" on the lake, say public health officials, is the primary cause of death among the 231 on-reserve Chippewas.

Georgina is a small, central Ontario community rife with contradictions. Although united by the centrality of Lake Simcoe in their midst and residents' seasonal preoccupations with fishing, the Town is also geographically and culturally divided by the lake. The Town proudly boasts the banner of "Ice Fishing Capital of Canada," and yet in 1998, Town Council approved a $600,000 harbour development project which will contribute substantially to the range of toxic chemicals, including mercury and DDT, already known to be contaminating lake catch (EAGLE Working Group 1995).[4] And while the Town's diversity is celebrated at events such as the annual pow wow at Sutton District High School, few mainstream community-development activities include representation from the Chippewas. In fact, it is quite common for the Chippewas to be completely overlooked in local planning initiatives. The 1997 York Region Health Services *Health Status Report 1991–1996*, for example, makes no mention of the health status of Island residents or of the unique challenges to healthy living faced by Chippewas both on and off the reserve. Moreover, while the many untimely and tragic deaths of Chippewas due to drowning and exposure on Lake Simcoe have become a part of Town lore, the Chippewas' present-day living conditions remain, for the most part, invisible. Only a handful of non-Native mainlanders have ever been to Georgina Island; most have no knowledge of how to get there or of the difficulties involved in having to transport all amenities from the mainland across the channel's notoriously unpredictable waters.

Our Standpoint in the Everyday World of Native / Non-Native Relations

Canada's historic maltreatment of its indigenous peoples is foundational to the contradictions that characterize relations in Georgina today. In this paper, we report on a project, which we initiated in mid-1996, broadly aimed at improving the quality of these relations. This project arose out of our concern for the historic disparity between Native and non-Native health care as it has taken shape within our Town. As long-time residents, we knew that many programs and services were simply not accessible to the peoples of Georgina Island. Equally central to our project, however, was our growing concern about the broad restructuring of health care in Ontario. We knew that health care reform was having a qualitatively different effect in the lives of women as compared to men in our community. We knew that women made up the majority of home care users, as well as the majority of paid health care workers and unpaid family caregivers. And we also knew that health care reform was having a qualitatively different effect in the lives of women resident on Georgina Island as compared to women resident on the mainland of Georgina.

In the pages that follow, we recount our efforts and the efforts of other local women to redress the inadequacy of health services among the Chippewas and the differential effects of health care reform in Ontario through the extension of our Town's mainland hospice services to Georgina Island. However, our aim is to provide more than a simple documentation of our experiences. Drawing on Dorothy E. Smith's (1987, 1990a and 1999) analytic procedures, where the exercise of power is examined as ruling practices in the everyday world, we endeavour to reveal how the inadequacy of health services among the Chippewas of Georgina Island is an accomplishment of relations of ruling.[5] Our aim is to make visible the kinds of ruling practices which determine the course of our lives at a local level, as well as the ways in which we, as white women,[6] are active in these ruling practices.

We build our argument from our standpoint in the everyday world of Native/non-Native relations. At the time of undertaking this project, we were responsible for the leadership of hospice services in our Town. One of us, Patricia Simpson, was the Executive Director of Hospice Georgina, and the other, Sheila Porte, was a member of Hospice Georgina's volunteer board of directors. Although differently situated—one of us, a resident of the mainland and of European heritage, and the other, a resident of the Island and of mixed European and Native heritage—as white women we share a sense of responsibility for the redress of historical and contemporary injustices manifest in our community. We also share an awareness of how relations of power and knowledge are organized in and through institutions and discourses in ways that make it possible for us to live these relations without reflecting on them. There is nothing from within our positions of privilege as members of the dominant group that reflects back on this privilege; it just is. Hence, our project—as the writing of this paper—has arisen out of our desire to name the social construction of our own power and privilege and the limitations of this power and privilege, as a way of contributing to the transformation of relations in the place where we live, work and raise our children.

We begin with an overview of the historical circumstances of our Town in our effort to reveal how we came to be where we are today. Drawing on the work of Harvey McCue (1978), we marshall evidence to show that the history of our Town is rooted in the violence of European imperialism. We argue that the legacy of European imperialism is today manifest in ways which are both ideological and material. We discuss, for example, the prevailing notion that residency on Georgina Island is entirely a matter of individual choosing, as well as the commonly held belief that all townspeople may be neatly accommodated in one of two groups—"white/mainland resident" or "Chippewa/Island resident." We also detail the material means by which the Island population's capacity to cope with life-threatening illness and grief has been curtailed. Finally, we link the history of Georgina and our imperial legacy with contemporary injustice in our Town taking shape in the form of Ontario's health care system restructuring. We raise questions about partnerships between mainstream and Native communities and ask whether (equal) partnership is, indeed, achievable, or if such an endeavour simply acts to reproduce a hierarchical relationship founded on the value dualisms of "white" versus "Native" and "professional health care" versus "traditional medicine." We conclude that, as white women, we are agents of "neocolonialist" power and are thereby active in accomplishing the imperial project which began in this country almost five hundred years ago, at the same time as we may be agents of change. In the final pages of our paper, we urge other, similarly situated women to consider their own everyday experiences as a standpoint from which to explore institutional practices operative in their lives. Such a methodological starting point, we suggest, offers a means of extending women's understandings of extra-local forms of social organization and how it is that these extra-local forms operate to order and control our lives and the lives of other, differently situated women.

How We Came to be Where We are Today

The Chippewas of Georgina Island have a long, documented history marked by the subversion of their pre-capitalist subsistence economy and the state's imposition of an elaborate and tightly regulated system of segregation running parallel to a correspondingly intricate plan for Native assimilation (Bourgeault 1991: 88). The Chippewa's history has been contorted by efforts on the part of British and French colonizers and their descendants to make First Nations peoples dependent upon them and their governments and other institutions. The Royal Commission on Aboriginal Peoples (1996)[7] has chronicled the human and social costs of the imperial project that has taken shape on Canadian soil. From the outset, this imperial project has involved violent, opportunistic encounters with pre-existing indigenous societies.

During the War of 1812, the Chippewas of Lake Simcoe were loyal to the British and contributed at least fourteen of their men to the British forces during the Battle of York in Upper Canada (McCue 1978: 6).[8] After the war, the Chippewas of Lake Huron and Lake Simcoe surrendered land on which the present day counties of Simcoe, Grey, Wellington and Dufferin are located, thereby enabling the British to establish new routes from Niagara to Michilmackinac and from York to Matchedash Bay to shorten the travel time between Montreal and Lake Superior (7). In return for $4,000 in 1815 and $1,200 in goods in 1818, the government took possession of almost two million acres of prime settlement land, including Holland Landing, which was considered strategically important for the movement of military personnel and materials (7). Then in 1830, at the behest of Lieutenant-Governor John Colborne, the Chippewas of Lake Simcoe were moved from Snake Island and the Cook's Bay area of Lake Simcoe to a stretch of land between Coldwater and Lake Couchiching. Colborne was charged with responsibility for implementing a policy of

Indian segregation and he delegated to Thomas Anderson, his newly appointed Superintendent of Simcoe and Matchedash, the task of promoting farming in an attempt to reduce the band's nomadic patterns. It was hoped that farming would make it easier for missionaries "whose tasks of conversions were weakened in the absence of established settlements" (9). In time, the Chippewas' successful farming of the "Coldwater Tract" caught the attention of the new Lieutenant-Governor, Sir Francis Bond Head, and he ordered the Chippewas off the land to make room for British settlers (Cowie 1997). By about 1839, Chief Joseph Snake had moved his band back to Snake Island, but by the mid-1870s, most of the band had relocated to its present-day location on neighbouring Georgina Island, where more arable land was available.

At the time of the Chippewas' relocation to Georgina Island, the water level around the sand islands that dot the channel between the mainland and the Island reserve was only ankle-deep and the Chippewas were able to walk back and forth from the mainland, herding their cattle and bringing wagon loads of goods across from Nolans' Landing (Cowie 1997: 6). However, the building of the Trent-Severn Waterway in the early part of this century changed all that and proved catastrophic to the Chippewa way of life. According to elders and other long-time residents, the water depth in the channel rose by up to fourteen feet, submerging the Chippewas' fields of wild rice, a main staple of their diet.[9] Farming gradually declined due to difficulties getting farm machinery across to the islands, and many band members were forced to seek employment on the mainland.

Today, the channel crossing remains hazardous to safe year-round movement. Storms come up suddenly on the lake and the water in the channel, which forty years ago froze to several feet deep, freezes today to only about twelve inches in thickness. In the past eighty years, since the completion of the first phase of the Trent-Severn Waterway, twenty-six Chippewas have died by drowning or exposure on the lake. In the past five years alone, an esteemed Chippewa physician, a respected teacher and two cherished women elders have succumbed to the perils of travel across the channel. On the night of December 30, 1998, when the Island car barge broke down with a full load of cars and their occupants aboard, the aging ferry had to be used to push the barge across the icy waters to the Island. Events such as this have become quite commonplace in our Town—so commonplace, in fact, that they rarely receive much local attention.

The seeming lack of noteworthiness of these common occurrences may be explained, in part, by the prevailing notion that residency on the Island is entirely a matter of individual choosing. This notion is reinforced through the seasonal presence of cottagers who come from as far away as Michigan and as nearby as Sutton to vacation on Island land leased from the band. Visitors who cross to the Island for the first time frequently romanticize the perils of crossing by boat or ice road; they often speak of "escaping" to the Island and of the so-called "simple life" as a proxy for progress and material wealth. Thus, the dangers of having to rely on the passenger ferry, car barge and ice road to get back and forth between the Island and the mainland are perceived as part and parcel of Island residents' choice of a more remote (read idyllic) place of residency and a slower paced (read originary) style of life made possible by being cut off from the mainland.

The history of settlement in Georgina helps us, as white women, to see how we came to be where we are today. The notion that residency on the Island is simply a matter of individual free choice is rendered false by the Island's history and by the present day realities of life on the reserve. Within the context of state segregation and regulation of Native peoples, what is understood as free choice is revealed to be coerced voluntariness. The dangers of travel to and from the Island are exposed as integral to systems of oppression and inequality which have developed over time in our Town as part of a nation-building project which has eclipsed the nationhood of Native peoples and from which we, as white women, have directly benefitted. The concept of free choice is an artifact of dominant ideology—both a product and producer of a social order in which the dominance of one falsely homogenized group, namely European colonizers and their descendants, is made possible through—and, in-deed, mutually constitutive of—the subordination of another similarly diverse, yet falsely homogenized group, namely the Chippewas.

Our colonizing "forefathers" (men were the most direct agents of empire) left us many legacies, most of them unfortunate, many of them destructive. One such legacy has been the collapse of rich, diverse identities into two monolithic and polarized groups, one marked "In-dian" and inscribed as inferior, the other denoted "settler" or "land owner" and engraved as superior.[10] The state's system of categorizing Native peoples is based on the assumption that the population can be broken down into a binary comprised of "Indians" and "non-Indians." And yet this type of "either/or" categorization cannot possibly accom-modate the complexities of lived experience. A white woman who lives on Georgina Island with her Chippewa husband and their children may identify as other than either white or Chippewa; a woman of mixed parentage may think of her identity as shifting over time (Zack 1994). Moreover, the designating of "Indian status" at the birth of a child is far from a straightforward process and is influenced as much by social relations within the band as by so-called blood percentages.[11] But the fact that the reality of life belies the either/or reductive manoeuver matters little. The Indian/non-Indian binary holds enormous sway because it is written over with other binaries which organize dominant modes of thought, such as animal versus human, nature versus culture, and body versus mind. These dualisms are deeply entrenched habits of thought which prop up systems of oppression and inequality and which have real material consequences.

Our Imperial Legacy
The material consequences of the imperial legacy of false dualisms have taken many different forms over time. Today, these consequences include a divided system of health care funding and delivery based on two interlocking assumptions: 1) that all persons living on-reserve are Native and all persons living off-reserve are non-Native; and 2) that one's identity is fixed and unchanging over time. While there is movement on both the federal and provincial fronts to consolidate health care funding and delivery,[12] today in Georgina, the prevailing bifurcated system continues to disadvantage Chippewas and their Native and non-Native family members.

The Community Health Centre on Georgina Island, which is funded by the Medical Services Branch of Health Canada, provides an array of health promotion and illness prevention programs and services for status (i.e., registered) Chippewas.[13] These programs and services range from blood pressure clinics to workshops on smoking cessation and sexually transmitted diseases. While the centre provides no active treatment, Chippewa residents with status can be assessed by health care practitioners, including a psychologist, a chiropractor and a massage therapist, who visit the Island on a pre-scheduled basis. It should be noted, however, that the provision of these services depends on these practitioners' willingness to negotiate the channel crossing. These same health promotion programs and health care treatment services are offered in locations throughout mainland Georgina, primarily in the urban nodes of Keswick, Sutton and Pefferlaw. These programs and services are directed at the non-Native population and are funded by the Ministry of Health of the Province of Ontario. By contrast, these mainland programs and services do not depend on practitioners' willingness to participate.

The individual differences within the communities and the broad diversity in the definition of residence have been reduced into two monolithic groupings—white/mainland resident versus Chippewa/Island resident. This is foundational to gaps in local health service delivery. Yet, like the dangers posed by the necessity of travel across the channel, the Chippewas' difficulties around access to health care are taken-for-granted features of life in Georgina. The fact that the Island is twenty minutes by car barge followed by forty minutes by land ambulance away from the nearest hospital—and this in only the most favour-able of conditions—warrants little attention. Even life-long residents of the area seem unaware that when a fully equipped ambulance is needed on the Island it has to make the trip from the Virginia Beach boat launch to the Island and back again by barge; if it misses the routine barge departure, there can be up to a half-hour delay on either side of the crossing. This means that when people on the Island are in the most acute need of medical treatment they can be up to two hours away from the nearest hospital.

The gaps in local health service delivery have the greatest effect on those who are chronically ill and permanently disabled. The situation of one elderly Chippewa man confined to a wheelchair offers a case in point. This man relocates on a seasonal basis between the mainland and his long- time home on Georgina Island. With each relocation to the main-land, he must be processed by the Province of Ontario's home care bureaucracy, which means that he and his son and daughter-in-law must make do until a home support worker has been assigned to his so-called "case." Sometimes the delay is just a few days; more recently, with the advent of the new Community Care Access Centre (CCAC) in York Region, it is up to two weeks.[14] Once assigned, the home support worker visits twice a day to assist him with bathing and other personal care, as well as preparation of his mid-day meal, relieving his daughter-in-law of these responsibilities. With each relocation to the Island, however, he depends on the availability of the Island's one health care aide. His daughter-in-law explains that when her father is on the Island, she makes arrange-ments to leave work every day at noon to check on him and prepare him his meal.

In another instance, the family of an elderly Chippewa woman who requires intensive nursing care is likewise caught in the gulf between two differently funded and differently oriented health care systems. The woman's daughters have provided her with loving, round-the-clock care for many months; one of them even quit her job to move back to the Island to care for her mother. Their brother, who lives close by on the Island, visits their mother, but only for short periods of time. Days have stretched into weeks, weeks into months, and the health of both daughters has begun to suffer. Long days filled with bathing, dressing and lifting their mother in and out of her wheelchair are followed by sleepless nights of turning, repositioning and changing bed linens. One daughter says she is "having trouble with her nerves" and is smoking more heavily since moving in with her mother. "Neighbours keep their distance," the daughters explain, adding that neighbours may be leery of the Hoyer lift and oxygen tank that have been moved into their mother's house. As well, there is no visiting nurse from the mainland who will agree to travel to the Island to relieve the daughters.[15] As a result, they have become reliant on the Island's community health nurse who drops by on her own time in the evenings to lend them a hand. Shortly after their mother's discharge from hospital, the daughters were told a physiotherapist from the mainland would visit to assess their mother. But six weeks have passed. High winds and rain have been making the channel crossing especially difficult; perhaps, they offer, this is why they have had no news, as yet, of the visit. In the meantime, their mother goes without the therapy she so desperately needs and the daughters have all they can do to help their mother with the necessities of daily living. These women do not want to move their mother away from her Island community, much less to a nursing home on the mainland several hours drive away. They say they "have seen too many elders leave the Island and never come back." But the daughters are faced with a difficult choice: they can continue to care for their mother at the risk of their own declining health, or they can separate their mother from her family and friends and the comfort of her home community and admit her to a nursing home on the mainland where she will be the only Native woman. Here we come to see how an apparently similar range of choices (to care at home or to admit to a nursing home) has a qualitatively different effect in the lives of women on Georgina Island compared to women on the mainland.[16]

Restructuring on the Backs of Women, Young and Old

The preceding two situations attest to women's caregiving responsibilities in Canadian society today where women bear the brunt of caring for ill and aging family members and friends. This fact is confirmed by the Canadian Study of Health and Aging (1994) and by a Statistics Canada report on Canadian caregiving."[17] According to the Statistics Canada (1997a) report, 19 percent of women between the ages of forty-five and sixty-four are caregivers compared to 11 percent of men in the same age group. Moreover, most of these women caregivers "already have many obligations, with the majority being married with children and having work commitments outside the home" (Cranswick 1997: 3). But not only do more women than men have caregiving responsibilities, women caregivers "are doing the more demanding tasks such as personal care" (4) compared to men caregivers who tend to have women in their lives to support them in their caregiving tasks.[18]

The greater responsibility of women for caregiving in our society is rooted in a dominant gender ideology that attributes to women a "natural" proclivity to empathy and caring. Consider the fact that 15 percent of women employed outside the home are also caregivers compared to 10 percent of employed men, and that 16 percent of unemployed women combine job search activities with caregiving duties as compared to 12 percent of unemployed men (Cranswick 1997: 3). But what is especially significant about prevailing gender ideology is that, while it seemingly pays tribute to women's caregiving capacities, it also attaches lesser value to women's labour. As a result, a woman is often seen as the obvious choice to assume the caregiver role within a family precisely because, compared to a man, she risks losing less income and fewer benefits, and stands to forfeit fewer career advancement opportunities when she takes on caregiving responsibilities that compromise her ability to seek or maintain employment. Moreover, since five times more women than men work part-time, women are generally seen to be more available than men to assume caregiving responsibilities. And although labour analysts speculate that women work part-time in order to juggle family and community responsibilities, a Statistics Canada report reveals that 34 percent of women who work part-time want full-time jobs (Crawford 1998b, Fast and Da Pont 1997).[19] The gender ideology which glorifies women's so-called instinctive caregiving capacities and which assigns lesser value to their labour places women in the position of assuming the burden of caregiving responsibilities; this, in turn, operates to keep women socioeconomically disadvantaged in our society. There are, of course, a host of other social relations—age and class, for example— which layer over and intersect with relations of gender and likewise come to organize women's lives.

In Ontario, the policies of the Progressive Conservatives under the leadership of Mike Harris have added to women's condition of socioeconomic disadvantage. The provincial Tories have downsized the public sector, which was an important component of women's employment gains during the 1970s and 1980s. It was primarily through the public service that women were able to narrow the wage gap with men from 66 percent in 1989 to 73.4 percent in 1996. But since the spring of 1996, 16,000 people have been eliminated from the provincial civil service payroll and there have been huge cuts to female-dominated fields such as nursing and social work. Women's progress is being undermined through the creation of new structures of production, including part-time work and other practices of work flexibility, that relegate women again to the lower echelons of the labour hierarchy (Benería 1997: 329). Thus, more and more women are being confined to work within the home, a point made poignantly with the addition, for the first time, of babysitting to the list of the top ten jobs most frequently cited by women for the year 1996 (Crawford 1998a: L2). A policy research paper recently published by the Canadian Research Institute for the Advancement of Women (CRIAW) confirms that the current thrust towards the "'deprofessionalization' of home care work" is contributing to Canadian women's vulnerability to poverty (Morris et al. 1999).

Health care restructuring under the provincial Tories is increasing the numbers of acutely and chronically ill people being cared for at home and thereby contributing further to women's burden. Shortly after taking office, and despite a pre-election promise not to cut health spending, the Tories decreased provincial grants to hospitals by $800 million and slashed funding to community-based projects addressing a broad determinant of health issues.[20] As a result, people are not only being released from hospital earlier and earlier with more and more surgery being done on a day-surgery basis, but they are being released into community environments unprepared for added responsibility for health matters. The impact on the home care system has been immediate and direct.

In July 1998, North York's Community Care Access Centre (CCAC), one of Ontario's forty-three new home care brokering agencies, reported that its nursing caseload for the year was almost double that predicted owing to "a growing number of acute care patients, 'mostly the elderly with chronic diseases' released by hospitals into the home care system" (Anderson quoted in Walkom 1998: B5). Since then, the Tories' promised health reinvestments have arrived in the form of funding to support a continuation of the historic dominance of institutional health care with its focus on acute care and biomedicine, including MRI machines, $32.8 million paid to eighty-one of the province's hospitals for "overflow" beds already in operation and a regional cardiac care centre at York County Hospital in Newmarket. In the meantime, the home care system continues to grow "leaner and meaner," and there is mounting pressure on women to pick up more and more caregiving responsibilities. During the winter of 1998, a seriously ill woman and sole-support mother who lives in Georgina had her home care curtailed, leaving her two young daughters to walk two kilometres to the nearest store to purchase groceries and push them home in a borrowed grocery cart. The woman expressed her frustration about this situation:

> There's no sidewalk and the snow is piled too high to push [the cart] through. It's not safe. But it's more than that. My girls shouldn't have this indignity. I worked all my life and now we just need some help.

There is mounting evidence that the provincial Tories' health care restructuring is occurring on the backs of women—young and old alike.

The Tories' restructuring agenda, which is being fuelled by their election promise of a balanced budget and a 30 percent reduction in provincial income tax rates, is having another trickle down effect which disproportionately touches the lives of women. Community-based groups are increasingly being called upon to step in and fill the gap left by the withdrawal or inadequate provision of publicly funded services with volunteers. Many people celebrate the use of volunteers as a so-called return to traditional community values. However, the specific ways in which volunteers are active within their communities reveal the inadequacy of this analysis. The distribution of volunteer work is not only tipped toward women (Cranswick 1997: 3, Denton et al. 1998: 17),[21] but the nature of women's and men's volunteer involvements differ significantly. According to a report on work environments in community-based health and social service agencies published by the McMaster Research Centre for the Promotion of Women's Health, it is women volunteers who do the work involving personal care (Denton et al. 1998: 6–7). And like caregiving within the family, this work exacts a considerable toll on women, with as much as 54 percent of home care volunteers in one study reporting "depression or burnout" (Denton et al. 1998: 78).

"Filling The Gap" in Georgina
By late 1996, the effects of the Tories' health care restructuring were being felt in Georgina and in Hospice Georgina. Hospice Georgina is a not-for-profit community agency based on the mainland providing care to people with life-threatening illness and their families. Hospice Georgina receives $12,500 in funding annually from the Ministry of Health. Volunteers from the mainland raise additional funds through local fundraising activities. Like other local hospices, Hospice Georgina works in affiliation with Palliative Care Services of York Region (PCSYR) which acts as a transfer agency and a regional trainer for hospice volunteers. Hospice Georgina has a part-time executive director who is responsible for the coordination of hospice services within the community as well as volunteer recruitment and support.

The number of calls for assistance to Hospice Georgina from overextended families had begun to climb dramatically and the situations of more and more families were near crisis by the time their request for help was received. One night, a Hospice visiting volunteer paid a late night call to a man who lived in a local trailer park with his wife who was near death. A neighbour had called and asked for a volunteer to come immediately. The volunteer's notes summarize what she encountered:

> Knocked on door, but no response. Entered and found Mr. ___
> crying at wife's bedside. Says he has been trying to feed her
> crushed Tylenol in yogurt (no elixir!) to ease her laboured breath-
> ing. She appears comatose. He has been alone x 4 days; no
> visiting nurse over weekend. Called doctor's office, but he is

away 'til Tuesday; does not think there is an on-call. Sat together and chatted; calmer; made pot of tea. Called priest.

It was around this time that York Region Home Care (now the CCAC) and local providers of care in the home began appealing to Hospice Georgina for respite for families of people with serious, but non-terminal, illnesses—a young woman and mother of a brain-injured teen who needed relief in order to do some banking; an ailing elderly woman and her husband who were housebound and needed some emotional support; the family of a severely disabled Chippewa woman on Georgina Island needing a day of respite to attend to business on the mainland. Hospice Georgina had twelve visiting volunteer caregivers at the time, all but one of whom lived on the mainland. Nine of these volunteers were each providing regular support to one local family; two of these volunteers were each providing support to two local families. As well, the then executive director of Hospice Georgina was working in cooperation with a school parent association and a group of women at a local church to provide meal preparation assistance to families in crisis. But it seemed there was never quite enough help to go around.

The situations of families on Georgina Island were especially acute. The premature deaths of four members of the Island community in just five short years had exhausted its available resources and depleted the Island population's capacity to cope with life-threatening illness and grief. Hospice volunteers from the mainland, many of whom were already overextended, were reluctant to regularly make the channel crossing. Even those willing to make the trip were unable to do so during times of the lake's freeze-up and thaw.

The Dilemma of Partnership

In early 1997, the members of the volunteer board of directors of Hospice Georgina—all of whom were local residents, some of whom were also recipients of hospice services or local health care practitioners—began discussing ways of building the Island population's collective capacity to care for families in crisis while, at the same time, forging a stronger link between the Island and the mainland. In consultation with the Hospice Georgina directors, we developed a general proposal for a joint project between the Chippewas of Georgina Island and Hospice Georgina, based on the principles of primary health care.[22] The proposal centred on establishing a partnership involving the extension of hospice services onto the Island and the provision of training for Island residents interested in becoming hospice visiting volunteer caregivers. We shared this proposal with the executive director of Palliative Care Services of York Region. PCSYR is funded by the Ministry of Health as a regional trainer in palliative care and as the manager of York Region's pain and symptom management teams. PCSYR also serves as a conduit for funds which flow from the Ministry of Health to palliative care agencies in York Region. The executive director of PCSYR suggested that we prepare funding proposals for submission to PCSYR and to the United Way of York Region.

We then proceeded to develop two brief funding proposals to append to our general proposal. In the first of these funding proposals, we requested $30,000 from the United Way of York Region under its Community Initiatives Funding to cover the cost of extending Hospice Georgina services onto the Island. The United Way provides this type of funding in the form of short-term operating grants for projects that address one of its designated "priority areas" for funding, which at the time included promoting ethnoracial diversity and building "community capacity" (United Way of York Region 1996: 4 and 1998: 8).

Our proposal met the United Way's two key criteria, which were non-duplication in the service being proposed and lack of alternative funding. The evaluation component of our proposal centred on the number of Islanders we anticipated training as volunteers and the population of the Island community to be served by these volunteers. We also addressed qualitative measures which centred on quality-of-life issues for Island residents; first and foremost among these was the necessity for very sick and dying people resident on the Island to leave their home community due to lack of in-home volunteer caregiver support.

These same project evaluation criteria were addressed in the second of our two funding proposals which was submitted to PCSYR. This proposal requested that PCSYR provide one of its routine volunteer training sessions on the Island. Hospice Georgina pays an annual fee to PCSYR for the provision of training for its volunteers, and so this proposal addressed only those additional costs to be incurred by PCSYR, such as the cost of educators' travel between the mainland and the Island.

We submitted our proposals in June 1997. Within two weeks, the Ministry of Health's long-term care coordinator expressed reservations about PCSYR's support for Hospice Georgina's alliance with the Chippewas and requested documentation detailing "outcome measures" for the partnership. She also directed the executive director of PCSYR to request a written statement from the Chippewas of Georgina Island tribal council indicating its support for the project. Although this request was made on two occasions, no such statement from the council was forthcoming. This may have been the result of miscommunication between Hospice Georgina and the tribal council; it may also have been an expression of the tribal council's resistance to the government's way of forging a partnership.

When the fall of 1997 arrived and we were still awaiting a response from PCSYR on its provision of training on the Island, we decided to proceed with developing an implementation plan while the weather still permitted crossing of the channel. We called a group together—residents, educators, health care practitioners and other interested people—for a discussion on the Island. At this meeting, a planning group was established with representation from hospice families and health care practitioners, from Island residents and mainland residents. In the meantime, we received a call of inquiry about our proposal from a member of the United Way's Citizen Review Panel. He asked us to explain how the planned partnership between Hospice Georgina and the Chippewas would lead to "improved efficiencies" and remarked, "Thirty thousand dollars seems like a lot of money to spend on a dying population."

In April 1998, Hospice Georgina received $15,000 of United Way Community Initiatives funding. But the expenditure of this money was immediately thrown into question when PCSYR recommended that an administrative fee in the amount of approximately $5000 be held back by Hospice Georgina to offset the cost of overseeing development of an administrative centre on the Island. After much discussion, the board decided to direct the full $15,000 to developing services on the Island. By this time, Hospice Georgina had a new executive director and, together with the board of directors, she commenced the process of hiring someone to coordinate the Island's hospice services. The job title for this position proved to be a contentious issue, with some people favouring the title "sub-coordinator." The title eventually selected was "Island coordinator," a title which nonetheless places the incumbent in a position of subordinancy to rather than partnership with the executive director.

In the fall of 1998, the board of directors and the new executive director decided to proceed with planning a training session for Island residents despite the lack of a formal expression of support from Palliative Care Services of York Region. Time was slipping by and the members of the Hospice Georgina board of directors felt a sense of urgency around the need to proceed with the project. The Island coordinator took charge of contacting speakers, booking meeting rooms and arranging the series of workshops. The tribal council covered transportation costs and the cost of producing teaching materials. The Island coordinator ensured that the teaching materials contained all the necessary components of the PCSYR *Core Concepts in Palliative Care* program as well as topics of special relevance to the care of Native peoples. In fact, many of the educators who teach in the PCSYR *Core Concepts* program taught in the Island training session. Nonetheless, when the session was completed, PCSYR was unwilling to provide the ten newly trained volunteers with certificates of accomplishment unless the phrase "from a Native perspective" was added to each one. This action was finally agreed upon despite the objections of some local organizers and some of the newly trained volunteers who felt this qualifier conveyed a negative message regarding either the quality of the training session or the level of care deemed adequate for residents of the Island. However, Hospice Georgina staff and volunteers knew that without the certificate of achievement, visiting volunteer caregivers could be placed in the position of having to assume additional personal liability for their provision of care to people with life-threatening illnesses.

Less than a year into the partnership between Hospice Georgina and the Chippewas of Georgina Island, the newly hired Island coordinator now coordinates the care of twenty-three people on and off the Island; this is more than twice the number whose care is coordinated by the Hospice Georgina executive director, who is based on the mainland. Lower numbers on the mainland are attributable, in large part, to personnel changes at the local CCAC which have required the executive director to rebuild relationships and communication channels between Hospice Georgina and the CCAC. And there are other inequities. The Island coordinator works up to forty hours a week and is paid for twelve hours a week at an hourly salary approximately two-thirds that of the executive director. An increasing percentage of the Island coordinator's time is allocated to meetings and committee work. Similarly, the executive director is working far in excess of the number of hours for which she is being paid, due to PCSYR and Ministry of Health requirements regarding the monitoring and reporting of "client" referrals and volunteer activities, and the demands of meetings and committee work. Moreover, the Island coordinator has a dual reporting relationship to uphold; she reports both to the Chippewas of Georgina Island tribal council and to the Hospice Georgina board of directors. All program funds are controlled centrally by the board of directors, and existing financial systems require both the Island coordinator and the executive director to pay out of their own pockets for many program expenses and then seek reimbursement.

The Hospice Georgina/Chippewas partnership is in its early stages, and board members and staff believe it holds much potential. They share a sense of commitment to this partnership as one which is providing a space in which to work out attitudes, beliefs, assumptions and aspirations, and which may ultimately lead to new relationships based on improved understanding. But the progress of the project raises difficult questions around the meaning of the word partnership and whether (equal) partnership is achievable in an environment in which one of the partners is perceived as having more legitimacy within the mainstream health sector, has more experience in the formal home care industry, has more internal authority, has more conventional networks to draw upon, has direct control of funds and so on. There is a real possibility for this partnership to "act as a cloak for ... neocolonialism" (Porter and Sadli 1997: 73), to reproduce a hierarchical relationship founded on the value dualisms of white versus Native and professional health care versus traditional medicine. Perhaps the potential for this to happen is even greater in this case because those affiliated with the dominant partner—that is, Hospice Georgina board members and staff—are predominantly women and so-called lay persons or direct providers of care, who are themselves considered marginal relative to other, more powerful decision-makers.

As central as dualisms are to prevailing systems of oppression and inequality, they are concepts which are, themselves, rooted in the imperial enlightenment and, therefore, are inadequate to the task of explaining, let alone critically opposing, the persistent legacies of imperialism. Anne McClintock argues this point in her challenging and thoroughly unforgettable book, *Imperial Leather,* in which she says that the notion of imperialism as "an inherently British project that impelled itself outward from a European centre to subjugate the peripheral territories of 'the Other'" falls short. Imperial power, McClintock (1995) argues, "emerged from a constellation of processes taking haphazard shape from myriad encounters with alternative forms of authority, knowledge and power" (15–16). Therefore, as white women, we are called upon to develop more sophisticated understandings of the overdeterminations of power and to seek to answer how power succeeds despite its provisionality and despite its constitution in contradictions such as those which characterize relations in our Town today.

The Everyday as our Problematic

A critical exploration that begins with our own experiences as residents of Georgina, and as a staff person and as a volunteer board member with Hospice Georgina, and moves out from there to examine the partnership between Hospice Georgina and the Chippewas reveals institutional processes which operate interdependently to organize, coordinate and regulate our lives and the lives of other women in our community. We come to see how our actions are mediated through institutions of power, such as the Ministry of Health, PCSYR and the United Way. We also see how professionalization reorganizes women's collective non-capitalist forms of organization into hierarchical strata, detaching us from local movements and connecting us, instead, to historically determined relations of ruling that extend beyond our community setting (Smith 1987: 217). We come to understand how our work is organized against us by textually mediated processes[23] in which we engage (Walker 1995: 78), how standardized and standardizing texts and bureaucratic processes, such as reports on volunteer hours and client numbers submitted quarterly by Hospice Georgina staff to PCSYR and the Ministry of Health, not only connect Hospice Georgina to the management system of government but also render women in our community invisible. These and other regulatory textual practices and related processes transform the lives of people who are ill and the women who care for them into abstracted categories through the use of non-descriptive language, like "volunteer" and "client," and figures which are held to be "factual," "objective" and "politically neutral" (Mueller 1995: 100). And yet, as Adele Mueller, drawing on the work of Foucault reminds us, "facticity is a social construction and not a direct relation to any 'real' phenomenon" (100). These texts and processes operate to eliminate the active presence of women as knowers and actors (Smith 1987: 15). Through them, women's knowledge of how to care for others, our judgment and will, is transferred to the practices of bureaucratic administration. Women's work and women's lives disappear from our view. We lose sight of the woman who quit her job to care for her mother; we are unable to see the elderly woman alone in her home with her ailing husband.

By using our own and other women's everyday experiences as a standpoint from which to explore the institutional practices that order and control women's lives, we are also helped to become more aware of social relations we cannot directly observe, but which organize our lives in important and consequential ways. We begin to understand how textual practices and bureaucratic processes connect the local, where we have come to know things as we experience them, with the extra-local which organizes our local setting (Mueller 1995: 99, Smith 1987: 3, 55–56, 98–99 and 1999: 49). The ordinary features of our lives and the lives of other women in our community are revealed to us as taking shape within a larger socioeconomic organization to which they are articulated (Smith 1987: 55–56, 88). Women's greater responsibility for caregiving within the home, women's greater involvement as volunteer providers of care within our community, and women's labour in volunteer-based agencies, which so often complement the allotted number of paid hours, are all tied to externalized and abstracted relations of economic processes. Our own and other women's increasing burden for the care of the ill and the dying in our communities is part of an economic world order operating to amass more and more capital in the hands of fewer and fewer people.

The recent works of Marie Campbell (1998) and Anna Yeatman (1994) shed additional light on the external relations of ruling that infuse and organize women's experiences within community-based organizations today. Yeatman's analysis of the international structuring of national social policies highlights the "performativity" of the postmodern state. Campbell, querying aspects of Canadian health care organization, attempts to specify particular performative practices. Performativity, according to Yeatman, is a principle which has come to replace paternalism in recent times as the basis for the state's control function (1994: 110). She discusses how performativity is operating today, within the context of the global political economy, to recompose relations between the state and the market (111) drawing our attention to the state and the market as differentiated aspects of the same fundamental social relation. The focus of Ontario Ministry of Health and PCSYR staff on what they commonly refer to as "outcome measures" is performative. This is evident in the emphasis placed on the provision of more and more hours of care provided by greater and greater numbers of (women) volunteers or the same number of (women) volunteers providing more and more hours of unpaid labour. These so-called outcomes are performing improved productivity and efficiency of the health care system. But as performance, they also mask a cost-shift from the paid economy to the unpaid economy, from governments to women in households, and obscure how community-based organizations act as extensions of the administrative processes of the state and market. Thus, we see that charitable, volunteer-based agencies, such as the United Way, are increasingly using language and drawing on themes lifted from the marketplace. The recently revised mission statement of the United Way of York Region, for example, emphasizes the importance of "obtaining maximum value from every dollar" (1998: 1).

Beginning from our own standpoint in the everyday world of Native/non-Native relations to explore the partnership between the Chippewas and Hospice Georgina helps us to understand how our everyday behaviours—behaviours which we commonly see as insignificant in the bigger scheme of things—in fact, perform the work of ruling. As Hospice Georgina board members and staff, we do not stand outside of relations of ruling but, rather, are integral to them (Smith 1987: 152). Through our routine administrative activities, state funding and other monies are allocated and the relations of volunteers to clients are organized in certain ways; certain courses of actions and certain experiences come to be treated as more legitimate than others. What is important to grasp here is that our activities are organized by and in turn organize, social relations that reproduce differences—such as those which characterize relations among Island and mainland residents in Georgina today—and thereby accomplish the work of ruling.

Coming to this awareness provides us with a platform for action founded on notions of the personal as political. We must begin by attending to the richness of the resources we bring to our understandings of our own lives, our families, our communities and our local organizations, and recognize the various ways in which we, as women, have been complicit in the social practices of our own silence. But as white women, we must also locate our own privilege and current material circumstances within a historical trajectory, thereby enabling us to trace power relations and, in the words of Dorothy Smith, "raising suspicion against time and its powers of separation" (1987: 23). Furthermore, we must reject old habits which have involved imposing our own interests and methodologies on those who do not inhabit our same sociohistorical spaces, for imperialism is not something that happened elsewhere, in some other time—a disagreeable fact of history external to our identities and current circumstances. We are not responsible for having established the imperialist relations that have marginalized and brutalized Native peoples since the time of European settlement. We are, however, responsible for acknowledging these relations, for exposing their destructive impulses and for laying bare how and where their contemporary forms operate in our lives today.

Notes

1. This paper is dedicated to the memory of Barbara Charles, Lillian Big Canoe and Wanita Big Canoe, whose courageous struggles inspired us to tell about our own experiences.
2. Georgina Island First Nation Reserve is comprised, in full, of a group of three separate islands—Georgina Island, Snake Island and Fox Island—which lie approximately two miles off the southeast shore of Lake Simcoe, plus the shoreline hamlet of Virginia Beach. Most of the on-reserve populace (231 people) resides on Georgina Island, which is the largest island of the three at 4.5 kilometres long and 3.2 kilometres wide.
3. Agatha Christie's 1939 novel based on the nursery rhyme "Ten Little Niggers" and of the same title, is set on Indian Island off the coast of Devon, England. The book was first printed in the United States under the title *And Then There Were None*. In 1965, it was reprinted in the U.S. by Pocket Books under the title *Ten Little Indians*.
4. The Jackson's Point Harbour Development project includes forty-six new transient boat slips with room for expansion to eighty-five slips, two breakwaters and a harbour centre building.
5. Our use of the term "relations of ruling" references "that internally coordinated complex of administrative, managerial, professional and discursive organization that regulates, organizes, governs and otherwise controls our societies" (Smith 1999: 49).
6. Our description of our identities as white is not intended to imply that our identities, or the identities of others, are necessarily static across time. For an

elaboration of this point, see Zack 1995. Our description of ourselves as white is both a reflection of our current identities and our way of drawing attention to the privileges attendant upon being of white or light coloured skin in a racialized capitalist patriarchal society.

7. The report of the Royal Commission on Aboriginal Peoples was released to the public on November 21, 1996. The five-volume report is the culmination of five years of research and hearings conducted in ninety-six communities across Canada. Its 440 recommendations include that a new Royal Proclamation be issued by Her Majesty the Queen, reaffirming the Royal Proclamation of 1763, which would recognize Aboriginal title and governance and commit the Government of Canada to introduce companion legislation to provide Canada's indigenous peoples with the authority and tools to structure their own political, social and economic future. The report also details dozens of initiatives to help Native peoples strengthen their own capacities in areas such as health and economic development.

8. We wish to pay special tribute to the work of Harvey McCue. His 1978 chronicle entitled *The Lake Simcoe Indians: A History from 1792–1876* is an important contribution to the history of our community and was especially valuable in the preparation of this paper.

9. In *I Remember ... An Oral History of the Trent-Severn Waterway,* author Daniel Francis notes that since World War II there have been a series on ongoing conflicts pertaining to water level along the course of the Trent-Severn Waterway. He says that "a growing number of cottagers in the reservoir areas have created another conflict. Vacationers want water levels in their lakes kept up so as not to interfere with swimming and boating" (1984: 41).

10. The procurement of Upper Canada by the English was due, in large measure, to the military support of the Iroquois confederacy (Hall quoted in Clubine 1991: 3). There followed a period of imperialist expansion by Europeans marked by a change in Native peoples' position from ally to subject of the Crown and the rise of an ideology of European superiority and the inferiority of different "races" (Ng 1993: 53).

11. Waldram, Herring and Young explain:
    We can identify two broad legal categories of Aboriginal peoples: those with Indian "status," and those without. "Status" or "registered" Indians are those individuals legally recognized by the federal government to be "Indians" for purposes of the *Indian Act*. First passed in 1876, the *Indian Act* was designed to facilitate the administration of programs to Indians, as well as the assimilation of Indians into mainstream Canadian society. (1995: 10)

12. In 1994, the Minister of Indian Affairs announced in the House of Commons the federal government's intention to dismantle the Department of Indian Affairs and Northern Development. The federal government's role in providing services to Native peoples is increasingly viewed as one of "funder" rather than "provider." But as well, a new relationship is emerging in which the provincial and territorial governments are increasingly interposed between the "special relationship" that has governed federal government/ First Nations relations. In 1991, the Province of Ontario issued a Statement

of Political Relationship acknowledging Native peoples' inherent right of self-government and committing the province to further negotiations to articulate this right. An Aboriginal Health Office was established within the Ministry of Health and, in 1993, a draft Aboriginal Health Policy was prepared which was the first of its kind in Canada (Waldram et al. 1995: 202–03).

13. The provision of health care in First Nation communities is seen to be the responsibility of the Government of Canada. Although the federal government does not accept any treaty obligations to provide health services, "native communities see the provisioning of health care as a historic right enshrined in either treaty, charter or as an obligation flowing from the seizure and occupation of lands" (Ontario Advisory Council on Senior Citizens 1993: 54).

14. Diana Gustafson in this volume uses the same theoretical lens to explore how actual work processes in CCACs facilitate the downloading of caring labour onto family members.

15. It is very common during the late fall, winter and early spring for visiting nurses based on the mainland to refuse to traverse the channel separating mainland Georgina from Georgina Island, citing dangerous water or ice conditions. This is frequently the case even on days when local resident traffic is flowing freely across the channel. Often there is a difference of opinion between the Town of Georgina municipal office and the Chippewas of Georgina Island band office regarding weather conditions and the safety of travel between the mainland and the Island.

16. Douglass Drozdow-St. Christian in this volume investigates how aging women in urban Ontario access appropriate health care services and how they understand their options since health care reform.

17. This 1997 report is based on data from the 1996 General Social Survey which involved the survey of 13,000 Canadians aged fifteen and older in ten provinces between February and December 1996.

18. What is defined as caregiving activity is determined by who is characterized as the caregiver (Keating et al. 1994). The Canadian Study of Health and Aging (1994) found that men tended to participate in short-term, clearly defined activities such as providing transportation and financial support, whereas women tended to coordinate family caregiving and provide more intimate, poorly defined, emotionally exhausting aspects of care. Less intimate activities, like providing transportation or financial support, were less often included in women's caregiving activities.

19. Gregor, Keddy, Foster and Denney in this volume describe the efforts of displaced Nova Scotia nurses to maintain their economic viability by accepting part-time and volunteer work.

20. The federal government's cut in its contribution to the provinces through the Canadian Health and Social Transfer cost Ontario $2.8 billion. The Harris government subsequently cut $800 million from universities, $2.1 billion from welfare and also reduced taxes by $5 billion a year. According to federal Minister of Health, Allan Rock, "Ontario is now receiving more under the Canada Health and Social Transfer (CHST) than it ever has. For 1999–2000, CHST for Ontario totals $10.9 billion in cash and tax transfers, which the

province may use for health care if it wishes" (Rock 2000).

21. Elizabeth Esteves in this volume examines how women's volunteer work is changing as hospitals address the new fiscal imperative.

22. The World Health Organization (WHO) identified primary health care as a favoured strategy to achieve *Health for All by the Year 2000* (WHO 1978b). The principles of primary health care include equitable accessibility of health services to all populations, public participation in the planning and operation of health services, increased emphasis on health services that are preventive and promotive rather than curative only, use of appropriate technology and intersectoral and interdisciplinary collaboration (Stewart 1995).

23. Dorothy Smith argues that the mediation of social relations by texts (written, printed, televised, computerized or other) is a key characteristic of our late-twentieth-century patriarchal capitalist mode of production. The textually mediated character of this mode of production, she says, enables social relations to be organized in abstraction from local settings, "hooked into" extra-local relations of ruling that are embedded in, and yet that transcend, the local setting (1999: 49).

11

The Impact of Canadian Health Care Reform on Recent Women Immigrants and Refugees

Sepali Guruge, Gail J. Donner and Lynn Morrison

Introduction

Every year, over 100,000 immigrants and refugees enter Canada of whom approximately 50 percent are women (Immigration and Citizenship Canada 1997). In spite of this influx, the particular needs and the input of immigrant and refugee women have been mostly ignored in various aspects of health care (Anderson 1985 and 1991, Beiser 1997, Boyd 1975, Guruge 1999, Lynam 1985). This lack of attention is especially relevant as Canada's health care system undergoes changes and reforms.

An overview of immigrants' and refugees' current health situation, including those aspects specific to women, is presented in the first part of this chapter. That immigrant and refugee women are already overburdened due to language, employment and immigration difficulties is highlighted. These difficulties are exacerbated by isolation from family and friends, cultural and functional adjustment to a new country and marginalization and discrimination. This chapter argues that some recent health care reform initiatives increase that burden. The discussion that follows focuses on the impact of three specific reform initiatives on the health of immigrant and refugee women: (1) the empowerment of patients and their active participation in care; (2) a shift in the focus of health care delivery from disease and disease treatment to health promotion and disease prevention; and (3) a shifting of care from hospitals and institutions to the home and the community. Lastly, some recommendations are made for easing the negative impact of immigrant and refugee women's encounters with these reform initiatives.

Immigrants' and Refugees' Current Health Situation

Fundamental inequities in health care persist, despite the relatively good health status of Canadians and despite the promises of equitable health care for all that are made in legislation such as the *Canada Health Act*, the *Canadian Multiculturalism Act* and the *Charter of Rights and Freedoms* (Beiser 1997, Guruge and Donner 1996). Indeed, the opportunity to achieve health is not equitable but, rather, is based on social conditions (Hay 1994). Inadequate housing and nutrition, lack of support systems, unemployment and underemployment can lead to poor health which may in turn restrict people's abilities to improve those immediate conditions. This circularity is particularly evident among immigrants and refugees, who use the health care system less than the mainstream population. Even when they do use it, they do not receive equal or quality care; in fact, immigrants and refugees, especially those who do not speak English, receive poor diagnoses, fewer diagnostic tests, over-prescription of medications and, at times, unnecessary treatments and procedures (Guruge and Donner 1996, Palmer 1991).

A web of factors contributes to this inequity and differential treatment in the Canadian health care system. These factors derive from two categories of sources: those that make it difficult for immigrants and refugees to access and use the health care system; and those that make it difficult for health care professionals to provide quality care to immigrants and refugees. This chapter addresses the factors associated with the first category, with attention to the needs of women immigrants and refugees. For a discussion of the factors associated with the second category, see Guruge and Donner (1996).[1] Although some of these factors that contribute to inequity and differential treatment are applicable to English- and French-speaking Canadian women, the context within which immigrant and refugee women access care and treatment results in more severe repercussions for them.

Factors that Restrict Access to Care and Treatment

Historically, women in North America generally have been neglected by the medical community. Health concerns specific to women (such as breast cancer, cervical cancer and menopause) have received minimal attention compared to health concerns specific to men (Holloway 1994). In areas such as cardiovascular disease and HIV/AIDS, women were excluded from research and drug trials. In too many cases, the results of studies of men were assumed to be equally applicable to women (Bell 1997, Holloway 1994, Smeltzer 1992). The impact of the neglect has been reflected in areas such as HIV/AIDS—nearly five million women were either ill or dead by 1992 (Reid 1992)—yet, the Canadian and

American case definitions for AIDS did not include women's symptoms until 1993.

Immigrant and refugee women have been doubly disadvantaged. First, studies that addressed women's issues focused mainly on women as an homogeneous group (Anderson 1985, Lynam 1985, Meleis and Rogers 1987) and neglected "additional ascriptive dimensions of their overall status" (Boyd 1975: 406). Second, studies of immigrants and refugees have addressed mainly issues concerning men or issues regarding women's participation in the workforce in terms of their labour and wage patterns. Only a few studies have been conducted about immigrant and refugee women's health in Canada (Anderson 1985, 1990, 1991 and 1997, Boyd 1975, Lynam 1985).

Immigrant and refugee women often are not included in various studies because of factors such as biases in referral networks, methods of recruitment, inadequate nutrition, lack of childcare and inaccessible study locations. Even when they are accepted as participants in studies measuring the effectiveness of various health interventions, the consent forms, questionnaires, interviews, measurement tools, scales and equipment often are not culturally or linguistically appropriate for them (Guruge 1999). This unsuitability and insensitivity can, in turn, arouse their suspicion of the research and diminish any incentive for them to participate or continue in such studies. The result is a lack of adequate evidence about whether immigrant and refugee women would benefit, come to harm or not be affected at all by various health interventions and treatments (Dresser 1992).

The Socioeconomic and Cultural Context
within which Care is Accessed
For many immigrants and refugees, the difficulties in dealing with an illness are exacerbated by the stress of leaving their homeland and establishing a home in a new country. The move may result in the disruption of lifestyles, loss of families and friends, loss of respect and social status, and loss of financial stability and employment. They also may face functional illiteracy, cultural disparity, social isolation, marginalization and racial discrimination (Anderson 1991, Guruge and Donner 1996, Lee 1994). When illness occurs, unfamiliarity with the Canadian health care system may increase an already chronic or acute state of stress. For instance, newcomers may not know how to register at a hospital emergency desk, how to enroll for services such as meals-on-wheels and prenatal care, or how to obtain aids and equipment. Although some may be unaware of existing services, others, particularly those who do not have their Canadian citizenship, may assume they are not eligible to use these services. No systems are in place to inform people about such

services and resources; thus, many are prevented from benefitting from the available resources.

Moreover, if newcomers do access such resources and services, they are not treated the same as white Canadian patients (Lea 1994). Patients are expected to adopt Canadian values and beliefs and to learn to speak English if they are to receive good care (M. Parent, personal communication, 1997). Although it would be ideal for newcomers to speak the language of their host country, the unfortunate reality is that many cannot. Immigrants, and especially refugees, may spend long hours in physically demanding jobs or work in several low-paying jobs just to meet their basic needs and to support other family members awaiting immigration clearance back home. They are often too tired at the end of the work day to attend English classes; indeed, learning English may not be one of their immediate survival strategies (Guruge and Donner 1996). Women may additionally be burdened with having to find childcare on a limited budget in order to attend English language instruction (Gleave and Manes 1990).

Even if newcomers do have the time, money and resources to attend English classes, learning a language is not an easy task for most (Gleave and Manes 1990), especially for older people. One of the authors knows of a woman in her late 60s from China who attended classes to learn English for ten years. Although she can read and understand English, she lacks confidence in speaking in English. This is not an isolated incident. Even if people are able to carry on a conversation about food or manage grocery shopping, discussing their health and understanding medical and nursing terminology can be extremely difficult for them. Moreover, during crises, emergencies, or accidents, people fluent in English tend to revert automatically to their first language. Therefore, "speaking English and being familiar with Canadian ways may be impossible and should not be a prerequisite to access to health care" (Guruge and Donner 1996: 37).

Employment Issues

The economic situation of many refugees may influence not only their access to and use of the health care system but also the priority they place on their health. Lee (1994) found that, although immigrants as a whole have a higher employment rate than native-born Canadians, this statistic disguises the high levels of underemployment. Most refugees work in several low-paying jobs, sic to seven days a week, for ten to twelve hours a day. For those who do not earn even the minimum wage, illness management can be a heavy burden. In a case known to one of the authors, an Indian Tamil woman living in Toronto who has a university degree in chemistry and speaks fluent English, works in an office earning less than $5 per hour. Although she frequently works more than eight hours per day she is never paid overtime wages. Often she cannot afford to pay for medications and other medical expenses for her daughter who has a chronic illness. Hers is not an rare situation. It is not uncommon to find qualified foreign-trained physicians working as technicians or orderlies in hospitals in Toronto (Lee 1994) or teachers working as store clerks (Waxler-Morrison 1990).

Often, foreign credentials are not recognized in Canada; additional course work or years of upgrading may be required. The money and time needed for these courses are rarely available to most refugees. They also may face differential treatment when seeking support from their superiors. In a case documented by Collins et al. (1999), a nurse with a diploma education wanted the time off to upgrade and obtain her bachelor's degree in nursing. She intended to fund herself. Her manager, who allowed this nurse's white colleagues to take time off without any conditions, told her that she could take time off from her work to attend classes, "only if it was a degree of her [manager's] choice at a university of her [manager's] choice."

Even if the opportunity exists to take additional courses or Canadian exams, professional jobs require Canadian experience—a circularity of reasoning which is hard to break if employers are unwilling to recognize foreign experience. Further, most often immigrants and refugees need to have better qualifications than English- or French-speaking Canadians to acquire prestigious jobs. Their lack of fluency in English may detract from their qualifications. At times, their accents or minor mistakes in their spoken English inhibit their ability to receive promotions and awards. In an extreme case, a Caribbean nurse was told to speak properly, purely based on her accent, even though English was her first language (Collins et al. 1999). Issues such as racism, discrimination and harassment at work are only beginning to be addressed. Although cases of racism in the nursing profession have been documented in Canada (Calliste 1993, Collins et al. 1999, Das Gupta 1993), further research about these issues is needed in other professional fields and employment areas.

Immigrant and refugee women's average income is much lower than that of their English- or French-speaking Canadian counterparts (Women and Mental Health Association 1987). When compared to most women in more prestigious positions, women in the lower echelons of the workforce lack control, freedom and independence at work (Anderson 1993). Consequently, they may find it difficult to organize their time to meet the requirements of illness management, such as negotiating time off for care and treatment or attending clinics and doctors' appointments during the workday. Anderson found that some of the immigrant women were hesitant to take steps to control their diabetes such as monitoring blood sugar levels, managing a special diet, eating on time or taking insulin at work. They feared that if their employers and co-workers found out, they would be fired, harassed or easily replaced.

Family Issues

According to a United Nations document, women are the "sole bread-winners in one third of the world's families," in addition to being the primary caretakers in the home (as cited in Browner and Leslie 1996: 260). Women have multiple responsibilities which are all too often managed at the expense of their own health. Further, an increase in participation in the workforce does not significantly improve newcomers' social status (Bloom 1985, Griffith 1985). For many immigrant and refugee women, their first job in Canada may also represent their first paid employment (Singer et al. 1996). Not only are they trying to deal with the stress of working outside the home, they are often also attempting to maintain a balance between the roles and expectations of their country of origin and those of Canada (Morrison et al. 1999).

Power imbalances can be created within households because the woman newcomer is sometimes the first to find employment and may become the sole breadwinner. Consequently, the husband's self-esteem, respect and status within and outside the home may be threatened. As a result of feeling emotionally frustrated husbands may discourage their wives from learning English or, in severe cases, they may resort to abuse and violence within the household (Gleave and Manes 1990, Lee 1994, Morrison et al. 1999).

Male violence against women is now acknowledged as a serious social issue but little money has been set aside for research or programs that address the causes of violence and the interventions that are specific to immigrant and refugee women.[2] Barriers that may prevent immigrant and refugee women from seeking help or cause them to remain in abusive relationships include lack of nearby family and friends, dependency on their husbands to receive Canadian immigration status and fear of deportation. Further, these women may believe that accessing services such as welfare or living in a shelter even for short time periods could jeopardize their chances of sponsoring family members to Canada. Also, linguistic and cultural barriers may prevent them from seeking help (Lurch 1991).

The point at which a woman is in the immigration process can have a huge impact on whether or how she will utilize health care. According to Gleave and Manes, those who are waiting to be accepted as refugees have no medical insurance "except for the federal emergency procedures which require lengthy paperwork" (1990: 64). Jimenez (1991) states that the Ontario Ministry of Health has not developed a policy to address the lack of health care services for women without immigration status. Although some community health centres offer health services to such women during their pregnancy, no health services are provided to women experiencing other health problems. In such cases, they may wait until their medical or psychiatric problems peak before they seek care, thus risking their lives. The irony is that, although refugees have equal opportunity to pay taxes with other Canadians, they do not have access to health care. For those who are eligible, simply knowing that they can access the health care system can decrease their stress and anxiety.

Linguistic and Cultural Issues

Another barrier to recent immigrants' and refugees' access to health care is the unavailability of culturally and linguistically appropriate resources, including health, illness and treatment information, appropriate methods of information delivery and appropriate interpretation services.[3] Research has shown that if culturally and linguistically appropriate services are available, immigrants and refugees tend to use even the normally least utilized mental health services (Meleis 1991, Vega et al. 1986). The following example indicates the importance not only of language but also of culture in health care. An *Indian* Tamil-speaking psychiatrist working in one of the downtown hospitals in Toronto had a considerable number of *Sri Lankan* Tamil-speaking patients who had been seeing her over a period of several years. They all suddenly left her for a *Sri Lankan* Tamil-speaking psychiatrist who started working in the same facility.

In addition, the assumption that anybody who can translate information will be adequate is neither appropriate nor ethical in many situations. In some instances, children have been used as translators to discuss their parents' health concerns or problems around such subjects as birth control, abortions and sexually transmitted diseases (Stevens 1993). One of the authors witnessed a situation in which a teenage boy was forced to ask his mother when her last menstrual period was. This family came from one of the South Asian countries where mothers do not discuss such issues even with their daughters. In other cases, women may not want their families' involvement in their care, or the "family may be the source of distress and women may need counselling apart from their families" (Anderson 1997: 13).

In the absence of family members or friends, non-health-care staff members have been used for interpretation. Using non-health-care staff who may lack of knowledge of medical and nursing terminology can lead to misunderstandings. This practice also can pose confidentiality issues (Anderson 1997). Patients may occasionally become the subject of community gossip (Poliakoff 1993). Thus, "a woman may be denied the opportunity of equitable access to services on a confidential basis. So the very structure of the health care system compromises the care a woman receives" (Anderson 1997: 13).

Clearly, a number of systemic barriers hamper immigrant and refugee women's access to health services. Given the centrality of immigrants to Canada's history and social progress it is vital that these barriers be addressed and eliminated as we move to reform the health care system in Canada.

Reform Initiatives to the Canadian Health Care System

Canada's health care system is considered to be one of the best in the world. However, it is not without its problems, and the need for change has been recognized. Since the mid-1980s, the health care systems in most provinces have been reviewed by independent commissions in order to suggest improvements. Largely as a result of these reviews, the most extensive round of health care reforms since the beginning of Medicare was undertaken (Evans 1993, Hurley et al. 1994). Canadian health care reform is being driven by multiple objectives which include cost-containment, concerns about the effectiveness or the appropriateness of some medical care, demands for greater patient participation in decision-making, and the need to improve overall efficiency (Evans 1993, Hurley et al. 1994). In order to achieve the primary objectives of increasing access to quality care that requires less costs, several reform initiatives are being implemented.

The three reform initiatives of special interest in this chapter are: (1) the empowerment and active participation in care; (2) the shift in focus from disease treatment to health promotion; and (3) moving care to the home and the community. Although many researchers from various backgrounds have proposed that these reform initiatives will improve the health care system, others, both health care professionals as well as patients, have raised concerns that they will negatively affect health care delivery (Ministry of Public Works and Government Services 1997, Skelton-Green and Sunner 1997). These initiatives will have a significant impact on women, not only because one in ten women work in health care and account for 80 percent of the health care workforce, but also because of the fact that women "provide the overwhelming majority of the unpaid care" (Armstrong 1997: 13). The following sections examine how these three reform initiatives could be particularly problematic for immigrant and refugee women.

Empowerment and Active Participation in Care

One objective of health care reform is to empower patients and foster their participation in care, which would increase their responsibility for their own health care and treatment. However, the values implicit in these goals can be quite foreign to patients from some cultural backgrounds. For instance, in some cultures decision-making is a collective process. Asking a woman from such a background to make her own decision regarding treatment may not only offend her family members but also place her in an uncomfortable position. Similarly, an emphasis on teaching the patient instead of the whole family may not always be effective. To some people from other countries the notion of empowerment may also involve issues such as dealing with the consequences of colonization and poverty or of fighting for their freedom.[4]

Immigrants and refugees need to be informed of the way the system works so that they can actively participate in care and avoid further stress and anxiety in the process. For example, in some countries, neighbours and the extended families are considered to be automatically a part of the caretaking group. It would not be unusual in such cultures for a woman to leave her children aged five to eight at home alone and expect the neighbours to look after them while she sought medical treatment. Although these newcomers may come from cultures that place a high value on childcare, they need to be informed that such behaviour is considered neglect in Canada. If the children were to be taken to the Children's Aid Society or if the women's actions were questioned, the ensuing devastation could precipitate ill health from stress. Thus, empowerment for some immigrant and refugee women may begin with being informed about health care, education, employment and child welfare policies, regulations and laws.

Moreover, health care and treatment as we know it in Canada often is not the norm in some developing countries. Some people may seek hospital care only when home remedies fail, while others may be unfamiliar with the roles and responsibilities of nurses, dietitians, pharmacists, physiotherapists and occupational therapists (Guruge and Donner 1996, Richardson 1990). In some Central American countries, for instance, nurses are not as respected as in Canada; rather, they are seen as menial hospital workers (Gleave and Manes 1990). Such a preconception would affect how immigrant and refugee women relate to nurses and how willing they are to receive advice and care from them. Still others may come from cultures that show high respect for health care professionals and expect them to make decisions on behalf of their patients who do not have the medical expertise. Thus, a physician who asks patients to make a decision about a medical procedure may be perceived as someone who lacks skills. This could result in the patient's seeking help elsewhere.

Further, decision-making may be difficult for some immigrants and refugees in a health care system that is quite foreign to them.

It may be ethnocentric for Canadian caregivers to expect active participation in care from immigrants and refugees. Patient roles and responsibilities, as well as caregiver roles, can differ from culture to culture. Among Chinese, who have closely-knit extended families, for example, passive participation may be expected of patients (Chin 1996). In some other cultures, older patients may depend on their children, or husbands on their wives, to care for them during their sickness (O'Hara and Zhan 1994, Turkoski 1985). Similarly, people from some Middle Eastern countries believe in complete rest and abdication of all responsibilities in order to save their energy for healing purposes. In these instances family members and health care professionals are expected to take care of them. (Meleis 1996). Although the empowerment of patients and their active participation in care can be seen as giving people more control over their lives, especially for those who value Western concepts such as independence and privacy, these goals may not be appropriate or applicable to everyone. Health care professionals, therefore, should ask themselves whether their expectations of patients' roles are realistic and reasonable and, more importantly, whether they are truly in the patients' best interests.

The Shift in Focus from Disease Treatment to Health Promotion

For some time, health care professionals have advocated shifting the focus from disease and treatment of disease to health promotion and disease prevention. Although this represents an important change in how care is viewed, consideration should be given to what an emphasis on health promotion and disease prevention means to recent immigrants and refugees. Are these concepts important to them? What kinds of health promotion actions should be initiated and what methods of information delivery should be used? Would these methods be culturally and linguistically applicable and appropriate?

Health promotion is a "multifaceted constellation of perceptions and self-initiated activities designed to enhance personal well-being and fulfillment" (Duffy et al. 1995: 23). Health promotion concepts and health promotion and disease prevention activities are deeply rooted in cultural beliefs and values (Choudhry 1998). In some Middle Eastern countries, health promotion activities include avoiding hot–cold or dry–moist shifts and wind and drafts, as well as staying warm and eating and resting well. Therefore, women of such backgrounds may make a priority of resting rather than going to an aerobics class. They may require clear information about the importance of ambulation, self-care and exercise as well as reinforcement of such information (Meleis 1996).

In Western society, health-promotion activities are often distinct from other activities of daily living. It may entail, for example, joining a fitness class or subscribing to a health magazine. Both activities have a single purpose, to promote and maintain health, that is separate from other activities. In some other countries, however, most women do not actively seek or participate in health promotion activities; rather, these activities are unconsciously integrated into their everyday lives (Choudhry 1998). In some Indian and Sri Lankan villages, women may walk for miles to get water from a well and walk back with one big pot of water on their heads and another on their hips. Similarly, laundry or shower taking are labourious undertakings because each requires that pots be cleaned manually and water drawn from wells repeatedly. Cutting and transporting wood for cooking purposes or tending to vegetable gardens requires strength and endurance. Such activities provide these women with sufficient exercise. Once in Canada, however, these women have access to washing and drying machines, indoor plumbing for showers and laundry and gas or electric stoves for cooking. Consequently, the exercise they derive from daily living is diminished. Running, using a stair-master or attending a fitness class may be bewildering alternatives to some of them.

Chen, Ng and Wilkins observe that immigrants are, by and large, a healthy group on their arrival in Canada for three reasons:

> [first] people in good health are generally more inclined than those in poor health to emigrate, [second] employability, which is a factor in granting permission to immigrate to Canada, requires a certain level of health, [and third] before they are admitted, potential immigrants undergo screening that ensures that they do not suffer from serious medical conditions. (1996: 33)

Although recent immigrants, especially those from non-European countries, tend to have better health than Canadian-born people, the prevalence of chronic illnesses and the long-term disability level of immigrants who have lived in Canada for over ten years tend to approach that of the Canadian-born population (Chen et al. 1996).

After arrival in Canada, immigrants and refugees may assign priority to needs other than health promotion, such as food, employment, money, immigration hearings and finding lawyers. For them, having the time, money and resources to pay attention to health and health promotion is something of a privilege. In addition, women's health promotion practices will vary according to their personal, familial and cultural background. Choudhry states that, like women in many other countries, "Indian women are socialized to willingly subvert their own needs to those of their husband, children and parents. Responsibility for the well-being of others, the patriarchy and their cultural norms hinder many from focusing on themselves" (1998: 273). Although some traditional practices, such as use of contraceptives, are changing under their new circumstances and exposure to Canadian values and beliefs, some practices, such as arranged marriages, remain (Morrison et al. 1999).

Lastly, Canadian health promotion programs that address immigrant and refugee women's health issues are not well developed. Evaneshko points out,

> [the] majority of health education programs have been one of two types: those developed by whites for use with white patients, or pre-existing white programs adapted to an ethnic group by layering a thin veneer of cultural information over the white-based format. (as cited in Tripp-Reimer 1989: 613)

In the case of diabetes, for instance, a patient may be told to curb her carbohydrate intake, that is, to eat half a cup of cooked rice or pasta per meal. However, this recommendation may be unrealistic for those who are used to eating two to three cups of pasta or rice two to three times a day. Eating rice is important to many people from countries such as China, Sri Lanka, India and Thailand. Moreover, changing to a dietary regimen of unfamiliar foods and ingredients is challenging, especially when one is dealing with the stress of living with a chronic illness. One of the authors is aware of patients with diabetes who continue to eat three cups of rice three times a day with self-increased doses of hypoglycemic agents or insulin. They may not tell health care professionals about this practice, because (1) they are embarrassed to say that substituting rice with anything else is not regarded as a meal, and (2) they do not feel comfortable with health care professionals whom they acknowledge as the experts but whom they believe do not understand the significance of certain foods in their diet and overall lifestyle. These reactions may sometimes lead them to avoid health care professionals altogether and use traditional healing methods or alternative therapies. These examples demonstrate why simply translating health promotion and disease prevention information may not be effective in the case of the immigrant and refugee patients.

Moving Care to the Home and the Community
The third reform initiative is the shift of care from hospitals and institutions to the community and the home. Some of the related initiatives that have been implemented as a result of this movement are early patient discharge, day treatment, outpatient care and home care management of

the chronically ill and the disabled. Moving care to the home may promote independence by giving control of patients' health, illness management, care and treatment to them and their families. However, the implicit and erroneous assumption underlying this shift is that all patients and their families have the ability to manage an illness at home and have the resources, including the time, money and commitment, to do so.[5] While these changes in health care delivery affect all Canadians, they have particularly problematic implications for immigrant and refugee women.

Although moving care to the home may curb hospital and institutional expenses, this move causes an increase in immediate costs and expenses for the family and the caregiver in the short term. Also, it can create long-term costs for both the care receiver and caregiver in the forms of stress, anxiety and strain on family relationships. The extra pressure on time and money can create conditions where care is impossible (Armstrong 1997) and can eventually lead to ill health, abuse, marital breakdown and psychological problems.

Most often women are the caretakers of families, regardless of their culture or religion. Armstrong says that they are the "lowest, lowest cost care providers," however, women are becoming less able to function in this role as more of them enter the workforce 1997: 26–27). In the case of immigrant and refugee women who are already working extra hours in low paying jobs, giving up their jobs may be impossible especially if they are the family's sole breadwinner. Others, who are already in abusive situations, may face further abuse and violence as a result of the anxiety, stress and emotional and financial strain the spouse may be undergoing.

In situations where the survival of the family depends on the employment of both parents in laborious, low income jobs, terminating that employment for one of them is impossible. So that the whole family is not jeopardized, caretaking responsibilities are often shifted to elderly members of the family. This may seem like a reasonable and practical solution to the problem but may add to an existing burden of physical limitations for the aged. If the woman of the household is sick and other female relatives are unavailable, the caretaking responsibility may fall on her children. This scenario becomes more complicated and difficult for those who are not eligible for health care because of the lengthy immigration process.

Even if women are able to manage relinquishing their employment or to keep working while taking care of a sick family member, they may not be able to take on the caretaking responsibility with skill and confidence. Armstrong notes, "most of the care being sent home has never been done there. Never before have people been sent home with oxygen tanks and catheters, feeding tubes and surgical bandages" (1997: 26–27).

For those who do not speak English or those who cannot understand the technical language in which most instructions are written, implementing a rigorous medication regimen or changing colostomy bags, needles or intravenous tubing may prove to be extremely distressing. Unless a woman is already working in a nursing or other health profession, she may be unable to undertake these tasks or have the time to learn the skills, thereby putting herself and her family member at risk (Armstrong 1997). Others may simply continue with their traditional healing practices since they may not be able to substitute what has become unmanageable and incomprehensible caretaking.

Similarly, others who are unfamiliar with the way the system works may feel helpless in emergency situations. In a case known to one of the authors, a woman who is fluent in English was home alone when her six-month-old baby had a seizure. Her first reaction was not to dial 911 but to run out to the hallway crying for help. This woman's husband, who has been working in Canada for fifteen years, had explained to her upon her arrival in Canada that she should dial 911 in case of an emergency. Instead she did what was customary for a young newlywed or new mother in her culture and went running down the hall expecting neighbours to help. Unfortunately, in Canada, neighbours have a tendency to avoid getting involved. Consequently this woman's husband blamed her for the crisis and the child's ensuing disability following the seizure.

In those situations where women are not fluent in English, the lack of language skills further hampers their ability to understand and manage a family member's illness and can further isolate them if they are the one who is ill. Anderson (1990) comments that immigrant and refugee women feel very much alone when dealing with the psychological impact of their illness. Often they do not have the strong social support system they would have had in their home country (Pilowsky 1991). The physical and emotional burden of caretaking may cause further health problems for women who may, in turn, need to seek health care themselves. If that is the case, shifting care to the home could be more costly by increasing the burden of illness on the system. Unless proper support is available to those who are taking care of sick people at home or in the community, patients will repeatedly enter emergency departments and, of course, with increasing complications. This situation is applicable to all Canadians, but can have particularly dire consequences for immigrants and refugees.

The question of how to allocate scarce resources may be the primary problem in illness management for low-income immigrant families. Paying rent and buying food for the family may be given greater priority than purchasing orthopedic pillows, food or vitamin supplements, or prescribed or non-prescribed medications. Immigrant and refugee families who are already struggling financially within a new environment and with a new language are not given adequate social support to alleviate the burden of illness. Moving care to the home increases that burden dramatically. The existing health and social services are not sufficiently meeting their needs. Although there are "health and social services to assist families with caretaking, the ongoing management and monitoring of illness become their responsibility" (Anderson 1990: 75). The benefits of home care to both the patients and their families are not contested when resources are adequate, but the needs of low-income families, single-parent families and immigrant and refugee families should be addressed.

Recommendations for Improving the Care Given to Immigrant and Refugee Women

It is generally well understood that one's health and wellbeing are not primarily determined by medical and institutional care. Rather, they result more from such determinants as adequate nutrition, housing, a clean and safe physical environment, having supportive and safe relationships, control over one's life, a positive childhood experience, meaningful and secure paid employment and sufficient income (Armstrong 1997). Therefore, focusing on active patient participation, moving care to home and community and emphasizing health promotion and disease prevention will not achieve the goals of health care reform if attention is not given to the determinants of health and wellbeing and the sociocultural context within which patients access and use the health care system.

The recommendations in the following section attempt to address some of the determinants of health for immigrant and refugee women. They are not presented as answers to all the socioeconomic, linguistic and cultural issues that immigrant and refugee women face. However, they do provide a place to begin to address a significant problem in Canadian health care delivery—how to make services accessible to refugees and immigrants.

The Development of Linguistically and Culturally Appropriate Services

- Develop the systematic use of cultural interpretation programs or personnel as opposed to translation services that lack knowledge of the subtleties of a culture. Toronto's Queen Street Mental Health Centre developed such a program using their own staff members as resource persons.

- Develop educational materials that are in specific languages and that incorporate cultural nuances. A Toronto community group working in the area of HIV/AIDS developed materials that include visual and verbal representations of specific cultural groups.
- Use health teaching and health promotion methods that are culturally appropriate and geared towards specific communities. Teaching methods, for example, should reflect each cultural group's ways of learning, such as using songs, stories or drama to disseminate information.
- Use first hand information. For example, asking patients with diabetes to bring in samples of their food would help health care professionals planning their meals to understand what patients consider as the most important types of food, their methods of preparation and the quantities they eat (Guruge et al. 1998).
- Mobilize the community to make resources available to address illness issues. For instance, Chinese meals-on-wheels could complement the standard meals-on-wheels (Guruge et al. 1998). Some social service organizations in Toronto address the needs of the Spanish-speaking community. Unfortunately, not all communities have such services and those that exist are in a vulnerable state and continuously subject to cutbacks.
- Use community television programs and community newspapers which disseminate educational materials to address issues and conflicts related to traditional approaches versus current Western approaches to managing illness and promoting health behaviours (Guruge et al. 1998).
- Ask ethno-specific professional associations to provide valuable academic, research-based and applied information for developing linguistically and culturally appropriate educational materials and programs.

The Participation And Representation Of Community Members

- Develop strategies to incorporate community leaders' knowledge and expertise in the process of developing, implementing and improving educational, therapeutic and preventive health promotional and healing activities. For example, community leaders may be employed to learn about the usual daily activities of women from a certain cultural group and to design ways of incorporating exercises and physical activities into these women's lives.

- Increase representation of immigrant and refugee women on the boards of directors of universities and colleges that train health care professionals. They are also under-represented on the boards of hospitals, health councils and provincial and federal ministries where policies that determine the level and type of changes to health care are developed (Ministry of Public Works and Government Services 1997). Community members' voices and opinions must be given equal value and consideration.
- Establish formal collaborative relationships between hospitals and community groups and programs to provide culturally and linguistically appropriate care to immigrants and refugees. Groups and programs such as Across Boundaries, Hong Fook Mental Health Service, Access Alliance and Women's Health in Women's Hands facilitate seminars to educate staff, students and volunteers working in psychiatry about relevant cultural and language issues (Williams 1999).
- Develop programs to assist immigrants and refugees with learning how to participate in and use the health care system as part of new Canadian orientation or citizenship programs.

Recognition of the Sociocultural Context within which Patients Access Health Care

- Pay particular attention to assessing the constraints, burdens and barriers in immigrant and refugee women's lives. The obligations and priorities in their lives should also be recognized (e.g., are they supporting a child in university or parents back home? Or are they already taking care of older parents or someone with a disability in the house?). Support and resources should also be made available to immigrant and refugee women to enhance their efforts to educate themselves and gain control of their health.
- Address women's needs in the workforce, which includes examining the existing ways of recognizing and accepting their credentials and being creative about where they can use their skills and expertise until they complete their upgrading. Certain community centres such as Toronto's World Tamil Movement offer free computer courses to members of their community. Universities, in collaboration with various government sectors, may be able to offer trained professionals to provide support and the necessary skills and expertise to various communities on a monthly or yearly basis. Corpora-

tions may be approached to donate their time and services rather than just funds.

- Make effective use of the knowledge and valuable resources of immigrant women. "There are no adequate policies to open new options for them. They are deprived of demonstrating their highest potential and their host societies are deprived of making use of that highest potential" (Meleis and Rogers 1987: 205). A trained doctor from Russia (who has not yet passed her Canadian-approved exams) could be employed with another Canadian doctor in a community centre frequented by Russian patients. This arrangement would allow the immigrant physician to participate in a somewhat similar capacity to her previous experience while learning the Canadian medical system. Further, the Russian patients' participation in the health care system would be facilitated as would the Canadian-trained doctor's learning about her patients' cultural and religious beliefs, attitudes and behaviours toward health, illness, care and treatment.

Coordination among Government Agencies and Services

- Coordinate all levels of government agencies in addressing not only the health issues of immigrants and refugees, but also their socioeconomic, language and cultural concerns as a whole. As Williams (1999) points out, collaboration among agencies such as the Municipal Task Force on Community Access and Equity, Canadian Heritage and Urban Alliance on Race Relations would ensure that health issues are not discussed in isolation of other factors.
- Develop links with family practitioners, lay practitioners and community leaders to facilitate early interventions, thereby reducing emergency hospital admissions as well as the delay in immigrants seeking care (Williams 1999).
- Establish links between health institutions and the communities they serve. Hospital health fairs that target various communities can promote hospital resources to these communities.

Research And Education

- Fund and support research that addresses immigrants' and refugees' health and health needs. Such research should focus on a comprehensive overview of the accessibility of services.

Further, funding applications for research addressing immigrant and refugee women's health should be promoted particularly if those research strategies could directly benefit the groups they are targeting. The Centre for Excellence in Research on Immigration and Settlement in Montreal is an organization which funds such research.

- Researchers should involve community members in developing research goals and the tools, measures and consent forms used in research examining health issues relevant to these communities.
- While doing research in communities, researchers might use the opportunity, where appropriate, to provide workshops or educate the community about recent developments in managing certain illnesses.
- Nursing and other health professional education programs should be "visit[ed] and revisit[ed]" (Donner 1998: 9) in order to better prepare culturally aware health care professionals. Donner identifies several elements and policies that should be implemented in order to ensure that the importance of culture, religion and language is recognized in nursing education:

    a) a "just admission standard with equitable access. [This policy should include] evidence of activity to recruit from those populations that were traditionally excluded.

    b) Recruit faculty who understand and support the principles of culturally sensitive care. This [policy should] include recruitment of faculty who represent the society in which we live, an equal opportunity for them to participate in administrative positions within the faculty, and ongoing opportunities for all faculty members to become educated and aware of the indicators of culturally sensitive care.

    c) A curriculum content that integrates cultural sensitivity into student assessments, evaluations and exams" (9).

- Promote culture care as a part of the continuing education of health care professionals in hospitals and community agencies. For example, the College of Nurses of Ontario (1999c) recently developed *A Guide to Nurses for Providing Culturally Sensitive Care*, which was distributed to all nurses in the province. This publication represents an important beginning in addressing the needs of the communities served by Ontario nurses. However, steps should be taken to ensure that this guide is used in everyday practice.

Workforce Related Issues

- Recruit and train staff with the language skills and expertise needed to provide care to those communities accessing services in each hospital. This training should also include information about traditional and complementary therapies that patients may be using interchangeably or at the same time.
- Designate "staff, time and financial resources to integrate an ethnoracial focus into all program activities" (Williams 1999: 5). Where this is not possible, staff assignments should be flexible so that their language and cultural skills and resources could be used effectively.
- Make efforts to understand not only overt but also subtle racist practices at the individual as well as the institutional level. Educate staff about racism at work through forums and workshops that address issues such as how to file complaints, who to contact in the process, what anti-racism strategies to use and ways of dealing with the Workers' Compensation Board (Calliste 1996).
- Develop guidelines and processes to address workforce inequities and harassment of employees by their colleagues or superiors. Ensure that those who are harassing staff or patients undergo training programs and that their actions and behaviours towards others at work be evaluated.

Conclusion

Health care reform initiatives may benefit many Canadians but for most women immigrants and refugees these initiatives have the potential to overburden an already stressful life. Women immigrants and refugees are already subject to underemployment, discrimination, competing priorities, disempowerment and abuse within relationships, coupled with an unfamiliarity with the Canadian health care system. Additionally, they must often contend with culturally and linguistically inappropriate information and health care situations. Consequently, recent reform initiatives may actually contribute to already existing inequities in health care rather than helping to reduce them. The recommendations provided in this chapter would be instrumental in meeting the basic health care requirements of immigrants and refugees. Their implementation is imperative in order to alleviate the potentially negative impact of Canadian health care reform initiatives on women immigrants and refugees.

Notes

1. Denise Spitzer in this volume explores factors from both sources in her study of childbirth experiences of immigrant and Aboriginal women.
2. Si Transken in this volume discusses the impact of cuts to staff and resources on services for women who have been sexually violated.
3. For a discussion of linguistic and cultural issues relating to the care of immigrant women during and after childbirth, see Spitzer in this volume.
4. See Simpson and Porte in this volume for a critical discussion of how the legacy of colonialism contributes to present-day problems in an Aboriginal community.
5. Diana Gustafson in this volume explores one factor that contributes to downloading the burden of care onto the shoulders of unpaid family members, usually women.

12

Aging Well:
Strategies for Wellbeing Among Older Women in a "Restructuring" Ontario

Douglass Drozdow-St. Christian

Introduction: Other Voices, Other Rooms

This chapter grows out of an ongoing study of aging, health, self-actualization and social connection among a group of older women living in several urban centres in southern and southwestern Ontario. This particular project began about five years ago, as part of a longstanding interest in how people make their own "healths"[1] within the cultural and institutional frameworks which condition their options and limit their possibilities. The project, which continues today, has expanded beyond this initial interest to explore how health, identity, community membership and the insidious ideologies of social death[2] can become strategies deployed by older and elderly women in the day-to-day practice of being meaningful and active agents, not only in their own lives, but in the lives of their communities.

Importantly, this chapter is not about victims, although being victimized by diminishing institutional support for health is something of which these women are acutely aware. But rather than simply taking the position of victim that circumstance attempts to dictate, the women I am writing about here have taken a different approach to their precarious and endangered position, an approach premised on direct resistance to victimology, which is at the heart of contemporary political discourse on marginalization. Indeed, in resisting, the women I introduce here give lie to the perspective that the only responses to institutional change are reactionary and submissive. The complexity of resistance cannot be overstated, as anthropologists have learned, sometimes to their dismay, in the last several decades.[3] The simple equation of domination-resistance has proven inadequate for understanding the action and reaction in relationships of unequal power. This is because degrees of cooperation, strategic withdrawal and open defiance, to name a few, can provide practical avenues through which to subvert domination (Comaroff 1985 and 1993).[4] In calling what these women are doing resistance, I am not suggesting that their taking action is a conscious reaction to domination and subordination. Instead, I am drawing attention to the way their individual rational responses to the official health care system produce the effect of resistance, even if that is not their conscious motivation. Some of these women are devising less individualistic responses that produce more overt expressions of resistance, but the line between these remains blurred. We need further study of the inherent pluralism in the engagement between patients and official health care structures in order to develop a clearer concept of resistance without consciousness, as well as to understand how this necessary pluralism of engagement may undermine the effectiveness of the dominating structures and processes. The risk remains of seeing every article of diversity as resistance, a risk we should assiduously avoid lest resistance end up a catch all concept which encompasses too much and so explains very little.

I also need to issue another important caveat, to temper the optimism that this chapter explores. Of the more than two hundred women I have interviewed over the last five years, the women I am speaking of here— twenty-seven in all—represent a small minority.[5] For the most part, social, political and institutional changes which have directly and often adversely affected the status and health of older women have exacerbated an already longstanding negative status associated with being female and elderly in Canada (Abu-Laban and McDaniel 1995, Marshall and McPherson 1995, see also Greer 1992). The majority of the women I have come to know over these years have been victimized in multiple ways by the restructuring of health and community care underway in Ontario, and many, though not all, see themselves as either witting or unwitting victims of these changes.[6] What this chapter explores are the reactions and pro-actions of a small group of older women who, in taking stock of the changes going on around them, have been able to reconstruct their healths in terms of something they themselves build. By beginning to step away from the institutional framework of official health care systems, they point toward a different model of health making which better uses self-reliance, but also recognizes the limits beyond which self-reliance is not sufficient. Their actions suggest new ways of engagement between individuals creating health and healthy communities and the larger institutions to which they can turn.

Making sense of something as complex and intimate as health and wellbeing is, at the microsubjective level, difficult. That is because the calculations, meanings and life histories of each individual vary. That is less a truism than it seems. Health has certain conventional meanings, and illness is experienced in ways which are comparable between individuals. But making sense of health and, in particular, making it sensible when it plays so central a part in defining our sense of personhood, needs to take account of lived experience. Specifically, we need to consider both the inner psychology of lived experience and the culturally conditioned frameworks within which individuals engage their worlds. This lived experience creates diversity out of what seems, on the surface at least, to be a singularity. My objective in the work I have been doing with older women in Ontario is to explore the diversities within this singularity from an ethnographic perspective.[7] Following them in their day-to-day engagements with their bodies, their friends and their community and with the institutions which serve them or to which they turn in the pursuit of service is an ongoing process. The goal is a detailed understanding of how this group of women make a sensible healthy world through their engagement with it.

The group of women on whose lives this discussion is based live in several large urban centres in southern Ontario. They range in age from sixty-one to ninety. Of the twenty-seven women in this group, seventeen live in their own homes or apartments, six live in retirement homes and four reside in nursing homes.[8] Of the twenty-seven, twenty-one are widowed, two have never married, two live with a male spouse and two live with female domestic partners. Only one of this group has a disabling disease, though it is not age-related. All twenty-seven consider themselves to be in good to excellent health, though as one put it to me "good health is one of those 'all things considered' things, isn't it." Unlike more than 10 percent of the larger group, none of the women in the group I write about here are on any psycho-active medication, except one who is taking low doses of a tricyclic antidepressant as part of a pain management protocol. Average Geriatric Depression Scale (Sheikh and Yesavage 1986) ratings for this group are well within the normal, non-depressed range, which contrasts markedly with American figures that suggest somewhat more than 20 percent of women over the age of sixty-five are characterized clinically as suffering from some degree of measurable depression (Miller 1997, Shua-Haim et al. 1997).[9]

The socioeconomic status of this group covers a broad range, from several women living solely on government pensions (including survivors' benefits) to two women whose income from annuities and other sources is in excess of $100,000. One woman in this group was homeless between 1991 and 1996, living in makeshift shelters, parks and other secluded urban areas during the warmer months and in church-run shelters during the winter. She now lives in a domestic partnership with another woman she met while living homeless in Kingston. The majority of the women in this group, as well as in the larger study group, would be classified as middle income according to Statistics Canada categories. About 15 percent fall below the current definition of the poverty line, a definition which is currently being revised upward as a result of political pressure on Statistics Canada. Three women in the smaller group are of African or Afro-Caribbean descent. All others are of European descent: nine trace their ancestors to continental Europe; the remaining fifteen are descended from families in the British Isles. Only one was not born in Canada.

Finally, twenty-five of the twenty-seven women in this group have children, and nineteen have grandchildren. Twenty-one of the women have living siblings, and two have at least one surviving parent. None are involved in direct care of either their siblings or their parent, although all but one with living siblings has regular contact with their brothers or sisters. The surviving parents of the two women in this group still live independently, including one surviving mother who is ninety-two years old.

As I noted above, all the women in this group are subjectively healthy. Objective measures of health, which is to say, catalogues of present or absent medical conditions, confirm the general good health of these women. While many are experiencing certain conditions related primarily to age and gender, such as osteoporosis, and while most have been treated for some chronic or inflammatory condition during the time I have known them, none in this particular group consider these illness events anything other than inconveniences. Even taking these conditions into account, they consider their personal health to be substantially better than that of the average woman of their cohort.[10] As this chapter explores, one of the reasons for this positive and optimistic self assessment of health is related directly to the actions these women, each in her own way, has taken in restructuring how they create and maintain their wellbeing.

The Times We Lived Through

Recalling life history is a time honoured way of creating a sense of self in the here and now, and the women in this group used life history recollection to position themselves and the kinds of experiences they are having today. Telling their life stories, an integral part of the process of telling me what they are up to today, has and continues to occupy much of the time we spend together. From these stories, we can draw some general observations about the lives these women have lived, without violating their privacy and confidence. What follows is analytic and interpretive, rather than direct and objective. I want to evoke the lives of these women rather than expose them. At the same time, I do not want to indulge that other artificiality of rendering my informants anonymous in order to take over the authority to speak about and for them. The line between appropriation and evocation is thin, and where I necessarily end up crossing it, I apologize. The violations are always in good faith.

All of these women were born in or near the cities in which they now live. They recall their home cities as places which have become "dirtier, bigger, more crowded, more dangerous, less friendly and strange." None of them see the changes in their home cities as positive although each in their way expressed affection for their cities and, with qualifications, for the people they knew and know. But city living, for each of them, has gone from being about neighbourhoods and a clear sense of belonging to a place to a sense of alienation and unfamiliarity which they find unsettling and unpleasant. " When I was growing up," one woman puts it, "we helped each other on and off the streetcar. Now I just stumble up and down the stairs like everyone else."

There is a deep sense of nostalgia for what they see as the deterioration of safety in the cities where they live. While violent crime continues to decline in most Canadian cities, crime targeting the elderly has increased (Doyle 1997, Statistics Canada 1994 and 1997b). This group of women are acutely aware of this change:

> There are so many of us now, I suppose the hoodlums just decided we are easier to attack. I mean, if you had to choose between me [a seventy-six year old woman who currently uses a walker when shopping] and my son [a professional football player], whose wallet would you steal? There certainly is danger in numbers, isn't there?

Another common theme in discussing how things have changed is decay. Quite often they point to how neighbourhoods have declined because the buildings and properties have been allowed to become shabby and unsafe. There is a pervasive sense that, during the course of their lives, the physical qualities of their urban landscape have degenerated. This contributes to a feeling that the city is no longer a safe place, that it is falling apart. Of greater importance for my purposes here, recollections of health, illness and caring mirror the same kinds of nostalgic recollections found in talking about the city itself.

This is reflected in particular in their accounts of how their experiences with personal physicians have changed over the years. "I don't know my doctor's first name, but I did, when my doctor was old John X. He was just John, and I was just Dolores.[11] My new doctor probably doesn't know my name either." The idea that relationships with personal doctors were personal relationships, something akin to a friendship, is something often expressed in my discussions with these women. Doctors were local and accessible. "My family doctor was my neighbour for twenty-five years" one woman recalls, "from when I was just a girl until, well, after my second baby, which is when he retired." This experience of knowing their doctors well was echoed in my conversations with most of the women in the group. Other health care practitioners including pharmacists[12] but not dentists,[13] were seen as neighbours and friends rather than professional contacts alone.

But I should make clear here that this is not some Arcadian nostalgia for bygone days. The positive recollections of community and health relationships are tempered with very pragmatic recollections of the cost of being healthy. Doctors, it is pointed out over and over again, used to cost real money, and fiscal considerations around seeking professional health care made these decisions more complex than they would later become, as medical care became generally socialized and tax funded. What they all remember positively is a sense of a personal relationship with their doctors and other health providers, a feeling that in spite of the economic decision-making that went into seeking care, the care was accessible. House calls by doctors, that dinosaur of urban health care, were evidence that doctors wanted to help and understood the vicissitudes of illness. "When I was five and my mother found I had a fever" one woman commented, "she would call Dr. X. and he would come to the house because who would take a five-year-old out in the snow with a fever of 105?"

While recalling with some fondness the personal quality of caring, they also remember the fears, especially of communicable disease, which punctuated their growing up. They talk about polio scares, about influenza outbreaks and about special concerns over tuberculosis, measles, chicken pox and whooping cough.

A positive change about which many women comment involves their feelings about hospitals. When younger, they tell me, hospitals were places of fear, of danger and perhaps of last resort. The cost of hospitalization itself marked for these women the seriousness of the illness or accident that made hospitalization necessary. With tax funded hospital access, the hospital became somewhat neutralized as part of their everyday health management which, while still serious, lost its connotations of fear and danger. Hospitals, they tell me, have become something friendly and ordinary, a common part of their overall health care. The friendliness and personal nature of expert health care they found with their doctors carried over to hospitals and did not change as hospital access became universal later in their lives. The hospitals of a few decades ago remained places where serious medical issues were addressed, but for these women, even that very serious level of care had a quality of personal engagement which they see as having declined more recently.

This is necessarily a sketch, but in broad outline, several themes in these women's recollections are clear. They recall greater accessibility, a more developed and enduring quality of personal caring by health care practitioners and a relationship between illness and healing that involved emotional and personal commitment by both experts and themselves.[14] They invested emotion, friendship and personal integrity in their relationships with professional health care providers because they felt that was possible in the context of health care delivery when they were younger. This is an important issue to bear in mind in thinking about health in the 1990s, and in particular the health of a growing aging population. Their expectations and experiences of health service over the decades have changed, sometimes in very fundamental but always important ways. Grasping these expectations and situating them within the institutional milieu in which health delivery is structured, policed and allocated is an essential component of any attempt to characterize health care restructuring. At the risk of repetition, there is no generic patient—no generic older female patient nor generic young male patient. Instead there are cohorts of patients with great internal variation and complexity, factors which health analysis has tended to elide.[15]

The Times We Are Living Now

Two key issues are striking when the women in this group speak of their health seeking activities today: the distancing of health care providers and the increasing reliance on large institutions such as hospitals and community care services, which they see as "depersonalizing," "arrogant," "too much interested in money," and "difficult to get to, to access."[16] Their comments focus on the officialization of health as an institutionalized service in which they, the patients, seem to have become lost and even forgotten. One informant told me:

> I remember when the butcher put in one of those little take-a-number machines. He was busy, we all took our turn, we all got our pork chops. But when the local hospital did the same thing, I couldn't help but wonder when having a heart attack had turned into getting a pork chop.

They see the gradual distancing that has taken place between them and their health care providers as not only negative and depersonalizing but as dangerous:

> I had my first heart attack—I've had three—in 1984. Each time, I have gone to the same hospital. But each time I have waited

longer and longer, with a machine in the room and nothing else. Every once in a while someone would come in and look at the machine and write something down and then go away, and you know, what is scary to me is that they looked at the machine and didn't look at me. I suppose as long as the machine kept blinking, they didn't need to look at me. But where was I, that is what I wanted to know. Who was sick, me or the machine?

Many of the women in this group have a very pragmatic sense of how this distancing has occurred. They recognize explicitly that political decisions about spending and resource allocation, coupled with changing population patterns, have all contributed to an increasingly bureaucratic and unresponsive institutionalized health care system. "I know there are more old people now than before, but I think the politicians have not kept up with that." This increasing reliance on health care institutions as they age is recognized as a problem which they feel has not been adequately addressed. And changes in recent years, including hospital closures, staff cuts and the consolidation of home services into a system most of them find impenetrable has led many of these women to recognize that the institutional health care system is not the sole problem. Rather, they see the nature of their relationship to the system and the history over the last thirty years of increasing reliance on this system as something which demands rethinking and rehabilitation.

A decline in reliability of the institutional health care system has led these women to recognize a need to not only renovate the health care system, but to revitalize and transform the way they themselves use it. Key to this is a sense of overdependence which they recognize traps them in the squeeze between political agenda and economic and social change. What these women bring to this rethinking is a fundamental and sophisticated understanding of how their own actions, rather than simple reactions, can shape a different way of doing health for themselves and for their communities.

"We gave them too much power, I think. We keep letting someone else decide what is good for us, and then when they let us down, we don't realize we let them let us down." The brunt of the criticism is shared by both politicians and health care providers. While each of these women has good things to say about some particular doctor or nurse or politician, they recognize that they have become enmeshed in a system which trades helplessness for universality, and the consequence of that helplessness, they understand, is a paralysis which makes it difficult for them to respond independently when the universality becomes decreasingly reliable.

> When I realized I couldn't do anything about the hospital clos-
> ing, or about my cancer doctor making me wait thirteen weeks to
> see him, I knew then that I was letting myself down if I didn't
> think of something to do.

Doing something, rather than being done to, is at the heart of this group
of women's response to changes in how health care is delivered.

The problem of waiting lists is one which comes up often in conversations with this group. Each has her own story of some troubling delay
in access to a service or a practitioner. In particular, they are concerned
with what they see as the inability of the hospitals in their areas to ensure
that timely emergency care is available. Older persons tend to make
greater use of hospital emergency services than their younger counterparts, in part a function of age-related health problems and in part a
matter of convenience. Many women tell me they once saw their emergency room as an extension of the services provided by the personal
doctor, a place they could go to when their doctor was not available and
a problem needed attention.

Two particular health concerns occupy them—cardiac and respiratory problems and fractures—and they see these two types of health
problem as requiring emergency intervention. These women are responding to lengthening waiting times in hospital trauma units, news
accounts of patients being forgotten on stretchers in back corridors, and
the repeating story of hospitals being compelled to turn away patients
from emergency centres because of lack of room or staff. Particularly
troubling for these women is their recognition these are the kinds of
urgent health interventions they are likely to require more often as they
continue to age.[17] Coupled with a concern that in order to obtain
emergency care they may need to be transported to some other city, away
from their network of family and friends, the "emergency room crunch"
tops the list of issues which concern them.

A different aspect of this issue relates to specialist care. While their
personal physician is readily available, they see specialists as difficult to
access. One woman having a suspicious uterine growth investigated told
me,

> I know I have to wait in line to see [the oncologist] but I can't see
> where that line ends. If I am so sick that I need a specialist, won't
> I be even sicker six months from now when I finally see him?

That concern over waiting lists couples with a suspicion that the objective
of the policy changes which have stretched specialist resources is a pay-
for-access system. Repeatedly, these women voiced the suspicion that the

crisis in specialist care was being manufactured by policy decisions in order to bring in a double system of care in which, should you be able to afford it, you could move to the head of a different line. This concern over the emergence of a two-tiered system based on ability to pay was expressed by more than 50 percent of the women in the larger study group, a suspicion which is reinforced for them by the ongoing disputes over fees between doctors' representative associations and the government.[18]

> I think it is only around the corner that the government will just say, well, we can't afford this anymore so here, you—I mean us— you pay. All this talk about business and economics and restructuring and closing hospitals, that's just the crisis they are making so that some other business can come in and take hospitals and doctors off the government's hands. That other business will be us, paying to live with our Visa cards.

What has become apparent over the period I have been working with these women is that they suspect the crisis in health care is a manufactured one. The women in this group see this in changes in the way their own personal physicians deal with patient appointments. The majority of women complain about their personal doctors going to a system of time limited appointments. One of the most articulate women in this group put it quite bluntly:

> First they start this five minute appointment thing and, then, they will start telling us if we need more time, they are going to charge us by the hour. And we will have to pay. So the choice will be hi, how are you, here's a prescription, goodbye, or an examination. And we will pay the difference.

Underlying this is the suspicion that restructuring, which claims to be addressing the health care crisis, is proceeding at the expense of a group which sees itself as the most in need of reliable health care and most vulnerable to changes. The reshaping of home care is an area where this sense of abandonment is felt acutely.[19]

Home care is something about which this group of women feel strongly because it connects with their concern about retaining their independence as they age. They see home care as the adjunctive service that will keep them in their own homes, help them retain their ability to function in their communities and serve as a networking resource that will connect them with the services they feel they will increasingly need as they age. Changes, most notably the amalgamation of all home care services into single regional bodies with, according to these women, increasingly restrictive access criteria, are viewed almost entirely negatively. "I liked the idea of one stop shopping when I first heard about it" an eighty-year-old woman told me, "until I realized that I was considered too healthy to even get into the store to look around, let alone shop."[20] One of the key drawbacks in the new system of administering home care is what one woman called "turning home care over to social workers." What strikes these women is that home care as it is now administered requires submission to a system of investigation and surveillance about which they are very suspicious. They see that they must first give up independence by giving over to the home care system their power to define themselves as needy or healthy. That is to say, the new system, which they see as overly bureaucratic and administratively cumbersome, only responds if they are willing to allow themselves to be defined as helpless. This undermines the very purpose of home care because, as one woman put it, "if I was bloody helpless, I wouldn't need home care because I wouldn't be at home, now would I?"

The other side of home care that troubles them is the fear that home care is being used to replace medical care. This group of women is deeply troubled by the shortening of hospital stays, a concern exacerbated by their sense that a bureaucratic home assistance system will be unable to effectively deliver the kinds of services they, individually, need. They see a kind of homogenization of service on the one hand and a degeneration of medical supervision during recovery on the other—two aspects of the home care system which put them most at risk.[21] In particular, they fear that the specific needs older, and especially older single, women face in recovering at home from an accident or illness will not be adequately addressed because the system of administering home care, having become large and institutionalized, will not be able to move with sufficient speed in the event of unexpected problems.[22]

One word that comes up often in discussing restructuring changes with this group of women is betrayal. They expected to age well, with a network of institutions in place to ensure that. They feel they were lead to expect this as a right that accrued to them over time. And responding to the changes they see going on about them, the deepest concern they have is that their expectations are being devalued precisely because they are old, and for many, because they are women.

The Times We Choose to Make

Health is a moment-to-moment orientation. Silent, asymptomatic bodies are the objective, and the good body is the body which says nothing—that is, healthy bodies are bodies which are, in a strange way, absent. Institutional health care systems require silent, absent bodies as a starting point, since bureaucratic intervention in health requires the bodies presented for care to be extraordinary. Silent, absent bodies are the gatekeeper mechanism which allows institutionalized health systems to function because they mark clearly the line between health and illness. For institutional health systems to work, the healthy need to be clearly marked from the ill, and control of this distinction needs to rest with the authority of the institution and its practitioners. The institution becomes the mechanism through which health and illness are defined, governed and surveilled. The individual must be transformed into a patient, and only the institution can have that authority because its very existence depends on its being the sole site at which health is defined. Silent acquiescent patients are a requirement of this system.

What I am suggesting in the following sections is that this group of women are challenging, in a fundamental and profound way, the authority of the institutional health system by retrieving for themselves the authority to define and produce their healths. The triumphs of this small group of women are greater than simply their sum. Their ideas represent a challenge to a health system premised on distancing, victimization, mortification and the mystification of health and illness. These women remain a minority which, in the five years I have been working with older women in Ontario, is showing few, if any signs of growing dramatically. Nonetheless their intervention into a process of health making, triggered by political and economic changes, needs to be read for implications beyond the slow small changes they are enacting in their own pursuit of control. This taking back of control, which underpins their actions, is an unintended but unavoidable consequence of the health system's breakdown in reliability, a reliability these women feel they have been coerced into expecting, only to have it transformed by forces over which they have no control. Making health care reliable and accountable to individual patients rather than to larger governmental structures is the path these women are exploring. In the process, they are remaking a relationship between health, personal integrity and community which exposes the critical contradictions embedded in the policy driven and authoritarian institutions of health surveillance and treatment delivery.

I have argued so far that two things combine in these women's relationships with their health. The first is a nostalgia for a different, more personalized kind of health care relationship. The second is that this group's thinking about their health focuses on the failure of reliability as well as the distancing between patient and provider over the last several decades. Key to this, for these women at least, is a sense of decreasing power and control over decision-making which becomes increasingly troublesome as they age.[23] Aging, they understand, is a period of increased health vulnerability, and the growing sense among this group is that an institutional health care system they had been compelled to rely on has, for primarily political reasons, begun to abandon them. Thus, they are drawn to reconceptualize the way they think about their health as a personal attribute and a personal responsibility.

But it is important to see this dissatisfaction as something more than reactionary. What these women are dealing with, and dealing with in often challenging ways, are deeper questions of authority and power, responsibility and rights, and a more holistic and social understanding of health as an ongoing practice rather than simply a state of existence. In what follows here, I review some of the ways in which this small group of women have responded to the challenge of change and restructuring in the health care system in Ontario. Specifically, I outline some of the strategies they are exploring to resolve the growing conflicts they see between what the institutional health system offers, or fails to offer, and what they see as an ideal and pro-active engagement between individuals, communities and institutions in the pursuit of health and wellbeing.

This group knows intuitively that the trade-off between institutional health care and individual health is a relinquishing of authority. They understand that for a bureaucratic health system to function, the patient needs to submit to its demands. The benefit to the patient is reliability, access and quality of care. As they see these benefits eroding, the balance of the exchange between the patient and the institution shifts even more in favour of the institution. In light of this, they are reorienting themselves toward creating their own wellbeing. This involves questioning and even withdrawing completely from this relationship of submission. This is expressed in several different ways.

It has long been recognized that institutional biomedicine requires some degree of mortification of the patient, as one of the strategies by which compliance is accomplished (Mechanic 1976 and 1994, Goffman 1959, 1961 and 1963). This institutionalized abjection is not a problem when the system meets the expectations of the patient, who can be said to enter into the relationship of mortification willingly, even if not articulately. As people perceive the reliability of the institution changing, however, they are less willing to abject the integrity of their personhood in exchange for care and healing. It is at the point of interface between authority and abjection that these women are beginning to express their growing dissatisfaction and their own move toward greater autonomy.

The cornerstone of this mortification is the presumed competence of the doctor or other caregiver. What became apparent in my conversations with these women was that the first step in reorienting their relationship to an increasingly unreliable health services system was to openly challenge the official caregiver's competence to decide on their behalf.[24] They are transforming the clinical encounter from one of submission and silencing to a strategic interaction (Goffman 1969) of collaboration or resistance.

The examination room is where the most important exchanges of authority and submission take place. It is the first place where some of the women in my group have taken steps to assert their new relationship with the health care system. The examination room, by its very design as well the as the protocols of isolation, waiting and the use of uniforms, sets up the space as one in which the patient gives in to the scrutiny of the clinical gaze. That gaze requires the patient's silence, excepting where the practitioner directly seeks diagnostic information. This selective silence effectively isolates the patient as a whole person for the purposes of diagnosis and therapeutic decision-making.

So the first point of contention the women in this group have engaged is a breaching of that silence. Quiescent cooperation is being replaced, in these examination encounters, with direct questioning and open resistance to the mechanics of the procedure. One woman said,

> I won't put on that stupid paper gown. After all, he [her doctor] doesn't wear one. And besides, I feel like I am just so much flesh in that thing. If he is going to talk to me about what is wrong with me, about what is bothering me or hurting me, he should talk to who I am and not just to some body with a mouth.

One woman talked about the "old poke, prod and command" approach of doctors she had dealt with in this way:

> There was a time when it didn't matter what I went for, I would put on this blue gown and lay on a table and he would feel this or grab hold of that, and mumble. Dr. X was a nice man, but when I was laying there, he would mumble and I would say things, and he would mumble. I never got everything out, because he would just mumble and then tell me to get dressed and he would leave the room. When he came back he would give me a prescription, and tell me, oh, you know, it was something with my stomach or with my blood pressure and I would leave. But I had not talked to him. Instead it was poke, prod and command. Not any more. If he won't talk to me, I just will go somewhere else. I want to tell

him what I am feeling and thinking, and he is going to listen before I am going to listen to him.

Whether doctors respond well to this is not clear, but of the twenty-seven women in this group, nine have changed personal physicians in the last five years, two of them more than once. And the most common reason for leaving their doctors for someone else was the failure or inability of the doctor to explain sufficiently and clearly their medical condition to them.[25] The decision to change doctors is another step toward restructuring how they maintain their wellbeing. In a sense, they want a relationship of shared information, a desire prompted for them by a recognition that doctors are not the infallible and reliable caregivers they once thought. While this reflects badly on doctors in some ways, it needs to be stressed that it is the mechanics of the doctor-patient relationship these women are turning against, rather than the actual doctors or the quality of care they provide. One woman made this clear when she told me,

> Dr. X has probably kept me healthy all my life, but times have changed and I have changed and he has not, and maybe he can't. I sometimes think he is trapped by his white coat and his white office and his white questions, you know. He can't get out but I think I can.[26]

A different side of the same issue involves challenging the parameters of consent. "You need this surgery" is no longer, for many of these women, sufficient explanation to justify their agreement. Instead, these women are asking for detailed and comprehensive explanations of their illnesses, of the treatment, of alternatives and especially of differential outcomes based on either choices in treatment or the choice to forego treatment. Treatment compliance is a thorny issue at the best of times, and throughout the larger study I encountered a number of cases where informants told me they make their own decisions about when to end a treatment and so on. This is an area of some concern, given that decisions about such things as drug dosages or stopping drug treatments before their prescribed end raise serious concerns about the effectiveness of many drug treatments. I am suggesting that for the women in this group at least, the issue is not the longstanding self-determination which has affected compliance. Rather, it is a different and more intensified order of demand and query where they are insisting on being full participants in the decision-making process by demanding complete information. They are challenging the limits of informed consent by defining it for themselves rather than according to the health or statutory system's requirements and expectations.

These aspects of the personal relationship between patients and doctors are only part of the ongoing changes in health making practice these women are devising. A different and broader order of practices and ideas link the personal health of each of these women to larger issues of community health and personal responsibility, things which this group sees as linked inextricably.

The first involves the question of home care. My informants observe a bureaucratization of home care services, services they consider essential to their continuing independence and good health.[27] Home care, which all but one have had experience with, was spread between both government programs and local non-governmental organizations such as church, ethnic or other community-based groups. Hospital coordinators often made the necessary arrangements for such things as housework assistance, visiting nursing care, meal preparation or delivery and so on. It was, many women told me, an inefficient system but one which worked since the means testing for each different kind of service was personal and, they felt, equitable. The amalgamation of these services under current restructuring has led, in their eyes, to a system of gatekeeping which is excluding them from services they feel they are entitled to, and in particular, services they once received. This new hierarchically structured evaluation and delivery system, still being put into effect as I write this, has left many of these women wondering how a pronouncement from a government policy official can possibly change them from being in need to being excluded from consideration for services.

In response to this, several of these women in different cities have looked carefully at the kinds of services they once received and at the kinds of services they feel are most effective in maintaining their home independence and/or convalescence. They have built this model of necessary service from their own experience and from the experiences of those around them, and have determined that bureaucratic structures, with what they see as intrusive and police-like means testing, are not appropriate to the kinds of needs they see themselves requiring. Armed with this understanding, many of these women have begun to establish networks of mutual caregivers from among friends and acquaintances. Such a network can provide all but the most technical in home care without subjecting them to institutional surveillance or denial of service. Bypassing the home care system, however, is not seen by these women as an advance or a better alternative but as a necessary response to a new system of evaluation and delivery which has failed to maintain continuity of either service or qualifying criteria. This is not, they insist, a better way but a necessary one, if they are going to continue to access assistance.[28]

In doing this, they are establishing networks of caregiving which can circumvent official home care services by tailoring assistance to specific personal needs. Some women have developed a network for sharing the work of preparing meals. Others have put in place a network for providing housekeeping assistance for people convalescing or in need of regular assistance due to diminishing mobility or other problems. Home visiting, simply to provide social contact for convalescents, or getting books from local libraries are also part of this. Some of these women have made arrangements to accompany each other to doctors' visits, in part to ensure they are keeping necessary appointments and in part to provide moral support in situations where someone's health is deteriorating.

Their objective here is to provide personalized home care, short of nursing care—although basic nursing assistance makes up part of this informal network of assistance—in response to a home care system which cannot or will not provide these services.

The idea of containing health care costs is important to these women, who recognize that no service can continue to grow unchecked. They respect efforts over the last decade or so to increase efficiency of service, but they are deeply suspicious of recent changes which they see as isolating the elderly and diminishing service for fiscal reasons rather than to increase efficiency and reliability. The need to take matters into their own hands is, as one woman said, "unfair and unrealistic but unavoidable." "This is our own downloading," she added.

This idea of downloading, a term that has gained considerable currency in recent years, is perhaps the underlying rhetoric behind a sense among many of these women that their actions need to be broader in scope than they have been. In order to safeguard their health and wellbeing, many feel they have to cast a wider net, a net that links their individual concerns to the wider issue of community health. This is consistent with findings in the larger group of women. Reaching their mature years seems to have brought with it a sense of greater community connection and a feeling of responsibility for community activism. While it is not possible to gauge how widespread this is, I think that a growing community and political activism on the part of older women is likely to continue, building as it does on the activism by seniors at a national level. But unlike the national activist organizations, what is striking here is a recognition of the need for local community activism, activism which at first sight may not appear directly related to health and illness. These actions stem from a belief that safety, community and neighbourhood connectedness are a responsibility for those around them and a sense that relying on "outsiders" is no longer an option. This is not a simple nostalgic revisionism, reflecting back to a time when people helped each other.[29] The complexity of the social organization of mass health care is not something done to people, after all, but something which people have collaborated in over the years. And the responses of this group of women continues that collaboration, though in directions which I do not believe planners in the health care restructuring process had anticipated. It is conventional to think of the aging as silently helpless, in spite of the history of activism on the part of many aging Canadians. This is reflected in the emotional management approach of many doctors towards their aging patients, something which seems to be unique to North America (Helman 1990, Palmore 1998). Activism by the aged, and indeed active aging itself, is still seen as deviant and even a problem to be medically managed (Counts and Counts 1985 and 1996).

These women, while only a small portion of the larger group I have worked with, need to be seen in the context of healthy and active engagement rather than as abnormalities in an otherwise slowly debili-tating aging population (Marshall and McPherson 1994, Hareven 1995, Turner 1995). Their suspicions, concerns and engagement with what they see as a decline in the level of support and opportunity they had expected would accompany their aging are not simply those of angry individuals disappointed by hospital cuts, but are reflective of a sophisticated process of re-engagement with the system they had relied on and which they now feel has failed them. They are engaging in a process which might be represented diagrammatically (see Figure 1).

Figure 1
Expectation Restructuring Model for Aging Women's Activism in Ontario (Adapted from Havelock 1973).

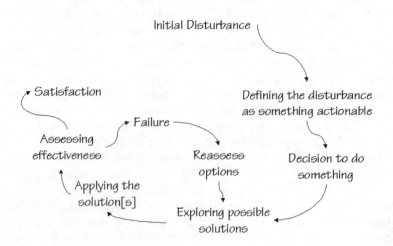

The model shows a rational response path in which some disturbance in expectations triggers a decision to act, followed by a reflection on the nature of the disturbance. It is this reflection on the underlying nature of what they see as the collapse of expectations which demands further investigation. Indeed, the first three steps in this rational response model need closer scrutiny if we are to understand how unmet expectations come to be recognized and what leads to the decision to act rather than simply to react. Since the objective of this chapter is to describe more than to analyze, and since the scope of such an analysis may well dwarf this chapter, I want simply to point out that theories and models of effective care vary between cohorts based on such things as gender, ethnicity, age, socioeconomic or political status, education level, and so on. I have only just begun the process of exploring this diversity but it is equally apparent to me that this diversity exists between individuals.

I want to conclude this section with a brief exploration of the issue of institutional residential settings and the attitudes the women in this group have begun to develop toward the option of moving into a retirement or nursing home. Going into a home, as it were, is seen by most of the women in my larger study group as a defeat. But among a smaller group, there is a sense in which seeking residential care can serve as a strategy serving their independence rather than as a submission in which they trade independence for relative security. They see residential care settings as sheltering them rather than isolating them.

Arguably, this is an overly optimistic view of residential care settings in Ontario, settings undergoing as much restructuring as acute health care facilities. The rigid social organization of these settings and the model of management which applies in most cases means the desire for shelter without isolation is as yet wishful thinking. But the sophisticated activist orientation of these women suggests a different restructuring that may occur as they respond to the often demeaning character of residential or nursing care facilities.

Therein lies the key to this entire section: exercising power and authority in defining and creating a healthy life. It's likely that I am not doing full justice to the scope of actions this group of women are exploring. There are things which, for lack of space I have not discussed, for example, the exploration of so-called "alternative" treatments, whether in seeking non-biomedical practitioners or in educating themselves about their healths, and using such things as diet, non-mainstream pharmaceuticals and so on. I have not discussed an effort by two women in a mid-sized community in southwestern Ontario to initiate a "grandchild" program through a local school, whereby high school students would be paired with elderly people in need of assistance.

Instead, I have sketched responses to what these women see as the changes which put them most at risk. This suggests two things: the first is to rewrite in some small way the perception that restructuring, or the health care system in general, produces only victims. I have tried to reorient how we see responses to institutional change in order to better look for the positive pro-active responses that emerge as possibilities for aging women and men alike. The second issue I suggest is that understanding any change, whether characterized as positive or negative in the institutional health care system, requires research from the patient upward rather than from the institution or policy downward. The engagement between patient and the health care system involves power and exchange, but it needs to be seen as multi-directional. The actions of this group of women may be small in scope and small in their impact on particular lives, but they are large and powerful correctives to an over-institutionalized view of health and aging which compel our attention and our own rethinking. Elderly women are, and will likely continue to be, isolated and abandoned by a health care system freighted with concerns for economic efficiency and bureaucratic control.[30] But they can and do occasionally resist and overturn that isolation and abandonment. Understanding the ways in which they do this is an issue that needs to be pursued.

Conclusion: *Aging Well is the Best Offence*

I describe here a group of women who are responding to aging, a changing health delivery system they feel has become less reliable, and a growing awareness that something important—their own authority to create a healthy existence—has been taken from them. I describe their efforts to reorganize their wellbeing by taking greater control of it. In the process, they have, sometimes explicitly but more often intuitively, rethought the very nature of health as an official or bureaucratized institution. They have inverted the conventional discourse of universal health care by interposing their own authority into a structure where loss of control is a major point of contention between official health practitioners and the people they service. In doing so, they point towards possible avenues of policy change, community and personal activism and the reorganization of reliance on institutional frameworks as responses to the slow, politicized transformation of the health care system in Ontario. This small group of women offer tantalizing suggestions for resisting the devaluation of their health needs. Their resistance includes stepping outside the official stream and creating a new network of health practice as well as using large institutions strategically rather than submissively. Thus, they are taking back authority and choice from the institutional framework which relies on their quiescent subordination. This action is at the heart of these women's resistance. In claiming an independent voice in making their own health, they effectively subvert the power of the institution to speak for their bodies, replacing it with a relationship of dialogue, conversation and, ultimately, cooperation.

The silent body of the conventional examining room, these women are suggesting, needs to be replaced by a questioning one. By questioning, the exchange of power and abjection in the therapeutic encounter may begin to approach the multi-directional flow of knowledge, control and participation these women seek. In this respect, then, these women direct our attention to issues about health, health care and power beyond the question of responding to diminishing or changing resources. I suggest that, perhaps only intuitively, they are asking us to think a new way of structuring health care premised on collaboration rather than submission and control.

Their actions, tentative as they are, recast health resources as something better developed from the ground up, from the patient up, rather than from policies downward. And in doing so, these women are discovering—or perhaps recovering is a better word—health resources which the over-reliance on official health policy has tended to obscure.

This chapter illustrates how several things conspired to produce this change. A combination of certain characteristics built into policy-driven health care systems and the recent policy changes which have reduced the capacity of the system to provide care create a tension in the relationship between patients and this system. This tension for these women at least, has led them to wonder aloud, and in practice, about what their relationship to this system should be. The decline in reliability they see as the result of policy changes which led to closures of facilities, staffing reductions and increased waits for both diagnosis and therapy undermines the authority of the health care system itself in such a way that, perhaps for the first time in their lives, they have found themselves in a position outside the system. This new outsider position has given them the perspective to critique the system itself. It is perhaps an irony that one consequence of political decisions regarding the "bottom line" commercialization of health care delivery has been the creation, at least among these older women, of a revitalized consciousness in which the power relations of the health care systems can be scrutinized and transformed. This is not a wide scale revolutionary change, but it is one which, though tenuous, points to a fundamental repositioning in which being stigmatized doubly as old and women, can be resisted by being old women and old healthy women.

But resistance, as a concept and a model, can prove a sticky trap. Whether it is appropriate to describe actions triggered by helplessness as a form of resistance is a complicated question. There is a process through which acts of necessity can create a crisis of consciousness out of which manifest resistance may emerge. Contemplating that requires contemplating what Spivak referred to as revolutions that as yet have no models (Landry and MacLean 1996). What these women are doing is perhaps best described as a signal that something is happening, a something which requires more thorough and wide ranging interpretation and analysis.

However, it is important to see these women's actions in the wider context of aging. Further analysis and interviews are needed if the accomplishments of these women are to translate into something more valuable than anomalous. That they stand outside the mainstream should suggest that the mainstream is more permeable and malleable than the official story of health and health care might lead one to think. Indeed, that these women are on the outside of that official story should suggest that a more careful and thorough analysis of health seeking and health making behaviour, from the patient up, is needed. That health policy relies on a monolithic and singular model of individual health is one of the many things the actions of these women challenge. Future research on the making of wellbeing as a personal project rather simply a compliance with some conventional ideology will, I don't doubt, reveal even more challenges to the received wisdom toward which these women's first provisional steps point.

Aging women in North America may well be unique among older women worldwide. Aging and gender in North America often conspire to render the already disempowered even more powerless, in contrast to other societies, where aging women have conferred on them, by their very status as aging women, increasing social power and importance (Counts and Counts 1985, Holmes and Holmes 1995). Perhaps these women, in tentative and speculative ways, are pointing toward a crack in that ideology of aging and disempowerment. Perhaps the slow degradation of a universal health care system has begun to widen that crack by destabilizing what was, for many of these women, the one thing they felt they could rely upon as they grew old—growing old well. By recognizing what they have given up to fit into the policy driven health care system and by realizing that the trade-off has left them vulnerable, these women are reclaiming some of that power in favour of a different kind of aging which confronts these disparities and failures head on. It is summed up best, I think, by the comment of one woman:

> You know that old saying that living well is the best revenge? Well, all things taken together, Douglass, I would change that to aging well is the best offence. That will get me through almost

anything. You're not very young, either. Remember that. Age well. That's how you win.

Notes

1. I am using this unusual formulation—healths—to flag the importance of seeing health behaviour, health status and health perceptions as dynamic and multi-factorial, on the one hand, and as highly idiosyncratic on the other. Each of us engages our bodies in multiple ways, and in the domain of health, this is especially true. Whether defined in terms of functional ability, the presence or absence of pain or other symptoms, appearance, or strength and endurance, to name a few, the subjective and objective experience of health is a pluralized and pluralizing phenomenology with highly particularistic and diverse qualities.

2. The concept of social death refers to culturally and institutionally conditioned patterns of disengagement through which the elderly or the ill withdraw from, or are excluded from, active and meaningful social presence. This may take the form of the removal of autonomy and volition in decision-making; in treating the aging or ill as, *de facto*, helpless; or, in extreme cases, the abandonment of the aging or the sick. Counts and Counts (1985) contains detailed discussions of this phenomenon in the context of Pacific societies. Marshall and McPherson (1995) discuss this in the Canadian context.

3. I want to thank Diana Gustafson for reminding me of the importance of this particular point.

4. Allocation of power and influence and strategies for women's resistance to the impact of reform are discussed by Simpson and Porte, Spitzer, and Transken in this volume.

5. The chapter focuses on positive responses to health care restructuring, and not, as is often the case, on victimization. This chapter speaks directly about a group of women selected out of the larger population. That selection was based on domain analysis of interview texts and the salient factors in perceptions of health care change, risk and reactions by subjects. All interview texts were coded using the Centers for Disease Controls simple text analysis program, EZText. Domain attributes were derived from focus group interviews and later modified based on preliminary single subject and life history interviews. A pile sort exercise allowed me to refine the domain analysis further, from which the coding for interview data were then derived. As this is an ongoing project, coding and recoding of interview data and re-analysis of interview texts and field notes continues. For the purposes of this chapter, this group of twenty-seven women have each expressed a high preference for pro-active response to health care change and changes in health risk. Unless otherwise indicated, it is this smaller group of women to which my discussion refers.

6. There are intriguing hints in the interviews of a method for using stigma and helplessness as a practical tool which some of these women deploy knowingly and to positive effect. Exploring this is beyond the scope of this chapter,

but I raise it to acknowledge that reaction and resistance, as well as collaboration and submission, come in many forms indeed.

7.   Methodologically, this research involves ongoing longitudinal interviewing, as well as what might be called open-ended socializing, under whatever conditions arise. I have shared Sunday dinners, attended the christening of grand and great-grandchildren, gone with some of them to doctors offices or hospitals, gone shopping or to church with them and spent entire days simply visiting with no other plan than to be a part of their daily rounds, whether in their own homes, in nursing homes, or other supervised living facilities and, in a few cases, during extended hospital stays. I have endeavoured to be either a participant or witness in the widest range of life activities conditions allow, and recently I have expanded the scope of this project, beginning field research with women living in rural and semi-rural settings. Participants have been drawn through an expanding "snowballing" network of contacts, and it should be clear no claim to anything other than an accidental sample is made here. As well as these traditional fieldwork techniques, I use protocols from the American Women Health and Aging Study (National Institutes of Health/National Institute on Aging 1995) to measure such things as life satisfaction, ability to meet daily functional demands, mobility and so on. The American protocols were chosen for expedience since they are available in a single published report. These protocols are combined with life history interviews and health domain salience interviews, using open-ended questions which are later coded for content. Fieldwork in urban settings is, in spite of its long history, not comparable to the traditional intensity of living among study subjects twenty-four hours a day for long periods of time. But it should not be seen as the "next best thing." By combining formal data collection techniques with more general participant observation over a long period, it is possible to achieve the same intensity of participation. As a fieldworker, I am not living with this group in a physical sense, but as a participant in both their personal lives and in the larger social and political community of Ontario, I am engaging their individual lives with a similar depth that is achieved in traditional fieldwork. On average, over the life of this project, I have spent about thirty hours with each participant.

8.   The nursing homes in which these women live are not twenty-four-hour nursing care facilities. Rather, they are like retirement homes, except that a nurse is on hand during the day and nursing assistance after hours is available on a fee-for-service basis. None of the women in this group live in a twenty-four-hour nursing care facility. Of the larger group of over two hundred women, only eighteen currently live in such facilities while another four live, for the moment, in hospital-based chronic care facilities.

9.   It is possible these low depression scores were a function of the context in which the instrument was administered, though test-retest using the same instrument produced consistent results for all the participants. It is worth noting that these women all scored somewhat above average on two anxiety instruments and one social anxiety instrument, though their scores would be considered sub-pathological. Both studies indicate, however, that for American women (uncorrected for racial or ethnic status and such things as urban-

rural dwelling), mild depression symptoms occur in 20–25 percent of community dwelling women over the age of sixty-five, a rate which increases to
over 30 percent for those living in nursing homes. It should be noted that the
reliability of this observation needs to be combined with some skepticism
over the DSM-IV definition of clinical depression (American Association of
Psychiatrists 1994), which is very broad. The instrument I use attempts to
correct for limited situational depression but it is known to show a high
incidence of false positives (Feher et al. 1992).

10. One reviewer of the original version of this chapter queried whether being
in "good health" had any effect on how the women in my larger study group
responded to health care system restructuring. Preliminary analysis of
interview data suggests a negative correlation between health status and
fears about the quality of health care available. In other words, the more
immediate the health concerns of participants, the greater the level of
concern that they will not receive adequate care. At the same time, this
heightened sense of fear appears to be coupled with feelings of relative
helplessness. One woman in the larger study group, who is experiencing a
resurgence of Lupus, a condition she had lived with for several decades,
sums up this feeling in her comment that "I'm just a sick old lady and no one
in those offices or hospitals cares that much about sick old ladies, so no one
is going to listen to me."

11. All names are pseudonyms, in keeping with ethnographic conventions of
ensuring privacy and reducing social risk for study participants.

12. It is interesting to note here that at least one major drug store chain in Ontario
is promoting their pharmacists as the neighbourhood professional who
knows your health needs best.

13. It is unclear from my preliminary analysis why dentists are not included as
health care providers. In an effort to define the domain of caregivers, I asked
respondents in the larger study group to arrange into two piles cards which
identified a range of health care workers. Fewer than 10 percent of this larger
group included dentists. In contrast, more than 75 percent included pharmacists and over 50 percent included home care providers such as visiting
homemakers. This appears consistent with conversations I have had over the
years with dentists, who often express concern that they are not taken
seriously as part of the health care professional continuum. This may be
generational, however, since in an accidental comparative test in which a
group of upper level undergraduate students (N=32, mean age 22) were
asked to sort the same list of possible health care professionals, I found that
more than 60 percent included dentists as health care professionals.

14. Doctors, nurses, pharmacists, nursing and non-nursing home care providers
are among the group of practitioners referred to when this group of twenty-
seven women recollects past relationships. That list is expanded somewhat
to include herbalists, chiropractors, nutritionists and, for ten of these women,
social workers, when they discuss their current engagement with health care
professionals.

15. See for example Health Canada's (Statistics Canada 1996 and 1998a) recent
reports on a longitudinal study of the health of Canadians, reports which
speak in generic terms about patient groups or categories but which avoid

the more complex questions of differential life course experience, the nature of expectations and their variation within cohorts and, most particularly, the personal intimacy within which health and illness are thought about and experienced by individual patients. The institutional milieu is a policy milieu, after all, but missing the exigencies of individual voice means missing the exigencies of lived experience, something which is at the heart of the health making studies on which this chapter is based.

16. A preliminary national study conducted by Health Canada (1998) found that a majority of practitioner and patient respondents experienced greater to substantially greater waiting periods for basic and intensive care services. These findings and the experiences of most of my informants contrast with two studies carried out during the same period by the Ontario Hospital Association (1998b and 1998c) which found significant and wide ranging decreases in waiting times and increases in service availability at Ontario hospitals. Such contradictory outcomes suggest that a systematic and rigorous set of criteria for measuring the effects of changes in service, including but not limited to accessibility and availability, has yet to be developed. Government and health institution assertions of improvement need to be subjected to more intensive critical scrutiny in order that a methodology applicable across jurisdictions and types of services might be developed.

17. This fear concerning the decline in availability and quality of emergency care at a time in life when they feel they are most likely to need it is shared by more than 80 percent of the larger study group, who expressed concern this kind of service has worsened in recent years. About 10 percent felt that emergency services had not actually worsened but, perhaps more telling, had always been inadequate. The remaining women in the larger subject group felt emergency services had always been adequate or had improved in recent years.

18. Jane Cawthorne in this volume examines how the dispute over fees plays out between obstetricians and midwives.

19. For a discussion of the ways the government goals of cost-containment and efficiency are reorganizing home care services, see Diana Gustafson in this volume.

20. Si Transken in this volume reflects on how the one-stop shopping approach to service delivery is impacting on social workers and the services they provide for women who have been sexually violated.

21. Simpson and Porte in this volume examine how systemic racism, an imperial legacy and geography isolate the Chippewas of Georgina Island.

22. The issue of convalescence following emergency care was one which came up in most interviews during this ongoing study. Many women expressed concern over a double burden that older patients face, that of seeing themselves as the most vulnerable to quality of convalescent care on the one hand, and of home-based convalescent care replacing in some way the acute medical care that they feel they will likely need at various points in their aging. Studies suggest this age and gender group, in general, have lower self-estimates of personal health, experience a greater sense of uncertainty and doubt, and have a higher likelihood of not following post-discharge treatment protocols than other groups (Ronayne 1985, Bours et al. 1998, Penrod

et al. 1998). Couple this general finding with the troublesome doubts they feel about the nature and quality of the home care system and I would suggest, based only on preliminary analysis, that while access to emergency care may be seen by most in this group as the most pressing and frightening issue in health care delivery restructuring, the changes in post-discharge care and their chances of recovery in a home-based convalescent setting is a persistent and even more deeply troubling concern.

23. The role of women in health decision-making is an important issue in the study of illness and wellbeing. Part of my larger project examines how women, from their multiple positions in families, in communities and as members of a devalued class, have long controlled the day-to-day practice of health decision-making. The institutional health care system has had to contend with this important role women take on when structuring its processes of authority and containment. The power women exercise in health decision-making and the constraints and challenges to that power are being explored in other cultural contexts but remains something of a lacunae in the medical anthropology and sociology of the industrialized countries (see Orubuloye et al. 1997, Sargent and Brettell 1996).

24. This challenge to authority needs to be seen in the context of medical training which has, as a key component, trained caregivers in the "rhetoric" of authority and competence through which they seek to enforce compliance (Haas and Shaffir 1987).

25. While my interview notes and subsequent questioning of one woman are not entirely conclusive, at least one doctor advised one of the women in this group to find another doctor, but it is unclear what this doctor's motivation was.

26. I was continually struck by the number of times the issue of doctors not listening to patients came up during my interviews with all the women in the larger study. This seems to be the most common complaint, with explanations ranging from "he does not care what I say" to "he has not time to listen to me, he has so many patients to see in one day just to pay his bills." Even women whose faith in their personal physician was substantial would often tell me that the doctor never listened to them when they tried to explain how they were feeling. Arguably, the most common front on which strained medical resources are being responded to is over the issue of compliance and miscommunication (see Myers and Midence 1998, Blackwell 1997, DiMatteo and DiNicola 1982).

27. The linking of independence and good health is something which runs through the majority of my interviews. While some in this smaller group are rethinking that connection, in general the most elderly women in the larger group equate a loss of independence with deteriorating health. As one woman from this larger group put it clearly, "when it is time for me to go to a home, I will know it is soon time for me to die. That is how sick I know I will be when that happens."

28. This is a good example of resistance without consciousness that I mentioned earlier. Compelled to take action in the face of changes in a service they see as essential, these women are taking necessary steps rather than politically aware ones. It should be noted, however, that these acts of necessity subvert

the amalgamation and bureaucratization of access to home care because they recover control from the institution. In particular, they take back control over the definition of need and of wellbeing. By doing so, these women's actions have the effect of resisting subordination to an institutional control and definition system they see as unwieldy and potentially dangerous. While the manifest intent of these actions is risk reduction, their latent effect remains resistance to subordination in a power nexus which is at the heart of the rationalization of publicly funded home care.

29. Indeed, if my interviews are any indication, most of the women in the larger study do not reflect back on earlier periods as times when people were more willing to help each other. That "golden age of neighbourliness" does not stand up to close scrutiny. While many women in the larger study group told me they certainly knew their neighbours better when they were younger, they almost all told me that did not mean their neighbours were any more willing to assist in such things as health care.

30. As I write this, a new example of the over-bureaucratization of health delivery is playing out in the press. A recent Ministry of Health directive requires the criteria for covering nutritional supplements to be enforced strictly and rigidly. This excludes many patients who formerly could get their supplements paid for. In phone interviews after this news story was reported, two informants discussed how it is exactly this kind of rigid policy control which deepens their suspicion that the aged and the chronically infirm are being "triaged" out of the health care system as an economic rather than medical efficiency.

13

Forget Reform–We Need a Revolution![1] Better Health for Canadian Women through Holistic Care

Farah M. Shroff [2]

The Canadian feminist movement has long advocated for change "by women, for women." In the future, change must come "through women, for all people," declares Ursula Franklin (1999), a physicist and social visionary who has worked for many years within the Canadian feminist movement. Franklin issued this challenge to people gathered at a symposium focused on designing research, policy and action approaches for eliminating gender inequity in health. Her words have powerful implications for everyone dedicated to reshaping the health care system.

In this concluding chapter, I take a step toward addressing that challenge by examining holistic care. This model could be used as a basis for promoting and improving the health of all Canadians. Integrated feminists and other critical scholars join a growing chorus of concerned citizens who question the dominant system of medicine in Canada. Approximately 75 percent of Canadians have used holistic medicine at one time or another (Ramsay et al. 1999). This suggests that it is time for the voices of the people the system claims to serve to be better heard.

I want to begin here by placing holistic care within the context of health reform in the new millennium. Health reform refers to a broad range of initiatives implemented at the national, provincial and local levels that are intended to reshape the health care system. These changes are not only happening in Canada, but in virtually every other part of the globe. In the South World, Structural Adjustment Programs, imposed by U.S.-based imperialist bodies such as the International Monetary Fund and the World Bank, are bleeding (already ailing) health care systems to a slow death (Werner et al. 1997). Women in the South bear the brunt of this drastic destruction to the infrastructure that once existed. All over the world, the dominant reform discourses of scarcity and efficiency (and their implementation) (J. Anderson, personal communication, November 1999) have a negative impact on women's formal and informal health care.

This has been the case in Canada. Joan Anderson (personal communication, November 1999) notes that in 1991, 10 percent of Canada's Gross
Domestic Product was spent on health care, but in 1998, due to cutbacks,
9.1 percent of the GDP was spent on health care. (One percent of $60 billion
is a significant amount of funds.) In 1995, the federal government
produced a budget that dramatically reduced health care transfer payments to the provinces. Anderson notes that, in 1999, the Canada Health
and Social Transfer appears to be infusing large amounts of money into
the health care system, but in fact, it is simply bringing the funding level
back to pre-1995 levels.

Throughout the 1990s, virtually every province in Canada commissioned large-scale reports to guide health care reform. Many of these
documents criticized health care systems for being inefficient (particularly in tertiary care settings), not valuing all cadres of the health workforce
and for leaving gaps in service provision. In my study of 243 government
documents pertaining to health care policy and design, I found that very
few (less than twenty documents) mentioned women's health as a high
priority (Shroff 1996). This kind of negligence is based on deeply rooted
patriarchal and sexist values held by those directing the health care
system. Government cutbacks and rising health care costs impact both
women and men but women have less financial resources to cope with
these changes (National Coordinating Group on Health Care Reform and
Women 2000). In B.C., Colleen Fuller (1999) concludes that a dearth of
publicly available information exists on women and health reform,
which makes it very difficult to evaluate the impacts of reduced federal
funding—the shift in emphasis from hospital-based to community-based
care, changes in the job picture, privatization, outsourcing, amalgamations and so forth. Armstrong and Armstrong's (1999) study entitled
Women, Privatization and Health Care Reform: The Ontario Case concludes
that these trends are putting women patients at risk and are adversely
affecting work environments for women health practitioners.

The preceding chapters in this book provide many concrete examples
of the far reaching and negative impact of health care reform on the lives
of various groups of women caregivers and care recipients. Taken together, these examples illustrate the need for changes that go beyond
reform—the need for a revolution in the way we act and think about our
individual and collective health and health care.

This chapter's contribution is to propose a revolutionary agenda for
transforming health care in Canada—one which builds on social justice
principles and validates holistic practices. I begin with a brief overview
of the dominant system of medicine in Canada. In this section allopathy
or the biomedical model of health care is criticized but nowhere do I
suggest that it be abolished. This system of medicine has many strong

points, particularly in regard to emergency and acute care services. Next, I define holistic health and trace its existence, first within a world context and then within Canada. This includes an overview of how many Canadians seek holistic health care and why they do. I weigh both the possibilities and pitfalls of the current way in which holistic care has been adopted in Canada. In doing so, I critique the New Age entrepreneurs who have co-opted the ideal of holism to serve distinctly non-holistic ends. Finally, I briefly outline a revolutionary agenda built on a foundation of social change and holistic multi-paradigmatic health care. Such change would require the political will to redirect some financial resources from high technology equipment, allopathic physicians' incomes and pharmaceuticals to social justice reforms and holistic health care.

Before moving on, let me position women in this discussion. Women are the main consumers and providers of health care.[3] These facts hold true for holistic health care as well—herstorically and currently, locally and internationally. Women are thus the leaders in holistic health care changes. In this chapter, women are presumed to be centre stage in this discussion.

Women's health is often reduced to reproductive health issues. This emphasis inadvertently reinforces the notion of women as breeders, and this is particularly true for women of colour (Davis 1981). Here, it is assumed that virtually all health issues are women's issues, and therefore, this chapter takes a broad-brush approach to women's health issues. Within an integrated feminist perspective, race, class, (dis)ability, sexual orientation, age and other factors are foregrounded, as appropriate, alongside gender. This anti-oppression lens encompasses feminist, anti-racist, leftist/neo-Marxist and other liberationist theories. Because the theoretical framework does not privilege gender as the only category of analysis, this chapter scrutinizes racism and capitalism as much as it does sexism.

The revolution in health calls for both individual action for wellness and structural changes that ensure more equitable resource distribution and attention to the political, social and economic determinants of health. Both holism and social justice are vital aspects of this call for "health for all." Furthermore, financial issues are paramount in Canadian health care debates, and fostering the resurgence of holism promises to facilitate a wiser allocation of health care dollars and resources. More importantly, holistic health care has the potential to improve the health status of Canadians.

A Brief Overview of Allopathic Medical Dominance in Canada

Allopathic medicine is the dominant form of medicine in Canada.[4] It has become so deeply embedded in the cultural bedrock of medical discourse that many Canadians accept allopathic medical ideas uncritically; there is a common-sense acceptability of the dominance of this system of medicine, and when many Canadians hear the word "medicine," they think of allopathic medical men in white coats.

Allopathy has a politically and legally enshrined monopoly over health care resources in Canada; it is the system of care that is (virtually) fully funded by the state in the form of medical insurance. A reductionist scientific approach, when applied to this system of medicine, reduces the human body to organs, tissues and cells. Concentrating on physical aspects of the individual human body, allopathic diagnostic techniques and treatments dismiss political, economic, social, emotional and psychological factors as significant aspects of health and wellbeing. This model of medicine tends to focus on disease and cure, on doctors' training and accomplishments, on science and technology, on objectivity and rationality. Allopathic medicine is professionalized, hierarchical, competitive, male-dominated and reflects the wider society in which it is embedded (Glendinning 1982).

All chapters in this book conducted, from different perspectives, a gender analysis of allopathy. Doris Grinspun, Janet Lum and Paul Williams looked at physician domination within Canada's health care system and its intricate ties to patriarchy. Sepali Guruge, Gail Donner, Lynn Morrison, Denise Spitzer, Patricia Simpson and Sheila Porte foreground racial and ethnic differences in the delivery of allopathic health care. As Elizabeth Esteves, Diana Gustafson and Douglass Drozdow-St. Christian point out, caring work most often falls onto the shoulders of women and an underlying assumption within the dominant health care system is that women will provide this service for little or no remuneration. The devaluation of women's work as health care providers, despite their dominance (in numbers) is examined by Si Transken and by Frances Gregor and colleagues. Jane Cawthorne goes on to illustrate how males, as the dominant force in the health care bureaucracy, perpetuate the devaluation of caring skills over technical knowledge derived from allopathic medicine. Similarly, as she points out, the fee-for-service payment schemes for physicians perpetuate inefficiencies and limit universal access to medical care.

I envision a system of health care that is holistically oriented and incorporates various systems of diagnosis and treatment, including ayurveda, traditional Chinese medicine and other bonafide systems of holistic care, as well as the most useful aspects of allopathy. Each system

of health care would be evaluated and the most useful aspects implemented in this holistic multi-paradigmatic system of care. This is different than the more common argument that allopathy and holistic health
care be practised side-by-side, an argument that fails to take into consideration existing power differences between allopathy and its holistic
counterparts. Here I envision a completely redesigned system that places
health promotion and disease prevention as the foundation.

Holistic Health Care in Canada

Holism is sometimes spelled as wholism which accentuates its semantic
connections to the word *whole*. The term *holistic* health care is used
throughout this chapter, instead of other commonly used terms such as
alternative and complementary. Briefly, the reason these other terms are
rejected is because referring to a health system as alternative sets it in
opposition to the dominant system and reinforces the primacy of the
biomedical model (allopathy). On the other hand, and in its favour,
alternative also implies that consumers of health care have choices and
that the dominant system may be replaced by other systems. The term
complementary health care implies that holistic health care may operate in
tandem with, and complement, allopathic medicine. The users of this
term tend to ignore the enormous philosophical, paradigmatic and
medical gulf that lies between holistic and non-holistic forms of care;
similarly, the fact that allopathic care is the sociopolitically and legally
dominant form of health care in Canada is also obscured by some users
of this term. This is not to state that holistic health care is *not* complementary to allopathic medicine, but that conscious efforts to bring these
systems together must be made with the idea of creating a brand new
approach to health care, not by *adding on* holistic care to the current
system.

Defining and Critically Contextualizing Holistic Health
Holistic thought forms exist in every part of the world and have existed
from the beginning of human existence. The world's history of medicine
is that of holistic health care. Holistic schools of thought vary in some
ways from region to region but are more similar than they are different.
The following principles unite them:

- entities and systems in the universe, including humans, exist
  as a unified whole (Cmich 1984);
- the parts of the whole are dynamically interrelated, and the
  individual cannot be separated from the social, cultural and

spiritual environment (Cmich 1984);
- the whole cannot be understood by the isolated examination of its separate parts (Cmich 1984);
- the whole is more than the sum of the parts (Cmich 1984);
- matter is interlinked, interconnected and dynamic; it is constantly changing and it is this transformation that denotes time (Verma 1995: 20); and
- malfunctions are understood and treated in the context of the social, cultural and spiritual environment; body, mind and soul are treated integrally (Verma 1995: 20).

Within holistic health perspectives, the body is understood in a unified manner. Injury to one part of the body may thus damage another, seemingly unrelated, part. Holistic principles maintain that the body has an innate capacity to heal itself and that the role of the physician is to first do no harm and second to assist the body in its natural tendency toward balance. Holistic health theory takes into account mind, body and spirit, and recognizes the interrelationship between human health and the social and physical environment. Holistic health theory, as defined here, is posited on the notion that life force, or *prana* (in Sanskrit), *chi* (in Chinese), *mana* (in Hawaiian), connects all life in the universe and that this energy is responsible for the life of all beings. Goldstein, Sutherland, Jaffe and Wilson (1988: 853) consider nine characteristics that typify holistic health care:

- an emphasis on the unity of the body, mind and spirit view of health as a positive state, not merely the absence of disease;
- concern with the individual's responsibility for his or her own health;
- an emphasis on health education, self-care and self-healing;
- a relationship between the provider and the client that is relatively open, equal and reciprocal;
- a concern with how the individual's health reflects familial, social and cultural environments;
- an openness towards using natural, "low" technology and non-Western techniques whenever possible;
- an emphasis on physical and emotional contact between the practitioner and the client;
- a belief that successful healing transforms the practitioner as well as the client; and
- acceptance of a spiritual component in the etiology and treatment of illness.

Goldstein and colleagues (1988) note that not all these characteristics are present each time the term holistic is invoked. They compare the above characteristics with the allopathic model which is posited on notions that health is viewed as the absence of verifiable pathology and that diseases arise from specific pathogenic agents. The allopathic model, they note, seldom considers social, spiritual or psychological aspects of health and illness as healing relies almost exclusively upon cooperation with a knowledgeable physician. Cures within allopathy, they state, usually involve goods and services such as procedures, drugs and hospital stays, which are controlled by physicians. Finally, Goldstein and colleagues (1988) assert that the patient's role is largely one of compliance in the allopathic model. They suggest that these basic characteristics make holistic health care and allopathic care quite different and that interest in holistic care is growing among health professionals and the general public.

It is precisely because of such growth and interest that holistic models also need to be considered critically. Howard Berliner and Warren Salmon (1985) point out that most systems of holistic health are overly concerned with the individual and her or his mind, body and spirit, but rarely examine the health connections to the larger social world. This is probably the most astute criticism of holistic health systems. Most systems of health care, including holistic ones, do not include social health as a major component. This lack of attention to social health is a serious gap in holistic health practices. Worse, within many systems of holistic medicine, patriarchal and class overtones are apparent.

In ayurveda, for example, some interpretations of *tridosha* theory (which notes different body/mind types amongst people) have likened *vata* (the air/ether type) to the Brahmin (the elite of the Hindu caste system) caste and portrayed *vata* people as noble, while *kapha* (the earth/water type) is portrayed as docile and slow, as the "ideal" Indian woman ought to be. In Chinese medicine, *yin* traditionally means the shady side of a mountain, but is also related with femaleness; under a patriarchal lens, yin and women are considered sinful. E.L. Ogden notes that "acupuncture is a system of non-absolutes, of energy balance. Energy is superficial or *Yang* and deep or Yin. Neither is good or bad as long as they are in equilibrium—either can be bad if in excess" (1976: 11). While this reasoned view (which states that neither yin nor yang is good or bad) is probably the original medical understanding, oppressive structures have affected modes of thinking. I found, in my readings of ayurvedic original texts, that these writings were not corrupted by hierarchical social structures,[5] but were changed to suit the needs of the rulers in more recent times, a reflection on the fact that medicine and politics have always been intricately intertwined. The dominant have interpreted and implemented holistic medicine to suit their needs and, therefore, within holistic medical philosophy and practice, there is a great need for equitable changes, particularly along gender, class and sexual orientation lines. Upper class, patriarchal and heterosexist interpretations of holistic health concepts abound in the literature. It is thus crucial to be as critical of holistic medicine as of allopathic medicine.

Berliner and Salmon (1985) attribute the popularity of holism to increasing dissent with the present system of medical care delivery. They claim that clients remain with holistic practitioners because of practitioner friendliness and interpersonal sensitivity. They believe that this positive rapport between practitioner and client is the major reason that clients go to non-allopathic practitioners. These kinds of communication issues are considered "soft" aspects of medicine and are not attributed as much importance as are "hard" aspects such as surgery. Unconvinced that holistic practices such as meditation, biofeedback and hypnosis produce health benefits, these authors suggest that most contain heavy doses of mysticism and charismatic elitism. This is possibly true of some New Age services such as shamanic healing, trance work and so forth. While these practices, within their cultural context, may provide a great deal of medical relief to the people who use them, some practitioners, in an unregulated environment, may appropriate and misrepresent holism as they have not received the appropriate training—which is often based on apprenticeships with the accomplished practitioners. This is dangerous, as are the claims made by some practitioners, masquerading as holistic healers, that they can miraculously *cure* diseases in order to lure vulnerable and ill people into paying huge sums of money for unproved therapies.

With such cautions in mind, the World Health Organization's (WHO) position on holistic medicine is noteworthy. The WHO (1978a) notes that traditional holistic medicine has intrinsic utility and should be promoted and its potential developed for the wider benefit of humankind. It notes that *holistic medicine is used by approximately three-quarters of the world's population.* The WHO concludes that holistic medicine should be evaluated, given due recognition and developed so as to improve its efficacy, safety, availability and wide application at due cost as well as that it is an integral part of people's culture and can and does freely contribute to scientific and universal medicine.

In summary, while it is clear that neither the allopathic nor the holistic model of care attends to social inequities, the latter embraces the emotional, mental and spiritual facets of the individual as well as the physical. It is partly for this reason that holistic care is popular. However, in my view, the holistic health care model could be improved and serve the needs of more people if race, class and gender analyses were taken into account. The health of the individual is clearly linked to her or his income, employment and security (from violence and emotional, social and physical harm). Understanding macro-factors such as capitalism, violence against women, pay inequities, workplace sexual harassment and so forth would add a great deal to micro-diagnoses of an individual's health, if only to bring more compassion from practitioners for those who are unjustly treated. At best, an analysis of social inequities on the part of practitioners could bring about a fully fledged public health movement which seeks to provide holistic care to all people, particularly those marginalized by oppressive social structures.

Popularity of Holistic Health Care in Canada

How Many Canadians use Holistic Care and Who are They?

Millions of Canadians report using holistic health care. A nation-wide study (Ramsay et al. 1999) revealed that almost three-quarters of Canadians have used at least one form of holistic health care in their lives. Another survey, conducted by the Angus Reid group in August 1997, showed that 42 percent of Canadians are currently embracing holistic medicines and practices and most have been doing so for at least the past five years. These results parallel those of the Canada Health Monitor telephone survey, which found that one in five Canadians aged fifteen years and over used at least one holistic practitioner within the last six months (Berger 1990, 1992 and 1995). Most consumers of holistic health care services have not given up on allopathic services. They use each system of medicine for treating different aspects of a chronic condition, such as HIV / AIDS, because they see results from a combination of different medical approaches. Alternatively, some Canadians treat their allergies or asthma using holistic approaches but go to an allopath if they break their leg, as they recognize that each approach has its successes in different areas. Generally, people find that what is missing in allopathic care can be found in holistic care.

Current survey data is likely underrepresenting the actual numbers of people turning to holistic health care practices. Statistical information is not easily compared because of differences in how data are collected. Each of the above surveys uses a different time frame (lifetime, past five years, past six months). Some researchers use narrower definitions than others when defining what constitutes holistic health practices. For example, people who practise yoga, tai chi, qi gong and some forms of martial arts are not counted among those engaging in holistic practices. Additionally, the definitions of holistic health care (or alternative health care, as most of the researchers call it) vary slightly, but most of the researchers asked about services that are not covered by medical insurance plans. This means that midwifery, which is now covered by a few provincial health plans, would not be included in some surveys, although many would consider midwifery to be a holistic health profession.

There are also uncounted numbers of people who use herbal medicine or other holistic therapies in their own homes and communities. In South Asian Canadian and Asian Canadian neighbourhoods, for example, traditional (holistic) medicines are sold in grocery stores and specialty herbal stores. Some estimates indicate that 20–25 percent of the general public use natural remedies such as herbs, garlic and vitamins to treat chronic problems (Cottrell 1995). Many food stores now carry bulk herbs such as Valerian (to assist with sleeping disorders), Echinacea (to treat colds and flus) and St John's Wort (to treat depression). Homeopathic remedies, particularly those used for common complaints such as pain and children's conditions such as teething, are easily available from regular pharmacies. The availability of these remedies may be higher today given the commercial success of the work of holistic health gurus Andrew Weil, Deepok Chopra and others.

Notwithstanding the limitations of statistical data, it appears that more women than men are turning to holistic healers and practices. According to one study on naturopathy, the typical client is female (approximately 75 percent), middle class (at least half earning more than $30,000 per annum) and university educated (approximately 63–65 percent) (Gort and Coburn 1988). A more recent study also reported a higher incidence of use among women with a post-secondary education living in Canadian cities (Berger 1995). The reasons for this are unclear.[6] It may be that women are attracted to the more client-centred, educational aspects of holistic medicine where power is shared more equitably between client and practitioner.

Most studies note that consumers of holistic health services tend to have some post-secondary education and many of these people live in urban centres. As well, people whose cultural traditions include the use of holistic health care tend to live in large urban centres, where their communities have congregated; traditional Chinese medicine, for example, flourishes in Toronto and Vancouver, where large Chinatowns exist.

While Earl Berger (1995) notes that baby boomers are the leaders in holistic health care consumption, another study found that those in the eighteen to twenty-four-year age group are most likely to use holistic health care. Income is not a significant factor in the consumer profile, as 54 percent and 55 percent, respectively, of the less-than-$20,000-a-year income group and the $60,000-to-$79,999-per-year income group report using holistic health care (Ramsay et al. 1999).

Collectively, Canadians use holistic health care 4.4 times per year and spend approximately $1.8 billion per annum on holistic health care (Ramsay et al. 1999). Chiropractic is the most popularly used system (36 percent having been treated chiropractically), followed by relaxation techniques (23 percent) and massage therapy (23 percent). Of those who had used holistic health care in the past twelve months, 88 percent found the care somewhat (40 percent) or very helpful (48 percent). This indicates that satisfaction with holistic health care is high (Ramsay et al. 1999).

Why are Canadians Seeking Holistic Health Care?

Almost half of Canadians (47 percent) used holistic health care because they experienced real and immediate results, in contrast to what they experienced from allopathic care (Ramsay et al. 1999). The Angus Reid survey (1997) reports the three most common reasons that people embrace holistic health practices are:

- they don't hurt you and may help a bit;
- regular medicines on their own aren't working; and
- alternative medicines are more natural.

Consistent with the above reasons, Ramsay, Walker and Alexander (1999) note that the most common reason for using holistic services is to maintain or improve general health and wellbeing. Canadians report visiting a variety of practitioners, including chiropractors, massage therapists, herbalists, naturopaths, reflexologists, acupuncturists and homeopaths (Berger 1992 and 1995). Many also seek advice from health food store staff and fitness or health instructors (Berger 1992). Those who use holistic practitioners consider lifestyle factors such as stress, exercise and smoking to be the most important factors affecting their personal health. Only 13 percent cited physiological conditions as causes of concern (Berger 1992).

Holistic Health as a Potential Solution to Canada's Most Pressing Health Problems

In 1986, the federal government report, *Achieving Health for All*, identified chronic conditions and mental health problems as the two biggest challenges facing Canadians. This points to the failure of allopathic medicine to treat and cure the most pressing and prevalent health problems of this era.

The diseases of the post-industrial era are those of the immune system. Environmentalists are ringing alarm bells about the extreme destruction of the planet. These trends are connected: the ecosystem is breaking down and the human immune system is deteriorating with it. Many immune system problems—anxiety, asthma, allergies, cancers, chronic depression, HIV / AIDS, chronic fatigue syndrome, lupus, mono-nucleosis, schizophrenia—are on the rise in North America today and some are affecting children at an excessive rate. Holistically, mental and physical health problems are considered to be intertwined.

Treating and curing some immune system problems has proven so difficult allopathically that it is quite common for mainstream treatment advice to include some holistic health care. Conventional AIDS treatment advice, for example, is to recommend anti-retro viral therapy along with Chinese medicine, naturopathy or another form of holistic health care. People with cancer are amongst those who utilize the services of holistic practitioners at a high rate, and it is estimated that 40 to 75 percent of Canadians with cancer use holistic health care to treat it (Brigden 1987, Knapp 1993).

Allopath N.S. Rao (1984) describes the three types of illnesses. First is chronic illness which includes conditions considered to be irreversible. Treatment is supportive as opposed to curative. Second is minor self-limiting disorders. These do not need active treatment, yet make up the bulk of allopathic doctor-patient relationships. Third are acute medical or surgical conditions in which timely intervention can cure or improve the quality of life. This category represents the smallest proportion of doctor-patient contact.

For both chronic and acute medical and surgical conditions, holistic care has great potential. For minor self-limiting disorders, holistic health promotion (amongst other things, this includes a healthy diet, restful sleep, meditation and practices such as yoga and tai chi) ought to avoid the need for people to seek expert care for such problems.

Indeed, many allopathic physicians are recognizing the value of holistic health care. In a study of 84 general practitioners in Ontario and 118 in Alberta (Verhoef and Sutherland 1995), 71 percent consider acupuncture useful or very useful; 59 percent consider chiropractic useful or very useful; and 55 percent consider hypnosis useful or very useful. However, physicians' knowledge about these services was very low. Willingness to refer patients to holistic practitioners varies from province to province, with Ontario physicians (65 percent) more likely than Alberta physicians (44 percent) to make such referrals.

The Medical Society of Nova Scotia, a provincial branch of the Canadian Medical Association, formed a complementary medicine section in May 1994 (LaValley and Verhoef 1995). In part, the section was founded in order to establish standards of accountability and ethics in holistic medicine. Its mandate is to promote and share information about clinical research, education and the practice of holistic medicine within allopathy. The section supports research which assesses the usefulness of holistic medicine for patient wellbeing and treatment. The members of the section acknowledge that allopathic medicine arises out of a different paradigm than holistic therapies. The five sub-specialties within the section include environmental medicine, bioenergetic medicine (including acupuncture and allied therapeutic techniques), homeopathy and homotoxicology, nutritional and botanical medicine, and intravenous nutrition and detoxification therapy.

William LaValley, the chair of the Nova Scotia Complementary Medicine Section, believes the creation of the section reflects the support of many family physicians for holistic medicine (Cottrell 1995). This was the first recognition by the Canadian Medical Association that holistic medicine requires their attention. In 1995, the B.C. Medical Association formed a sub-committee to examine nonconventional medicine. A similar process in the Northwest Territories is working on ways to integrate Aboriginal healers into the dominant medical system.

Not all physicians support the move toward holistic systems of care in Canada. Ian Goldstine, past president of the Manitoba Medical Association said, "What happened with the Nova Scotia medical society isn't happening here. My personal view is that chiropractors don't just want to look after your back. They want to be your family physician" (Cottrell 1995: 34). He cites stories of chiropractors who want to treat children and perform adjustments for asthma and ear infections. This, he claims, is dangerous. He argues that only the family physician is capable of providing all the primary care required by patients. These sentiments are not uncommon among family physicians, whose scope of practice overlaps with that of some natural practitioners. For some physicians, moving toward holistic health care represents competition for patients and a potential reduction in their incomes and their social status.

Holistic health and allopathy emerge from fundamentally distinct paradigms. While allopathic physicians are competent to practice allopathy they are not, without appropriate training, competent to practice holistic therapies. In fact, a significant amount of unlearning of reductionist thinking is a prerequisite for gaining an appreciation of holistic health care philosophy. Because the badge of MD reassures many Canadians that they are receiving the best care, some consumers may be fooled by allopaths posing as holistic health experts. Training and formal education must be standardized and regulated for allopaths interested in holistic care treatments.

Future Directions: Problems and Possibilities

Earl Berger, who conducts the Canada Health Monitor Survey notes that "[t]his is a very dissatisfied society," and "people are searching for a different way of living and alternative medicine is part of that search" (as cited in Chisholm 1995: 35). Many people report using both an allopathic physician and a holistic practitioner. This suggests that some Canadians already pick and choose from various systems of health care according to their needs.

This section focuses on the potential for health benefits, as well as some drawbacks, of the current way in which holistic care is adopted in Canada and includes a discussion about the relevance of social movements. Highlighted are realistic and pragmatic changes (as well as utopian hopes for a better future) that could occur in this country if there were enough political will to put a reasonable ceiling on doctors' incomes and to curtail the purchase of high technology equipment and pharmaceuticals. Savings from these items alone would allow for billions of dollars to be directed toward health promotion, community development, support for parents, equal pay for work of equal value, genuine and significant commitments to end violence against women, free feminist psychotherapy and holistic health care, to name just a few.

A Platform for Change

As noted in the previous section, some allopathic physicians are lobbying for change. Other changes are occurring within specific health-related institutions. For example, the National Cancer Institute of Canada estimates that approximately 40 percent of cancer patients try to cure themselves with some form of "unorthodox" treatment (Chisholm 1995). Doctors' Hospital in Toronto offers massage, acupuncture and relaxation techniques to mental health consumers and is funding research on acupuncture as a treatment for alcohol and drug addiction. Toronto East General Hospital's outpatient clinic offers Therapeutic Touch, which emanates from an old concept called laying-on of hands. Similar treatments are offered in a variety of clinics all over Canada. Since 1991, the University of Alberta has offered a two-hundred-hour continuing education certificate in acupuncture for health professionals. The University of Saskatchewan created a similar program for anaesthetists. Private companies, such as Husky and Atlantis Aerospace in southern Ontario, have hired naturopathic physicians to provide care for their employees (E. Flood, personal communication, 1995). While Canadian general practitioners do not appear to be in the forefront of holistic medicine, there is considerable acceptance of it. Marja Verhoef and Lloyd Sutherland (1995) note that 54 percent of Canadian physicians referred to holistic practitioners. Similar studies in other countries put the referral rate at 90 percent in the Netherlands and 58 percent in England (Verhoef and Sutherland 1995).

In the fall of 1993, the National Institute of Health in the United States announced that it would fund research in the following areas: ayurvedic medicine for the treatment of Parkinson's disease; yoga for heroin addiction and obsessive-compulsive disorder; acupuncture for treating depression; hypnosis for healing broken bones; music therapy for people with brain injuries; massage therapy for patients with AIDS, post-surgical patients and people with bone marrow transplants; and biofeedback for pain control and diabetes (Alternative Medicine: The Facts 1994).

It is significant that such an important funding body in the U.S. decided to fund holistic medical research. This type of research funding is not yet widely sanctioned by equivalent groups in Canada, such as the Canadian Institutes of Health Research (CIHR) and its member groups such as the Medical Research Council and the National Health and Research Development Program. However, these changes are possible if citizens organize and demand that holistic research is conducted, holistic health policies are formulated and holistic health care is implemented. Given their popularity, integrating holistic medical practices into the health care system should be part of policy reform. Impartial, fair assessment of holistic health care services and the practitioners who provide them should be integrated into practitioner peer review programs run by provincial licensing authorities and professional organizations. These assessments must be based on holistic paradigms. Separate colleges should be established for each system of holistic health care and all other measures that provide for the self regulation of these professions should be put in place.

Holistic health research, especially for treatments and cures of some of the most pressing illnesses of this era, should also be part of this agenda. Additionally, allopathic physicians ought to become familiar with holistic therapies, inform their patients that they are available, be able to discuss them, be non-judgmental and direct patients to appropriate sources of care and information. Most importantly, allopathic physicians ought to respect people's choices to seek the care that is in their best interest.

Infusing more money into health care is not necessary—$60 billion is sufficient for a nation with the relatively small population of Canada. What is necessary is a change in funding allocations. Canadian health ministries must muster the political will to seriously examine how this huge amount of money is being (mis)spent and demonstrate the courage to redistribute it so that it benefits all women, men and children equitably. The current imbalance in expenditure is simply illogical.

To illustrate, the total budget of the B.C. Ministry of Health was approximately $6 billion in 1992–3. Of that, 45.3 percent went to hospital care and 25.4 percent went to medical services, not including $49 million given to the B.C. Medical Association for insurance premiums, pension plans and malpractice insurance. Glen Cassie of the Association of Naturopathic Physicians of British Columbia asserts that only 1 percent of the budget is spent on so-called supplementary care, which includes registered massage therapists, chiropractors, naturopaths, physiotherapists and others. He also states that *these practitioners see approximately 30 percent of the consumers of health care in the province* (G. Cassie, personal communications, July 27 and 31, 1995).

Nothing short of a radical redesign of health care in Canada will rectify this situation. There are too many vested interests in maintaining the status quo.

Social Movements and Holism
Many social movements, while not directly advocating for holistic health, are advocating for changes that would bring about a more holistic society. This section names just a few social movements that are relevant to holism in general.

Avowedly non-religious movements and many quasi-religious movements make a connection between wellbeing and spirituality. Groups such as Alcohol Anonymous (and their off-shoots such as Narcotics Anonymous, Adult Children of Alcoholics, etc.) have very large followings.

Since the early 1980s, the environmental movement has been growing in popularity in Canada and is evidenced by the growth of the Green Party and non-partisan ecological community-based groups. There is also a growing consciousness amongst Canadians of the need to eliminate various toxic products, such as styrofoam, to waste less water and to purchase products which do not pollute the earth. Among other milestones, the 1962 publication of Rachel Carson's book, *Silent Spring*, launched the modern era of environmental concerns, with an emphasis on reducing garbage and pollution. Reliable information about the devastation of the world's forests, water sources, air and soils has prompted many Canadians into taking some action in their daily lives. Women have been at the forefront of this movement, organizing small neighbourhood recycling groups, as well as large groups such as the Western Canada Wilderness Committee. Advocating for biodegradable housecleaning products, composting and other easily accomplished environmentally friendly acts, women have shown great leadership in this area. Recently, partly due to education in schools (by mostly women teachers), youth are teaching the older generation about environmental issues (M. Joyce, personal communication, 1995). The four Rs include reduce, reuse, recycle and most importantly, rethink. Rethinking the ways in which people treat the earth has a great deal of holistic potential, and some parts of the environmental movement incorporate holistic thought-forms, such as the interconnectedness of all life. Protecting the earth, animals and plants has shown some environmentalists about the medicinal benefits of herbs and other holistic therapies.

As mentioned above, the association between cancers and environmental pollution are also being made by environmentalists, particularly by women's environmentalist groups examining breast cancer, for example, the Women's Educational Environmental Development group (WEED) in Toronto. Others are discovering that the environment and human health are intricately connected, because clean air, water and soil are necessary for the survival of all species. The environmental movement is not new to earth-based cultures, such as First Nations peoples, who have ancient philosophies that encourage stewardship of the ecosystem.

The spread of Buddhism, Taoism, First Nations' spiritualities and other earth-based cosmologies is also contributing to changing attitudes towards holism. These philosophies discuss the connection between all forms of life and inherently support holistic health care. Some Buddhist monks, for example, are specialized in spiritual healing. Meredith McGuire asserts that "today's spiritual movements are one expression of the dissatisfaction with the limitations of compartmentalized medicine" (1993: 148). She argues that holistic medicine's growth is directly related to dissatisfaction with allopathic medicine. There is also probably a sector of the population which is interested in holistic medicine in a more positive sense (not as a reaction to allopathy), in that they believe in its intrinsic value for health care.

First Nations holistic healing traditions are experiencing a revival. Elders and medicine people are applying a variety of traditional techniques for the treatment of alcoholism, drug addiction and mental health imbalances. In Alberta, Poundmaker's Lodge, a treatment centre for First Nations people, incorporates traditional holistic healing practices and encourages political analyses of racism and colonialism to assist people in empowering themselves. The Nechi Institute is another such treatment centre in Alberta. In Ontario, the Anishanabwe Health Centre uses some holistic First Nations healing traditions.

The women's movement is a highly diverse movement, and many feminists are also part of other movements. Ecofeminists, spiritual feminists and women's health activists are probably the ones most actively involved in holism. The recent upsurge of personal healing work within the women's movement is also drawing from holistic concepts.

A small but growing holistic health movement is evidenced in Canada by the large attendance (mostly by people of the middle classes) at vegetarian food and holistic health fairs, by consumer demands for healthier food choices and by the growth of health food stores. The radio show, "The Well Street Journal," on community channel C.I.U.T. in Toronto is an example of popular community support for holistic health; the weekly show centres on emotional, mental and physical aspects of healing, using a variety of natural modalities. A large number of free magazines on the subject, for example, *Alive, Common Ground, Shared Vision* and *Vitality,* are quite successfully marketed across Canada. They are supported by hefty advertising and distributed on stands in stores, cafes and other venues. In Toronto, the Learning Annex, an organization which offers educational courses on a variety of subjects, regularly offers seminars by holistic health experts.

In the early 1990s, a group called "Citizens for Choice in Health Care" formed in the Toronto area. They are devoted to lobbying for holistic health care, primarily with the purpose of gaining legitimacy through legislation. At a fall 1992 introductory meeting of this group, I saw a turnout of over sixty people and a membership list of hundreds. Included in the crowd were many seniors, some people with chronic illnesses and some holistic health practitioners.

The growth of the environmental movement, joined with the feminist, peace and other people's movements, may be the most powerful force in integrating holistic health within Canadian society. Organized people's movements have the potential to lead policy innovation.

There is need for cautious scrutiny of the shift toward holistic practices. A case in point is the relatively recent New Age movement[7] in North America. While there appears to be a genuine search for healing and wholeness, especially in helping people with chronic illnesses, family dysfunction and a variety of other difficulties, some aspects are appropriationist, individualistic and materialistic. For example, some services offer clients an opportunity to learn relaxation, meditation or a variety of techniques for health and healing without acknowledging and contextualizing these sources as derived from South World or First Nations communities. False gurus, shamans and medicine men, many of whom do not come from the cultures in which these traditions originate, claim to have original knowledge and are appropriating it and profiting from it. Those who can pay—often at high rates—are their only clientele. By commodifying and selling ancient health care this way, the New Age entrepreneurs profit and some people benefit, but at a great disservice to the communities from which they emanate. Within the context of European-American social, cultural, political and economic domination of the world, such trends perpetuate a colonial tradition of theft from the South World.

In a women's "healing circle" I attended in Toronto, an entrepreneur offered the group an opportunity for a weekend retreat in which we could "pop our blocks." She explained that she worked in a fast-paced business milieu, that her stress levels were very high and that she had little time to relax and deal with her emotional distress. She offered us the opportunity to cathartically release stress by spending several hundreds of dollars so that we could re-enter the world of capitalism and become rich. Her spiel was replete with promises of "being clear" in order to live in the fast lane and make money. In these settings, holistic health is promoted to people in the upper echelons of society so they can function better with less stress so as to better conduct their business (possibly exploiting the work of others). Warren Salmon asserts that "the dictum that the individual must exert greater responsibility for health [is] an easier set of tasks for the 'worried well' of middle-age and middle-class than for other social groups" (1984: 257). He notes that middle-class people have the discretionary income to purchase services from "entrepreneurs who have turned a cosmic ecological concern into a sales package marketed to aid coping with a stressful social existence" (1984: 257).

Janet McKee (1988) points to another critique of the shift toward holistic health care. In a review of the literature, she notes that many researchers are critical of the holistic health approach because it provides an individualistic solution to problems of health rather than a focus on changing the social causes of illness. Many sociologists claim that "the victim-blaming ideology promoted by the holistic health movement tends to shift the burden of blame for health problems from the social system to the individual" (McKee 1988: 775). This critique could be levelled at virtually all systems of medicine because none of them encompasses a social and political view of the determinants of health. In itself, it is not a solid enough argument to dismiss holism. Rather, it emphasizes the need to incorporate both individual and social efforts if visions of health for all are to be achieved. Most individuals do have some control over their lives. A healthy society is made up of people making personal efforts to be healthy, as well as social efforts to eliminate barriers to health.

Towards a Healthier Future

Michel Foucault envisions that in

> a society that was free at last, in which inequalities were reduced, and in which concord reigned, the doctor would have no more than a temporary role, that of giving legislator and citizen advice as to the regulation of his [sic] heart and body. There would no

longer be any need for academics and hospitals. (1973: 33–34)

While tertiary care institutions, both allopathic and holistic, will probably always be necessary for the sick, the greatest promise of holistic health care lies in the self-knowledge and self-care for health promotion and disease prevention. Chellis Glendinning explains:

> [t]o heal is to become whole. To move beyond the narrow view of women as weak, dirty and ineffective; to realize how wellbeing is determined by sexism (and racism and classism, as well) in a male-dominated culture; to take control of our bodies and lives—these are fundamental political acts. (1982: 292)

Similarly, gaining legitimacy for holistic health care in Canada is fundamentally a political issue.

Social Justice Changes for Health
The revolution in Canadian health care would include, first, the following social justice approaches to guaranteeing universal access to the determinants of health:

- guaranteed basic income for all citizens;
- adequate housing for all citizens;
- accessible education from preschool to post-secondary levels;
- accessible childcare and other social and educational supports for families;
- violence prevention programs that are designed for young children, especially boys, and are informed by integrated feminist theory;
- treatment programs for batterers and victims;
- a clean environment: unpolluted air, water, soils;
- responsible electronic and print media motivated by social justice principles;
- rewarding and well paid domestic and non-domestic work for all citizens;
- social and material supports for people with disabilities, seniors and the young.

This is clearly an unfinished list. People with vision could add many other points to it. The list also appears utopian. However, it is important to acknowledge that these fundamental changes would make an enormous difference to our health status. It is also important to recognize that in revolutionary Cuba, Nicaragua and elsewhere, for limited periods and in certain places, many items on this list were realized.

Eliminating poverty would be the single most powerful way of improving health; doing so would entail a breakdown of capitalist social structures. Perhaps the complete abolition of capitalism will not occur in Canada in the next generation, but it is realistic to imagine that a much more supportive social safety net could be provided. The welfare system and "employment insurance" are currently failing millions of Canadians who are in need of them. By using community development approaches to changing these systems, it would be possible to significantly decrease poverty in Canada. Likewise, all of the other items on that list are possible to achieve in Canada. Political will, driven by citizens, is key to making them happen.

Holistic Multi-paradigmatic Health Care

The other part of the revolutionary agenda for health is the creation of a holistic multi-paradigmatic health care system that begins with a focus on encouraging and fostering mental and physical wellness. Ayurvedic health care, from India, is one example of a system that has been designed to do this. Because it is not possible within the space constraints of this limited chapter to expound fully on ayurvedic medical concepts, readers are encouraged to turn to the works of Lad (1984), Tiwari (1995), Lad and Frawley (1986) and other accomplished ayurvedic scholars for further information.

Ayurveda literally means science/knowledge of life. Briefly, an ayurvedic focus on wellness includes a balanced approach to life. Maintaining a balanced state of mind is accomplished through positive social relations and routine attention to personal mental health; meditation, yoga, music, dance, other art forms and various related practices are recommended in ayurveda. A healthy diet is also a foundation of wellness. Ayurvedic theory is highly sophisticated in terms of its recommendations for food intake. Dietary suggestions, like all ayurvedic health advice, are based on the particular *prakriti* (basic mind/body constitution) of each individual, and each food is categorized into *prakritis* as well. There are very few "one size fits all" approaches within ayurveda, as seven basic *prakritis* exist. Contrary to what may seem a corollary to this, ayurvedic food regimes are not strict. Eating a certain food that is not considered beneficial within a particular ayurvedic recommendation can usually be remedied by the use of simple digestive aids such as fennel or cardamom seeds.

According to ayurvedic theory, the kitchen is the pharmacy and the pharmacy is the kitchen. Likewise, food is medicine and medicine is food. These ideas alone are revolutionary. For people to consider health within reach—through food—is to do away, at least for most healthy people, with a huge industry of pharmaceutical products that are aggressively peddled as health-producing products.

A series of health-promoting daily routines within ayurveda are also accessible. Scraping the tongue first thing in the morning, for example, has the obvious benefit of oral hygiene and is also a useful habit for keeping track of changes occurring within the digestive tract. Rinsing the mouth after every meal is another simple suggestion that keeps dental health high. These two easy-to-do routines are carried out by millions of people in India. Tongue scrapers are thus easily available in Indian markets. Dental research indicates that the teeth of Indians are generally very healthy; a diet low in sugar and other caries-producing agents, combined with constant attention to dental cleanliness, are the keys to this success.

Ayurvedic medicine also includes a wide variety of other health-promoting recommendations such as massage, yoga, exercise and intake of herbs, vitamins, minerals. Besides health promotion and disease prevention, ayurveda has a vast cornucopia of treatment options that include general medicine and surgery. This system of holistic health care has therefore incorporated in appropriate ways various reductionist techniques into its treatment regimens.

A holistic multi-paradigmatic system of care could build on some of the ideas from ayurveda, traditional Chinese medicine, First Nations health care and various other bonafide health traditions that have proven value. It would incorporate the most valuable aspects of allopathic medicine as well.

To make a multi-paradigmatic system of care women-centred, Canadian midwifery could be used as an existing example. The midwifery model of woman-centred care was tailored for pregnant, birthing and post-partum women. Virtually all elements are relevant for the care of women at other stages of health and illness. Informed choice, for example, is a vital component of care for women who are seeking treatment options for a life-threatening disease like cancer. Women need to be informed by health care providers of the benefits and risks—from an evidence-based perspective—of each treatment option. Applying the midwifery model has the potential to make significant changes in other parts of the health care system.

Concluding Thoughts

Canadian health reform has had many impacts on women. As the authors of this book point out, most of these impacts have been negative. Caring has been assigned negligible status within the health care system, and women's work, in general, is devalued within patriarchal, capitalist economies (Armstrong et al. 1993, Doyal 1997). Similarly, women care recipients have been undervalued and mistreated.

In concluding this book on women and health reform, this chapter attempts to illustrate the need for health reform that is both women-centred and holistic. The history of medicine in Canada is that of holism, starting from First Nations peoples. Allopathic medicine has only had a stronghold on the Canadian public for less than one hundred years. While allopathic medicine is useful for the treatment of acute and emergency care needs, holistic health care appears to be more promising for health promotion and disease prevention, as well as for mental health care and chronic conditions, which constitute a majority of the nation's health problems (Epp 1986). Evidence that holism is re-emerging is found in several social movements, including the environmental, spiritual, women's and holistic health movements. Almost three-quarters of Canadians have used at least one form of holistic health care in their lives (Ramsay et al. 1999), which is consistent with figures that indicate that approximately three-quarters of the global population uses traditional holistic health care (WHO 1978a). This reckoning does not take into account those Canadians who are engaged in self-care practices using holistic means, and so the figure is probably higher.

As Ursula Franklin (1999) was quoted as saying at the outset of this chapter, change in Canadian health care must come "through women, for all people." Change is possible! A revolutionary agenda for improvements to Canadian health status includes changes based on social justice as well as on holistic multi-paradigmatic health care principles. Strong citizens' voices, based in holistic practices and social justice movements, have the potential to transform Canadian health care.

Notes

1. The term *revolution* here refers to large-scale social change: a reconstruction of social values, structures and institutions. This is revolution in the Marxist sense. Reform, in my view, is the constellation of changes that is occurring in Canadian health care—a constellation which is not particularly revolutionary.
2. I would like to acknowledge the support of my beloved partner Roozbeh,

who helped to care for our playful baby Zubin, while I wrote this chapter. Motherhood should not take away these opportunities from women and I feel fortunate to be able to continue doing other kinds of work while I am still breastfeeding Zubin.

3. Women are the main consumers of health care partly because our reproductive functions have been medicalized (in some cases, for sound reasons, but not for the majority of healthy women). Thus we visit physicians for menstrual disorders, pregnancy, childbirth, post-partum concerns, menopausal concerns. Generally women take the young, elderly and others to the doctor and are, therefore, the health care brokers of most families. Women also constitute the majority of formal health care providers.

4. Allopathy or allopathic medicine are the terms that I generally use in reference to the dominant system of medicine in Canada. Its word roots: *allo* means other and *pathy* means disease or pathology. Literally, then, allopathy is the system of medicine that creates another disease. As a Western European term, it is often used in contrast to homeopathy: system of medicine that creates a *similar* disease.

5. I read of the original ayurvedic medical texts, *Carakasamhita* and *Sushrutasamhita*, and did not notice oppressive social discourse. I was reading a version translated into English from the original Sanskrit. Given that Sanskrit scholarship is flourishing both inside and outside India, I have every reason to believe that these translations were true to the original text.

6. However, the women's health movement has made it clear that many Canadian women are fed up with sexism in allopathic service delivery. Women have been raped and abused by their psychiatrists and other practitioners. Our health concerns are often not taken seriously and we are regularly under-diagnosed for serious health issues such as HIV/AIDS (Shroff 1991). It is no surprise that women are looking elsewhere for diagnosis and treatment of our health concerns.

7. The New Age movement is diverse. So these observations are made in general, with recognition that there are potentially significant differences within this group.

References

Abbott, P., and W. Claire (eds.). 1990. *The Sociology of the Caring Professions.* New York: The Falmer Press.

Abel, E.K. 1995. "'Man, Woman, and Chore Boy:' Transformations in the Antagonistic Demands of Work and Care on Women in the Nineteenth and Twentieth Centuries." *Milbank Quarterly* 73, 2.

Abel, E.K., and M.K. Nelson (eds.). 1990. *Circles of Care: Work and Identity in Women's Lives.* Albany, NY: State University of New York Press.

Abts, D., M. Hofer and P. Leafgreen. 1994. "Redefining Care Delivery: A Modular System." *Nursing Management* 25, 2.

Abu-Laban, S.M., and S.A. McDaniel. 1995. "Aging Women and Standards of Beauty." In N. Mandell (ed.), *Feminist Issues: Race, Class and Sexuality.* Scarborough, ON: Prentice Hall.

Adams, J. 1998. "Province Enters Baby Doctor Crisis." *Calgary Herald,* October 12.

Aiken, L., H. Smith and E. Lake. 1994. "Lower Medicare Mortality among a Set of Hospitals Known for Good Nursing Care." *Medical Care* 32, 8.

Aikens, A.M. December 9, 1996. *The Ontario Coalition of Rape Crisis Centres Response to the Ontario Women's Directorate's Framework for Action on the Prevention of Violence against Women in Ontario.* Ontario Coalition of Rape Crisis Centres.

Alberta Health. December 1993. *Health Goals for Alberta: Progress Report.* Edmonton, AB.

Alberta Health Planning Secretariat. December 1993. *Starting Points: Recommendations for Creating a More Accountable and Affordable Health System.* Edmonton, AB.

Alberta Society of Obstetrics and Gynecology (ASOG]. n.d. *Alberta Society of Obstetrics and Gynecology: Issues and Solution Fact Sheet.* Edmonton, AB.

"Alternative Medicine: The Facts." 1994. *Consumer Reports* (January).

American Hospital Association. 1992. *Hospital Statistics (1991–1992).* Available from the American Hospital Association, Chicago, IL.

American Psychiatric Association (APA). 1994. *Diagnostic and Statistical Manual of Mental Disorders* (4th ed.), Washington, DC.

Anderson, J.M. 1985. "Perspectives on the Health of Immigrant Women: A Feminist Analysis." *Advances In Nursing Sciences* 8, 1.

——. 1990. "Home Care Management in Chronic Illness and the Self-Care Movement: An Analysis of Ideologies and Economic Processes Influencing Policy Decisions." *Advanced Nursing Science* 12, 2.

——. 1991. "Immigrant Women Speak of Chronic Illness: The Social Construction of the Devalued Self." *Journal Of Advanced Nursing* 16.

——. 1993. "On Chronic Illness: Immigrant Women in Canada's Work Force—A Feminist Perspective." *Canadian Journal of Nursing Research* 25, 2.

——. 1997. "Speaking of Illness: Issues of First Generation Canadian Women— Implications for Patient Education and Counselling." Unpublished manuscript.

Angus, D. 1992. "A Great Canadian Prescription: Take Two Commissions and

Call Me in the Morning." In R. Deber and G. Thompson (eds.), *Restructuring Canada's Health Services System*. Toronto, ON: University of Toronto Press.

Angus, D.E. 1998. "Health Care Costs: Canada in Perspective." In D. Coburn, C. D'Arcy and G.M. Torrance (eds.).

Angus, J. 1994. "Women's Paid/Unpaid Work and Health: Exploring the Social Context of Everyday Life." *Canadian Journal of Nursing Research* 26, 4.

——. 1993. "Women's Health-Care Work: Nursing in Context." In P. Armstrong, J. Choiniere and E. Day (eds.).

Angus Reid Group. 1997. *Angus Reid Survey*. http://www.angusreid.com/media/content/pdf/pr970901_1.PDF

Armstrong, P. 1994. "Closer to Home." In P. Armstrong, H. Armstrong, J. Choiniere, G. Feldberg and J. White (eds.).

——. June 1995. "Privatizing Care." Paper presented at the 30th Annual Meeting of the Canadian Sociology and Anthropology Meetings, Montreal, PQ.

——. 1997. "Privatizing Care." In P. Armstrong, H. Armstrong, J. Choiniere, E. Mykhalovskiy and J.P. White (eds.).

Armstrong, P., and H. Armstrong. 1984. *The Double Ghetto: Canadian Women and their Segregated Work*. Revised edition. Toronto, ON: McClelland and Stewart.

——. 1994a. "Health Care as a Business: The Legacy of Free Trade." In P. Armstrong, H. Armstrong, J. Choiniere, G. Feldberg and J. White (eds.).

——. 1994b. Health Care In Canada. In P. Armstrong, H. Armstrong, J. Choiniere, G. Feldberg and J. White (eds.).

——. 1999. *Women, Privatization and Health Care Reform: The Ontario Case*. Available from National Network on Environments and Women's Health at York University (NNEWH), York University, Toronto, ON.

Armstrong, P., H. Armstrong, J. Choiniere, E. Mykhalovskiy and J. White (eds.). 1997. *Medical Alert: New Work Organization in Health Care*. Toronto, ON: Garamond Press.

Armstrong, P., J. Choiniere and E. Day (eds.). 1993. *Vital Signs: Nursing in Transition*. Toronto, ON: Garamond Press.

Armstrong, P., J. Choiniere, G. Feldberg and J. White. 1994. "Voices From the Ward: A Study of the Impact of Cutbacks." In P. Armstrong, H. Armstrong, J. Choiniere, G. Feldberg and J. White (eds.).

Arnup, K., A. Levesque and R.R. Pierson with M. Brennan (eds.). 1990. *Delivering Motherhood: Maternal Ideologies and Practices in the 19th and 20th Centuries*. London and New York: Routledge.

Arnup, K., A. Levesque and R.R. Pierson (with Brennan, M.) (eds.). 1990. *Delivering Motherhood: Maternal Ideologies and Practices in the 19th and 20th Centuries*. New York: Routledge.

Aronson, J. 1999. "Women's Experiences of Receiving Home Care: Responsive Community Care?" Paper presented at the Canadian Research Institute for the Advancement of Women Conference on Feminist Definitions of Caring Communities and Healthy Lifestyles, Sudbury, ON.

Assanand, S., M. Dias, E. Richardson and N. Waxler-Morrison. 1990. "The South Asians." In N. Waxler-Morrison, J. Anderson and E. Richardson (eds.).

Badgley, R.F., and S. Wolfe. 1992. "Equity and Health Care." In C.D. Naylor (ed.), *Canadian Health Care and the State*. Montreal, PQ, and Kingston, ON: McGill-Queen's University Press.

Baines, C., P. Evans and S. Neysmith (eds.). 1998. *Women's Caring: Feminist Perspectives on Social Welfare.* Second edition. Toronto, ON: Oxford University Press.

Bakker, I. (ed.). 1996. *Rethinking Restructuring: Gender and Change in Canada.* Toronto, ON: University of Toronto Press.

Bart, P.B., and E.G. Moran (eds.). 1993. *Violence against Women: The Bloody Footprints.* Newbury Park, CA: Sage.

Beiser, M. 1990. "Mental Health of Refugees in Resettlement Countries." In W.H. Holtzman and T. Bornemann (eds.), *Mental Health of Immigrants and Refugees.* Austin, TX: Hogg Foundation for Mental Health, University of Texas.

——. 1997. "Multiculturalism and Health Care." *Profile—Newsletter of the Royal Society of Canada* 5, 1.

Beiser, M., P. Johnson and D. Roshi. 1994. *The Mental Health of Southeast Asian Refugees Resettling in Canada.* Report submitted to Canada Health and Welfare, National Health and Development Program.

Bell, N.K. 1997. "Protocol 1076: A New Look at Women and Children with AIDS." In D.C. Umeh (ed.), *Confronting the AIDS Epidemic: Cross-Cultural Perspectives on HIV/AIDS Education.* Trenton, NJ: Africa World Press.

Benería, L. 1997. "Capitalism and Socialism: Some Feminist Questions." In V. Nalini et al. (eds.), *The Women, Gender and Development Reader.* Halifax, NS: Fernwood Publishing.

Benoit, C. 1998. "Rediscovering Appropriate Care: Maternity Traditions and Contemporary Issues in Canada." In D. Coburn, C. D'Arcy and G.M. Torrance (eds.).

Berger, E. 1990. *Canada Health Monitor Survey #4.* (July / August). Toronto, ON: Price Waterhouse.

——. 1992. *Canada Health Monitor Survey #12.* (March / June). Toronto, ON: Price Waterhouse.

——. 1995. *Canada Health Monitor Survey #16 (Summer).* Toronto, ON: Price Waterhouse.

Bergman, R. 1994. "Re-engineering Health Care." *Hospitals and Health Networks* 68, 5.

Berliner, H., and W. Salmon. 1985. *A System of Scientific Medicine: Philanthropic Foundations in the Flexner Era.* New York: Tavistock Publications.

Bernard, M. 1994. "Post-Fordism, Transnational Production, and the Changing Global Political Economy." In R. Stubbs and G. Underhill (eds.), *Political Economy and the Changing Global Order.* Toronto, ON: McClelland and Stewart.

Bhaskaran, H. 1993. *An Indo-Canadian Community Assessment Study.* Edmonton, AB: Edmonton Board of Health.

Bigelow, B., and M. Arndt. 1994. "Great Expectations: An Analysis of Four Strategies." *Medical Care Review* 51, 2.

Blackwell, B. (ed.). 1997. *Treatment Compliance and the Therapeutic Alliance.* Amsterdam: Harwood Academic Publishers.

Bloom, F.T. 1985. "Struggling and Surviving: The Life Style of European Immigrant Breadwinning Mothers in American Industrial Cities 1900–1930." *Women's Studies International Forum* 8.

Blume, S.E. 1990. *Secret Survivors: Uncovering Incest and its Aftereffects in Women.* New York: Ballantine.

Bolaria, B.S., and R. Bolaria (eds.). 1988. *Racial Minorities, Medicine and Health.* Halifax, NS: Fernwood Publishing.

——. 1994. *Racial Minorities, Medicine, and Health.* Halifax, NS: Fernwood Publishing.

Bolaria, B.S., and H. Dickenson (eds.). 1988. *Sociology of Health Care in Canada.* Toronto, ON: Harcourt Brace Jovanovich.

——. 1994. *Health, Illness, and Health Care in Canada.* Second edition. Toronto, ON: Harcourt Brace & Co.

Bourgeault, R. 1991. "Race, Class and Gender: Colonial Domination of Indian Women." In Jesse Vorst et al. (eds.), *Race, Class, Gender: Bonds and Barriers.* Revised edition. Toronto, ON: Garamond Press in co-operation with the Society for Socialist Studies.

Bours, G.J., C.A. Ketelaars, C.M. Fredericks, H.H. Abu-Saad and E.F. Wouters. 1998. "The Effects of Aftercare on Chronic Patients and Frail Elderly Patients when Discharged from Hospital: A Systematic Review." *Journal of Advanced Nursing* 27, 5.

Boyd, M. 1975. "The Status of Immigrant Women in Canada." *Canadian Review of Social Anthropology* 12.

Brandt, G.B. 1985. "Organizations in Canada: The English Protestant Tradition." In P. Bourne (ed.), *Women's Paid and Unpaid Work: Historical and Contemporary Perspectives.* Toronto, ON: New Hogtown Press.

Brigden, M. 1987. "Unorthodox Cancer Therapy and your Cancer Patient." *Postgraduate Medicine* 81, 1 (January).

Brink, P. 1976. *Transcultural Nursing: A Book of Readings.* Englewood Cliffs, NJ: Prentice Hall.

Broad, D. 1997. "The Casualisation of the Labour Force." In A. Duffy, D. Glenday and N. Pupo (eds.), *Good Jobs, Bad Jobs, No Jobs: The Transformation of Work in the 21st Century.* Toronto, ON: Harcourt Brace & Co.

Browner, C.H., and J. Leslie. 1996. "Women, Work, and Household Health in the Context of Development." In C.F. Sargent and C.B. Brettell (eds.).

Bubel, A., and D. Spitzer. 1996. *Documenting Women's Stories: The Impact of Health Care Reform on Women's Lives.* Report prepared for the Edmonton Women's Health Network.

Buchwald, E., P.R. Fletcher and M. Roth (eds.). 1993. *Transforming a Rape Culture.* Minneapolis: Milkweed.

Burstow, B. 1992. *Radical Feminist Therapy: Working the Context of Violence.* Newbury Park, CA: Sage.

Cade, B., and W.H. O'Hanlon. 1993. *A Brief Guide to Brief Therapy.* New York: W.W. Norton and Company.

California Healthline. 1999. "Home Health: Study Says Companies Avoid Sickest Patients." *California Healthcare.* Washington, DC: National Journal Group Inc.

Calliste, A. 1993. "Women of 'Exceptional Merit': Immigration of Caribbean Nurses to Canada." *Canadian Journal of Women and the Law* 6, 1.

——. 1996. "End the Silence of Racism in Health Care: Build a Movement against Discrimination, Harassment and Reprisals." Report of a conference held May 25–26, 1995, Ontario Institute for Studies in Education, Toronto, ON.

Cameron, D., and E. Finn. 1998. "Ten Deficit Myths." In L. Ricciutelli, J. Larkin and

E. O'Neill (eds.), *Confronting the Cuts: A Sourcebook for Women in Ontario.* Toronto, ON: Inanna Publications and Education Inc.

Cameron, S., M. Horsburgh and M. Armstrong-Stassen. October 1994. *Effects of Downsizing on RNs and RNAs in Community Hospitals.* (Working paper #94-6). McMaster University, Quality of Nursing Worklife Research Unit, School of Nursing, Hamilton, ON.

Campbell, M.L. 1998. *Research on Health Care Experiences of People with Disabilities: Exploring the Everyday Problematic of Service Delivery.* Manuscript submitted for publication.

Campbell, M., and R. Ng. 1988. "Program Evaluation and the Standpoint of Women." *Canadian Review of Social Policy* 22.

Canadian Nurses Association. 1998. *The Quiet Crisis in Health Care.* A Submission to the House of Commons Standing Committee on Finance and the Minister of Finance. Ottawa, ON.

Canadian Panel on Violence against Women. 1993. *Changing the Landscape: Ending Violence—Achieving Equality.* Ottawa, ON: Minister of Supply and Services Canada.

Canadian Society of Obstetricians and Gynaecologists. n.d. *The Obstetrical Crisis in Canada.* [Brochure]. Toronto, ON.

Canadian Study of Health and Aging. 1994. "Patterns of Caring for People with Dementia in Canada." *Canadian Journal on Aging* 13, 4.

Carpio, B., and B.B. Majumdar. 1991. "Putting Culture into Curricula." *Canadian Nurse* 87, 7.

Carver, V., and C. Ponée (eds.). 1989. *Women, Work, and Wellness.* Toronto, ON: Addiction Research Foundation.

Cawthorne, J. 1998. [Interview with Dr. Paul Martyn.] Unpublished Raw Data. November 16.

Chaplin, J.P. (ed.). 1975. *Dictionary of Psychology.* Revised edition. New York: Dell.

Charmaz, K., and D.A. Paterniti (eds.). 1999. *Health, Illness, and Healing. Society, Social Context, and Self: An Anthology.* Los Angeles: Roxbury.

Chatterjee, M. 1989. "Competence and Care for Women: Health Policy Perspectives in the Household Context. In M. Krishnaraj and K. Chanana (eds.), *Gender and Household Domain: Social and Cultural Dimensions.* New Delhi: Sage.

Chen, J., E. Ng and R. Wilkins. 1996. *The Health of Canada's Immigrants in 1994–95.* (Health Reports. Cat. No. 82-003, 7, 4). Ottawa, ON: Statistics Canada.

Chin, J. 1990. "Epidemiology: Current and Future Dimensions of the HIV/AIDS Pandemic in Women and Children." *Lancet* 336.

——. 1996. "Chinese Americans." In J.G. Lipson, S.L. Dibble and P.A. Minarik (eds.), *Culture and Nursing Care: A Pocket Guide.* San Francisco: University of California San Francisco Nursing Press.

Chisholm, P. 1995. "Healers or Quacks? Therapies Once Viewed as Fringe are Becoming Mainstream." *Maclean's,* September 25.

Choudhry, U.K. 1998. "Health Promotion among Immigrant Women from India Living in Toronto." *Image: Journal of Nursing Scholarship* 30.

Clayton, H. June 1990. *Community Development and Indian Health.* Presentation to the Canadian Public Health Association Conference, Toronto, ON.

Clubine, C. 1991. *Racism, Assimilation and Indian Education in Upper Canada.*

Unpublished manuscript. Ontario Institute for Studies in Education, University of Toronto.

Cmich, D.E. 1984. "Theoretical Perspectives of Holistic Health." *Journal of School Health* 54, 1.

Coburn, D. 1993. "State Authority, Medical Dominance and Trends in the Regulation of the Health Professions: The Ontario Case." *Social Science Medicine* 37, 2.

Coburn, D., C. D'Arcy and G.M. Torrance (eds.). 1998. *Health and Canadian Society Sociological Perspectives*. Third edition. Toronto, ON: University of Toronto Press.

Cole, G., and C. Brown. 1988. "Product-Line Management: Concept to Reality." *Journal Topics on Health Care Financing* 14, 3.

College of Nurses of Ontario. 1993. *Annual Report*. Toronto, ON.

——. 1994. *Statistical Profile of Registered Provisional Nurses*. Toronto, ON: Registration Department, Statistics and Research Section.

——. 1996. "A Guide to Working with Unregulated Care Providers." *Communiqué* 21, 2 (April).

——. 1998. *RN Entry to Practice Competencies Project Report*. Toronto, ON.

——. 1999a. *Annual Overview: 1998–1999*. Toronto, ON.

——. 1999b. *Information Resources/System Development Department*. Toronto, ON.

——. 1999c. "A Guide to Nurses for Providing Culturally Sensitive Care." *Communiqué* (June).

Collins, E., R. Hagey, U. Choudhry, R. Lee, A. Calliste, J. Fudge, J. Turritin, S. Guruge and S. Henry. 1999. *Research towards Equity in the Professional Life of Immigrants: A Study of Nursing in the Metropolis*. Unpublished raw data.

Comaroff, J. 1985. *Body of Power, Spirit of Resistance: The Culture and History of a South African People*. Chicago: University of Chicago Press.

——. 1993. "The Diseased Heart of Africa: Medicine, Colonialism and the Black Body." In S. Lindenbaum and M. Lock (eds.), *Knowledge, Power, and Practice: The Medical Anthropology of Everyday Life*. Berkeley: University of California Press.

Congress of Black Women of Canada, Toronto Chapter. 1995a. *End the Silence on Racism in the Healthcare Field*. A Conference for Black Nurses and Other Healthcare Workers, May 25–26, Ontario Institute for Studies in Education, Toronto, ON.

——. 1995b. *Report on Racism in Health Care*. A Conference for Black Nurses and Other Healthcare Workers, May 25–26, Ontario Institute for Studies in Education, Toronto, ON.

Connell, R.W. 1990. "The State, Gender, and Sexual Politics: Theory and Appraisal." *Theory and Society* 19, 5.

Connelly, M.P., and M. Macdonald. 1996. "The Labour Market, the State, and the Reorganization of Work: Policy Impacts." In I. Bakker (ed.).

Corea, G. 1985. *The Mother Machine*. New York: Harper and Row.

Cottrell, K. 1995. "The Age of Alternatives." *Chatelaine* 68, 7 (July).

Counts, D.A., and D. Counts. (eds.). 1985. *Aging and its Transformations: Moving toward Death in Pacific Societies*. Lanham, MD: University Press of America.

——. 1996. *Over the Next Hill: An Ethnography of RVing Seniors in North America*. Peterborough, ON: Broadview Press.

Courtois, C.A. 1988. *Healing the Incest Wound: Adult Survivors in Therapy.* New York: W.W. Norton and Company.

Coutts, J. 1997. "Ontario Doctors Endorse Salary Deal." *Globe and Mail,* June 2.

Cowie, E. May 1997. *Chippewas of Georgina Island First Nation Community Profile.* Chippewas of Georgina Island First Nation.

Cranswick, K. 1997. "Canada's Caregivers." *Canadian Social Trends.* [Catalogue 11-008-XPE]. Ottawa: Statistics Canada.

Crawford, T. 1998a. "Female Workers Face a Growing Uncertainty." *Toronto Star,* September 5.

——. 1998b. "Part-Timers Yearn For More." *Toronto Star,* September 5.

Das Gupta, T. 1993. *Racism and Paid Work.* Toronto, ON: Garamond Press.

——. 1996. "Anti-Black Racism in Nursing in Ontario." *Studies in Political Economy* 51.

Davis, A.Y. 1981. *Women, Race and Class.* Toronto, ON: Random House.

Demetrakopoulos, A., J. Grant-Cummings, V. Keyi, S. Nagpal with L. Ritchie and N. Sharma. 1997. "Health Policy." In N. Sharma (ed.), *The National Action Committee on the Status of Women's Voters' Guide* Toronto, ON: James Lorimer.

Denton, M., I.U. Zeytino_lu, S. Webb, K. Barber and J. Lian. April 1998. *Healthy Work Environments in Community Based Health and Social Service Agencies: Stage Two Report: Volunteer Questionnaire Findings.* (MRCPOWH Technical Report Series #6). Hamilton, ON: McMaster University.

Dickinson, H.D. 1996. "Health Reforms, Empowerment and the Democratization of Society." In M. Stingl & D. Wilson (eds.).

DiMatteo, M.R., and D.D. DiNicola. 1982. *Achieving Patient Compliance: The Psychology of the Medical Practitioner's Role.* New York: Pergamon Press.

Dinh, D.K., S. Ganesan and N. Waxler-Morrison. 1990. "The Vietnamese." In N. Waxler-Morrison, J. Anderson and E. Richardson (eds.).

Donner, G. 1998. "Culture Care in Nursing Education." *Culture Care Nursing Interest Group Newsletter.* Toronto, ON.

Donovan, M., and G. Lewis. 1987. "Increasing Productivity and Decreasing Costs: The Value of RNs." *JONA* 17, 9.

Doyle, D.P. 1997. "Aging and Crime." In K. Ferraro and F. Kenneth (eds.), *Gerontology: Perspectives and Issues.* Second edition. New York: Springer Verlag.

Doyal, L. 1997. *What Makes Women Sick?* New Brunswick, NJ: Rutgers University Press.

Dresser, R. 1992. "Wanted: Single White Male for Medical Research." *Hastings Center Report* 22, 1.

Dua, E., M. Fitzgerald, L. Gardner, D. Taylor and L. Wyndels (eds.). 1994. *On Women Healthsharing.* Toronto, ON: Women's Press.

Duffy, A., and N. Pupo. 1992. *Part-Time Paradox: Connecting Gender, Work and Family.* Toronto, ON: McClelland and Stewart.

Duffy, M.E., R. Rossow and M. Hernandez. 1995. "Correlates of Health-Promotion Activities in Employed Mexican American Women." *Nursing Research* 45.

EAGLE Working Group. February, 1995. *EAGLE Project: Environmental Analysis of Georgina Island First Nation.* Ottawa, ON: Assembly of First Nations.

Ehrenreich, B., and D. English. 1979. *For Her Own Good: 150 Years of the Experts*

Advice to Women. New York: Anchor Books.

Ellis, P., and P. Gaskin. 1988. "Executive Briefing: Sunnybrook's Matrix Organizational Model—Marching Ahead." *Healthcare Management Forum* 1, 2.

Enkin, M., J.N.C. Keirse and I. Chalmers (eds.). 1989. *A Guide to Effective Care in Pregnancy and Childbirth.* Oxford: Oxford University Press.

Epp, J. 1986. *Achieving Health for All: A Framework for Health Promotion.* Ottawa, ON: Ministry of Supply and Services Canada.

Epstein, L. 1992. *Brief Treatment and a New Look at the Task-Centred Approach.* Third edition. New York: Macmillan.

Evans, P.M. 1998. "Gender, Poverty, and Women's Caring." In C. Baines, P. Evans and S. Neysmith (eds.).

Evans, R.G. 1993. "Health Care Reform: 'The Issue from Hell.'" *Policy Options* 14.

Family Service Centre of Ottawa-Carleton. 1997. *A Response to the Framework for Action on the Prevention of Violence against Women in Ontario.* Ottawa, ON.

Fast, J., and M. Da Pont. 1997. "Changes in Women's Work Continuity." *Canadian Social Trends* [Catalogue 11-008-XPE]. Ottawa, ON: Statistics Canada.

Feher, E.P., G.J. Larrabee and G.T.H. Crook. 1992. "Factors Attenuating the Validity of the Geriatric Depression Scale in a Dementia Population." *Journal of the American Geriatric Society* 40.

Flynn, M. 1991. "Product-Line Management: Threat or Opportunity for Nursing? *Nursing Administration Quarterly* 15, 2.

Foucault, M. 1973. *The Birth of the Clinic: An Archaeology of Medical Perception.* (A.M. Sheridan Smith, Trans.). New York: Vintage Books.

Francis, D. 1984. *I Remember... An Oral History of the Trent-Severn Waterway.* Peterborough, ON: Friends of the Trent-Severn Waterway.

Franklin, U. 1999. "Keynote Address." Paper presented to the Made To Measure: Designing Research, Policy and Action Approaches to Eliminate Gender Inequity National Symposium, Halifax, NS, October.

Frideres, J.S. 1988. "Racism and Health: The Case of the Native People." In B.S. Bolaria and H. Dickenson (eds.).

Fuller, C. 1999. *Reformed or Rerouted? Women and Change in the Health Care System.* Available from the B.C. Centre of Excellence for Women's Health, Vancouver, BC.

Furman, B., and T. Ahola. 1992. *Solution Talk, Hosting Therapeutic Conversations.* New York: W.W. Norton.

Gadd, J. 1997. "A Drift to the Bottom." *Globe and Mail,* June 21.

Gadow, S. 1985. "Nurse and Patient: The Caring Relationship." In A.H. Bishop and J.R. Scudder (eds.), *Caring, Curing, Coping: Nurse, Physician, Patient Relationships* Birmingham, AB: University of Alabama Press.

Garteig, L. 1995. "Health Meanings and Dynamics among Urban Residing Native Women." Unpublished master's thesis, University of Alberta, Edmonton, AB.

Gaut, D. 1984. "A Philosophic Orientation to Caring Research." In M. Leininger (ed.).

Gil, E. 1988. *Treatment of Adult Survivors of Childhood Abuse.* Walnut Creek, CA: Launch Press.

Gilligan, C. 1982. *In a Different Voice.* Cambridge: Harvard University Press.

Glazer, N.Y. 1993. *Women's Paid and Unpaid Labour: The Work Transfer in Health Care and Retailing*. Philadelphia: Temple University Press.

Gleave, D., and A.S. Manes. 1990. "The Central Americans." In N. Waxler-Morrison, J. Anderson and E. Richardson (eds.).

Glendinning, G. 1982. "The Healing Powers of Women." In C. Spretnak (ed.), *The Politics of Women's Spirituality*. Garden City, NY: Anchor Books.

Graham, H. 1983. "Caring: A Labour of Love." In J. Finch and D. Groves (eds.), *A Labour of Love: Women, Work and Caring*. Boston: Routledge.

———. 1993. "Social Divisions in Caring." *Women's Studies International Forum* 16, 5.

Grahame, P.R. 1998. "Ethnography, Institutions and the Problematic of the Everyday World." *Human Studies* 21, 4.

Griffith, D. 1985. "Women, Remittances and Reproduction." *American Ethnologist* 12, 4.

Glenday, D. 1997. "Lost Horizons, Leisure Shock: Good Jobs, Bad Jobs, Uncertain Future." In A. Duffy, D. Glenday and N. Pupo (eds.), *Good Jobs, Bad Jobs, No Jobs: The Transformation of Work in the 21st Century*. Toronto, ON: Harcourt Brace.

Goer, H. 1995. *Obstetric Myths Versus Research Realities: A Guide to the Medical Literature*. Westport, CT: Bergin and Garvey.

Goffman, E. 1959. *Presentation of Self in Everyday Life*. Garden City, NY: Doubleday.

———. 1961. *Asylums: Essays on the Social Situation of Mental Patients and other Inmates*. Garden City, NJ: Doubleday.

———. 1963. *Stigma: Notes on the Management of Spoiled Identity*. Englewood Cliffs, NJ: Prentice Hall.

———. 1969. *Strategic Interaction*. Philadelphia: University of Pennsylvania Press.

Goldstein, M.S., C. Sutherland, D.T. Jaffe and J. Wilson. 1988. "Holistic Physicians and Family Practitioners: Similarities, Differences and Implications for Health Policy." *Social Science and Medicine* 26, 8.

Gort, E., and D. Coburn. 1988. "Naturopathy in Canada: Changing Relationships to Medicine, Chiropractic, and the State." *Social Science and Medicine* 26, 10.

Gottlieb, L. 1994. "Some Reflections on the Nurse Practitioner Movement: Potential Danger, Exciting Possibilities." *Canadian Journal of Nursing Research* 26, 4.

Gray, S. 1994. "Hospitals and Human Rights." *Our Times* 13, 6.

Grayson, J.P. December 1993. *A Report on Survey of Laid Off Hospital Workers*. Unpublished report submitted to Health Sector Training and Adjustment Program. Available from the Institute for Social Research, York University, Toronto, ON.

———. 1997. *An Evaluation of HSTAP's Support of Training*. Toronto, ON: York University Institute for Social Research.

Greer, G. 1992. *The Change: Women, Aging and Menopause*. New York: Knopf.

Gregor, F. June 1995. "Health System Reform and the Nursing Profession: A Critical Analysis." Paper presented at the 30th Annual Meetings of the Canadian Sociology and Anthropology Association, Montreal, PQ.

Gregor, F., S. Foster, D. Denney and B. Keddy. 1998. "Feeding the Hand that Bites You: Explaining Nova Scotia Nurses' Support for Health Care Reform in the Face of Job Displacement." Paper presented at the 4th International Qualitative Health Research Conference, Vancouver, BC.

Guldner, C. 1995. *An Introduction to Solution Oriented Brief Therapy*. Workshop conducted at the Human Sexuality Post-Conference, University of Guelph, Guelph, ON.

Guruge, S. 1999. "Effectiveness of Preoperative Teaching and Demographic Characteristics of Studies' Participants: A Meta-Analysis." Unpublished master's thesis, University of Toronto, Toronto, ON.

Guruge, S., and G. Donner. 1996. "Transcultural Nursing in Canada." *The Canadian Nurse* 92.

Guruge, S., R. Hagey and R. Lee. 1998. *The Importance of Culture-Based Explanations: A Chinese Example.* Unpublished manuscript, University of Toronto, Toronto, ON.

Gustafson, D.L. 1996. "The Impact of Hospital Downsizing on Registered Nurses Displaced from Full-Time Employment." Unpublished master's thesis, Brock University, St. Catharines, ON.

———. 1998a. Home Care or Caring at Home: Before and after Reform. Unpublished manuscript, Ontario Institute for Studies in Education, University of Toronto. Toronto, ON.

———. 1998b. "Reframing a Story of Job Displacement: One Nurse's Responses to Hospital Downsizing." *Canadian Woman Studies Journal* 18, 1.

Haas, J., and W. Shaffir. 1987. *Becoming Doctors: The Adoption of a Cloak of Competence.* Greenwich, CT: Jai Press.

Hagey, R. 1989. "The Native Diabetes Program: Rhetorical Process and Praxis." In J. Morse (ed.), *Cross-Cultural Nursing: Anthropological Approaches to Nursing Research.* New York: Gordon and Breach Science.

Halloran, E. 1983. "RN Staffing: More Care—Less Cost." *Nursing Management* 14, 9.

Hancock, W.M., P.L. Flynn, S. Derosa, P.F. Walter and C. Conway. 1984. "A Cost and Staffing Comparison of an All-RN Staff and Team Nursing." *Nursing Administration Quarterly* 8, 2 (Winter).

Hareven, T.K. 1995. "Change Images of Aging and the Social Construction of the Life Course." In M. Featherstone and A. Wernick (eds.), *Images of Aging: Cultural Representations of Later Life.* London: Routledge.

Harris, M. 1998. "Reforms Have Taken Root, Ontarians Forged Revolution." *Sudbury Star,* March 21.

Hartz, A.J., H. Krakauer, E.M. Kuhn, M. Young, S.J. Jacobsen, G. Gay, L. Muenz, M. Katzoff, R.C. Bailey and A.A. Rimm. 1989. "Hospital Characteristics and Mortality Rates." *New England Journal of Medicine* 321, 5.

Harvey, S., J. Jarrell, R. Brant, C. Stainton and D. Rach. 1996. "A Randomized, Controlled Trial of Nurse-Midwifery Care." *Birth* 23, 3 (September).

Havelock, R.G. 1973. *The Change Agent's Guide to Innovation in Education.* Englewood Cliffs, NJ: Education Technology Publications.

Hay, D. 1994. "Social Status and Health Status: Does Money Buy Health?" In B.S. Bolaria and R. Bolaria (eds.).

Hay, L.L. 1987. *You Can Heal Your Life.* Carlsbad, CA: Hay House.

Head, W. 1985. *An Exploratory Study of Attitudes and Perceptions of Minority and Majority Group Healthcare Workers.* Toronto, ON: Ontario Ministry of Labour.

Health Canada. 1998. *Summary Report: Waiting Lists and Waiting Times for Health Care in Canada: More Management!! More Money??* (May 25, 1999) [http://www.hc-sc.gc.ca/ hppb/nhrdp/wlsum5.htm]

Health Sector Training and Adjustment Program. 1997. *'96–'97 HSTAP Annual Report*. Toronto, ON.

Health Surveillance, Alberta Health. 1997. *Reproductive Health: Pregnancy Outcomes Alberta, 1985/86–1995/96* [ISSN 1480-1876]. Edmonton, AB.

Helman, C. 1990. *Culture, Health and Illness*. Second edition. London: Wright.

——. 1991. *Body Myths*. London: Chatto and Windus.

Hesterly, S., and M. Robinson. 1990. "Alternative Caregivers: Cost-Effective Utilization of RNs." *Nursing Administration Quarterly* 14, 3.

Heyssel, R., R. Gaintner, I. Kues, A. Jones and S. Lipstein. 1984. "The Johns Hopkins Experience." *New England Journal of Medicine* 310, 22.

Holloway, M. 1994. "Trends in Women's Health: A Global View." *Scientific American* (August).

Holmes, E.R., and L.D. Holmes. 1995. *Other Cultures, Elder Years*. Second edition. Thousand Oaks, CA: Sage.

Hungry Wolf, B. 1982. *The Ways of My Grandmothers*. New York: Quill.

Hurley, J., J. Lomas and V. Bhatia. 1994. "When Tinkering is Not Enough: Provincial Reform to Manage Health Care Resources." *Canadian Public Administration* 37.

Immigrant Women of Saskatchewan (IWS). 1993. *Immigrant Women of Saskatchewan Community Wellness Grant Program: Towards a Wellness Model for Immigrant and Racialized Women*. Saskatoon, SK: Saskatoon District Board of Health.

Immigration and Citizenship Canada. November 4, 1997. *1996 Census: The Daily Report*. Statistics Canada.

Islam, S. 1989. "The Socio-Cultural Context of Childbirth in Rural Bangladesh." In M. Krishnaraj and K. Chanana (eds), *Gender and Household Domain: Social and Cultural Dimensions*. New Delhi: Sage.

Jackson, E. 1993. "Whiting Out Difference: Why U.S. Nursing Research Fails Black Families." *Medical Anthropology Quarterly* 7, 4.

James, S. 1997. "Regulation: Changing the Face of Midwifery?" In F.M.C. Shroff (ed.), *The New Midwifery: Reflections on Renaissance and Regulation*. Toronto, ON: Women's Press.

——. 1998. "Registered Midwives—So What?" *Birth Issues* XIII, 2.

Jary, D., and J. Jary. 1991. *The Harper Collins Dictionary of Sociology*. New York: Harper Collins.

Jeffery, R., and P. Jeffery. 1993. "Traditional Birth Attendants in Rural North India." In S. Lindenbaum and M. Lock (eds.), *Knowledge, Power and Practice*. Berkeley: University of California Press.

Jenson, J. 1996. "Part-Time Employment and Women: A Range of Strategies." In I. Bakker (ed.).

Jimenez, M. 1991. "Having My Baby." *Healthsharing* 12, 3.

Kanhere, U. 1989. "Differential Socialisation of Boys and Girls: A Study of Lower Socio-economic Households among Gujarati Caste/communities in Ahmedabad." In M. Krishnaraj and K. Chanana (eds.), *Gender and Household Domain: Social and Cultural Dimensions*. New Delhi: Sage.

Kastes, W. 1993. *The Future of Aboriginal Urbanization in Prairie Cities: Select Annotated Bibliography and Literature Review on Urban-Aboriginal Issues in the Prairie Provinces*. Winnipeg, MB: Institute of Urban Studies, University of

Winnipeg.

Kavanagh, K.H., and P.H. Kennedy. 1992. *Promoting Cultural Diversity: Strategies for Health Care Professionals*. Newbury Park, CA: Sage.

Kealey, L. (ed.). 1979. *A Not Unreasonable Claim: Women and Reform in Canada*. Toronto, ON: Women's Press.

Keating, N., K. Kerr, S. Warren, M. Grace and D. Wertenberger. 1994. "Who's the Family in Family Caregiving?" *Canadian Journal on Aging* 13, 2.

Keddy, B., F. Gregor, D. Denney and S. Foster. 1999. "Theorizing about Nurses' Work Lives: The Personal and Professional Aftermath of Living with Health Care 'Reform.'" *Nursing Inquiry* 6.

Kitzinger, S. (ed.). 1988. *The Midwife Challenge*. London: Pandora.

Knapp, C. 1993. *Magic or Medicine?*. [Video]. Produced By Primedia Productions Ltd. with Cine-Medic Co-Productions. Toronto, ON: Channel Four/CUIT Television.

Knaus, W., E. Draper, D. Wagner and J. Zimmerman. 1986. "An Evaluation of Outcomes from Intensive Care in Major Medical Centers." *Annals of Internal Medicine* 104.

Kramer, M., and C. Schmalenberg. 1988a. "Magnet Hospitals: Part I: Institutions of Excellence. *JONA* 18, 1.

——. 1988b. "Magnet Hospitals: Part II: Institutions of Excellence." *JONA* 18, 2.

Kuhn, T. 1962. *The Structure of Scientific Revolutions*. Chicago: University of Chicago Press.

Kulig, J.C. 1996. "Insight, Experience and Expertise: Including Front-Line Workers in Decision Making." In M. Stingl and D. Wilson (eds.).

Kurian, G. 1989. "The Indo-Canadian Family: Changes, Challenges and Choices." In *Multiculturalism and the Indo-Canadian Family in Transition*. Proceedings of the National Conference of the National Indo-Canadian Council. Ottawa, ON.

Lad, V. 1984. *Ayurveda, the Science of Self-Healing: A Practical Guide*. Twin Lakes, WI: Lotus Press.

Lad, V., and D. Frawley. 1986. *The Yoga of Herbs: An Ayurvedic Guide to Herbal Medicine*. Twin Lakes, WI: Lotus Press.

Laidlaw, T., C. Malmo and others. 1990. *Healing Voices: Feminist Approaches to Therapy with Women*. San Francisco: Jossey-Bass.

Landry, D., and G. Maclean. 1996. *The Spivak Reader: Selected Works of Gayatri Chakravorty Spivak*. London: Routledge.

Lather, P. 1991. *Getting Smart: Feminist Research and Pedagogy With/in the Postmodern*. New York: Routledge.

LaValley J.W., and M.J. Verhoef. 1995. "Integrating Complementary Medicine and Health Care Services into Practice." *Canadian Medical Association Journal* (CMAJ), 153, 1.

Lea, A. 1994. "Nursing in Today's Multicultural Society: A Transcultural Perspective." *Journal of Advanced Nursing* 20.

Leatt, P., L. Lemieux-Charles and C. Aird. 1994. "Program Management: Introduction and Overview." In P. Leatt, L. Lemieux-Charles and C. Aird (eds.), *Program Management and Beyond: Management Innovations in Ontario Hospitals*. Ottawa, ON: Canadian College of Health Service Executives.

Lee, R. 1994. "Passage from the Homeland." *The Canadian Nurse* (October).

Leininger, M. 1978. "The Phenomenon of Caring: Importance, Research Questions and Theoretical Considerations." In *Caring: An Essential Human Need.* Proceedings of the National Caring Conference, Thorofare, NJ: Slack.
——. 1980. "Caring: A Central Focus of Nursing and Health Care Services." *Nursing and Health Care* 1, 2 (October).
——. 1991. "The Theory of Culture, Care, Diversity and Universality." In M. Leininger (ed.), *Culture, Care, Diversity and Universality: A Theory of Nursing.* New York: National League for Nursing Press.
Liu, L., G. Slap, S. Kinsmen and N. Khalid. 1994. "Pregnancy among American Indian Adolescents: Reactions and Prenatal Care." *Journal of Adolescent Health* 15.
London Sexual Assault Centre. February 5, 1997. *Statement to the Ontario Government about Violence against Women.* London, ON.
Lurch, M.A. 1991. "Where Does the Torturer Live?" *Healthsharing* 12.
Lynam, M.J. 1985. "Support Networks Developed by Immigrant Women." *Social Sciences & Medicine* 21.
Maher, J., and M. Riutort. 1998. "Canadian Health Care: A System in Peril." In L. Ricciutelli, J. Larkin and E. O'Neill (eds.), *Confronting the Cuts: A Sourcebook for Women in Ontario.* Toronto, ON: Inanna Publications and Education, Inc.
Mahoney, J. 1997. "Doctors' Deal Could Cost $1-Billion." *Globe and Mail,* May 16.
Maltz, W. 1992. *The Sexual Healing Journey: A Guide for Survivors of Sexual Abuse.* New York: Harper Collins.
Marks, L. 1995. "Indigent Communities and Ladies Benevolent Societies: Intersections of Public and Private Poor Relief in Late Nineteenth Century Small Town Ontario." *Studies in Political Economy* 47.
Marshall, V.W., and B.D. McPherson (eds.). 1995. *Aging: Canadian Perspectives.* Peterborough, ON: Broadview Press.
Masuda, S., and J. Ridington. 1992. *Meeting our Needs: Access Manual for Transition Houses.* Toronto, ON: Disabled Women's Network.
Mattson, S. 1995. "Culturally Sensitive Perinatal Care for Southeast Asians." *JOGNN* 24, 4.
Mauss, M. 1990. *The Gift: The Forms and Reason for Exchange in Archaic Society.* (W.D. Halls, Trans.). London: Routledge. (Original work published 1925).
McClintock, A. 1995. *Imperial Leather.* New York: Routledge.
McCue, H.A. May, 1978. *The Lake Simcoe Indians: A History From 1792–1876.* Unpublished manuscript.
McDaniel, S.A., and E.M. Gee. 1993. "Social Policies Regarding Caregiving Elders: Canadian Contradictions." *Journal of Aging and Social Policy* 5, 1/2.
McGee, P. 1992. *Teaching Transcultural Care: A Guide for Teachers of Nursing and Health Care.* London: Chapman and Hall.
McGuire, M.B. 1993. "Health and Spirituality as Contemporary Concerns." *The Annals of the American Academy of Political and Social Science* 527 (May).
McKee, J. 1988. "Holistic Health and the Critique of Western Medicine." *Social Science and Medicine* 26, 8.
McKelvey, M., and L. Bohnen. 1998. *Ontario Health Legislation: An Annotated Guide.* Aurora: Canada Law Book.
Mechanic, D. 1994. "Promoting Health: Implications for Modern and Developing Nations." In L.C. Chen, A. Kleinman and N.C. Ware (eds.), *Health and Social*

Change in International Perspective. Boston: Harvard School of Public Health/ Harvard University Press.

Mechanic, D., with L. Aiken et al. 1976. *The Growth of Bureaucratic Medicine: An Inquiry into the Dynamics of Patient Behavior and the Organization of Medical Care.* New York: Wiley.

Meleis, A.I. 1991. "Between Two Cultures: Identity, Roles and Health." *Health Care for Women International* 12.

——. 1996. "Arab Americans." In J.G. Lipson, S.L. Dibble and P.A. Minarik (eds.), *Culture and Nursing Care: A Pocket Guide.* San Francisco: University of California San Francisco Nursing Press.

Meleis, A. I., and S. Rogers. 1987. "Women in Transition: Being versus Becoming or Being and Becoming." *Health Care for Women International* 8.

Menzies, H. 1996. *Whose Brave New World? The Information Highway and the New Economy.* Toronto, ON: Between the Lines.

Messing, K., B. Neis and L. Dumais (eds.). 1995. *Invisible: Issues in Women's Occupational Health.* Charlottetown, PEI: Gynergy.

Mhatre, S.L., and R.B. Deber. 1998. "From Equal Access to Health Care to Equitable Access to Health: A Review of Canadian Provincial Health Commissions and Reports." In D. Coburn, C. D'Arcy and G.M. Torrance (eds.).

Midwifery Regional Implementation Committee. October 1996. *Midwifery Services in Alberta.* Edmonton, AB: Alberta Health.

——. June 1997. *Report of the Working Group on Midwifery Remuneration.* Edmonton, AB: Alberta Health.

Miller, M.D. 1997. "Recognizing and Treating Depression in the Elderly." *Medscape Mental Health* 2, 3 (May 25). [http://www.medscape.com/medscape/psychiatry/journal/1997/ V02.n03/mh16.miller/mh16.miller.html]

Miller, S.D., M.A. Hubble and B.L. Duncan (eds.). 1996. *Handbook of Solution-Focused Brief Therapy.* San Francisco: Jossey-Bass Publishers.

Mineyard, K., J. Wall and R. Turner. 1986. "RNs May Cost Less than You Think." *JONA* 16, 5.

Ministry of Public Works and Government Services. 1997. *Canada Health Action: Building on the Legacy.* Report for the National Forum on Health. Volumes 1 and 2. Ottawa, ON.

Mishra, R., G. Laws and P. Harding. 1988. "Ontario." In J.S. Ismael and Y. Vaillancourt (eds.), *Privatization and Provincial Social Services in Canada: Policy, Administration and Service Delivery.* Edmonton, AB: University of Alberta Press.

Mitchell, P., S. Armstrong, T. Simpson and M. Leutz. 1989. "AACN Demonstration Project: Profile of Excellence in Critical Care Nursing." *Heart and Lung* 18, 3.

Mitchenson, W. 1991. *The Nature of their Bodies: Women and their Doctors in Victorian Canada.* Toronto, ON: University of Toronto Press.

Morris, M., J. Robinson, J. Simpson, J. with S. Galey, S. Kirby, L. Martin and M. Muzychka. 1999. *The Changing Nature of Home Care and its Impact on Women's Vulnerability to Poverty.* Ottawa, ON: Status of Women Canada.

Morrison, L., S. Guruge and K. Snarr. 1999. "Sri Lankan Tamil Immigrants in Toronto." In G.A. Kelson and D.L. Delaet (eds.), *Gender and Immigration.* London: Macmillan Press.

Morse, J. 1989. "Cultural Variation in Behavioural Response to Parturition:

Childbirth in Fiji." In J. Morse (ed.), *Cross-Cultural Nursing: Anthropological Approaches to Nursing Research.* New York: Gordon and Breach Science.

Moscovitch, A., and G. Dover. 1987. "Social Expenditures and the Welfare State: The Canadian Experience in Historical Perspective." In A. Moscovitch and J. Albert (eds.), *The Benevolent State: The Growth of Welfare in Canada.* Toronto, ON: Garamond Press.

Mueller, A. 1995. "Beginning in the Standpoint of Women: An Investigation of the Gap between *Cholas* and 'Women in Peru.'" In M. Campbell and A. Manicom (eds.), *Knowledge, Experience, and Ruling Relation.* Toronto, ON: University of Toronto Press.

Myers, L.B., and K. Midence. (eds.). 1998. *Adherence to Treatment in Medical Conditions.* Amsterdam: Harwood Academic Publishers.

Nackel, J., and I. Kues. 1986. "Product-Line Management: Systems and Strategies." *Hospital and Health Services Administration* 31, 2 (March–April).

Nance, T. 1995. "Intercultural Communication: Finding Common Ground." *JOGNN* 24, 3.

Nankpi, T. 1994. "Perception of Social Support among Immigrant Punjabi Sikh Mothers in Edmonton." Unpublished master's thesis, University of Alberta, Edmonton, AB.

National Coordinating Group on Health Care Reform and Women. 2000. *Women and Health Care Reform.* Canadian Women's Health Network (CWHN), Winnipeg, MB.

National Institutes of Health/National Institute on Aging. 1995. *The Women's Health and Aging Study.* Bethesda, MD.

National Nursing Competency Project. 1997. *Final Report of the National Nursing Competency Project.* Available from the Canadian Nurses Association, Ottawa. ON.

Neander, W.l. 1988. "The Cultural Context of Infant Feeding among the Northern Alberta Woodlands Cree." Unpublished master's thesis, University of Alberta, Edmonton, AB.

Neuwirth, G. 1987. "Socioeconomic Adjustment of Southeast Asian Refugees in Canada." In J. Rogge (ed.), *Refugees: A Third World Dilemma.* Totowa, NJ: Rowman and Littlefield.

New, P.K., and W. Watson. 1983. "Pathways to Health Care among Chinese-Canadians: An Exploration." In P.S. Li and B.S. Bolaria (eds.), *Racial Minorities in Multicultural Canada.* Toronto, ON: Garamond Press.

Neysmith, S.M. 1998. "From Home Care to Social Care: The Value of a Vision." In C. Baines, P. Evans and S. Neysmith (eds.), *Women's Caring: Feminist Perspectives on Social Welfare.* Second edition. Toronto, ON: Oxford University Press.

Neysmith, S.M., and J. Aronson. 1997. "Working Conditions in Home Care: Negotiating Race and Class Boundaries in Gendered Work." *International Journal of Health Services* 27, 3.

Ng, R. 1993. "Racism, Sexism, and Nation Building in Canada." In C. McCarthy and W. Crichlow (eds.), *Race, Identity and Representation in Education.* New York: Routledge.

——. in press. "Toward an Embodied Pedagogy: Exploring Health and the Body through Chinese Medicine." In G.J.S. Dei, B. Hall and D. Goldin-Rosenberg (eds.), *Indigenous Knowledges in Global Contexts.* Toronto, ON: University of

Toronto Press.

Niblett, V. 1997. "The Humble Bed Bath." *College Communiqué* 22, 4 (December).

"No Card, No Care: Province Gets Tough on Health Card Fraud." 1998. *Sudbury Star,* February 28.

Noddings, N. 1984. *Caring: A Feminine Approach to Ethics and Moral Education.* Los Angeles: University of California Press.

Norris, E. 1995. "Achieving Professional Autonomy for Nursing." *Professional Nurse* 1, 1 (October).

O'Brien, M. 1981. *The Politics of Reproduction.* New York: Routledge and Kegan Paul.

Ogden, E.L. 1976. "Acupuncture as an Adjunct to Homeopathy." *British Homeopathic Journal* 65, 20.

O'Hanlon, P.H., and W.H. O'Hanlon. 1991. *Rewriting Love Stories: Brief Marital Therapy.* New York: W.W. Norton.

O'Hara, E.M., and L. Zhan. 1994. "Cultural and Pharmacologic Considerations when Caring for Chinese Elders." *Journal of Gerontological Nursing* 20.

O'Neil, J.D., and P. Gilbert. (eds.). 1990. *Childbirth in the Canadian North: Epidemiological, Clinical and Cultural Perspectives.* Winnipeg, MB: Northern Health Research Unit, University of Manitoba.

O'Neill, E. 1998. "From Global Economies to Local Cuts: Globalization and Structural Change in our own Backyard." In L. Ricciutelli, J. Larkin and E. O'Neill (eds.), *Confronting the Cuts: A Sourcebook for Women in Ontario.* Toronto, ON: Inanna Publications and Education, Inc.

Ontario Advisory Council on Senior Citizens. 1993. *Denied Too Long: The Needs and Concerns of Seniors Living in First Nation Communities in Ontario.* Toronto, ON: Publications Ontario.

Ontario Council of Hospital Unions/Canadian Union of Public Employees (OCHU/CUPE). March 1995. *When Patients Don't Matter: How Government Cuts are Undermining Health Care.* Toronto, ON.

Ontario Health Services Restructuring Commission. 1998. *Metropolitan Toronto Health Services Restructuring Report, 1997.* Toronto, ON: Ontario Ministry of Health.

Ontario Hospital Association. 1998a. *Hospital Report 1998.* Toronto, ON.

——. 1998b. *Barriers to Integration.* Toronto, ON.

——. 1998c. *The Hospital to Home Interface.* Toronto, ON.

Ontario Human Rights Commission. May 6, 1994. *Minutes of Settlement between Ontario Human Rights Commission and Valda Christian, Sue Dillon, Janet Edwards, Lana Henry, Sharon Luddington, Annette Wilmot, Hazel Washington and Ontario Nurses' Association and Northwestern General Hospital.* Toronto, ON.

Ontario Ministry of Health. 1989. *Health Professions Legislative Review. Striking a New Balance: A Blueprint for the Regulation of Ontario's Health Professions.* Toronto, ON.

——. 1991. *Hospital Statistics, Daily Census Summary: 1990–1991.* Toronto, ON.

——. 1993. *A Healthier Ontario: Progress in the '90s.* Toronto, ON.

——. 1994. *Managing Health Care Resources: Meeting Priorities.* Toronto, ON.

——. 1999. *Hospital Statistics, Daily Census Summary: 1998–1999.* Toronto, ON.

Ontario Nurses' Association. October 1996. Presentation to the Metro Toronto

Anti-Racism, Access and Equity Committee. Toronto, ON.

———. 1997a. "CNO Responds to Petition about New Standards for Nursing." *The ONA News* 24, 1 (January–February).

———. 1997b. "Re: Quality of Service and Unregulated Workers." *The ONA News* 24, 1 (January–February).

———. 1997c. "Patient Care Eroded by Lack of Nurses." *The ONA News* 24, 3 (April–May).

———. 1998. "Ontario Human Rights Commission Takes up the Fight for Grad Nurses." *The ONA News* 25, 1 (January–February).

Ontario Women's Directorate. n.d. *Prevention of Violence against Women, It's Everyone's Responsibility* [Pamphlet]. Toronto, ON.

Orubuloye, I.O., F. Ogunthimehna and T. Sadiq. 1997. "Women's Role in Reproductive Health Decision Making and Vulnerability to STD and HIV/AIDS in Ekiti, Nigeria." *Health Transition Review* 7 (supplement).

Ottawa-Carleton Community Coalition. 1997. *Ottawa-Carleton Community Response to the Framework for Action on the Prevention of Violence against Women in Ontario* Ottawa, ON.

Overall, C. 1993. *The Future of Human Reproduction.* Toronto, ON: Women's Press.

Palmer, H. 1991. "It's a Start." *Healthsharing* 12, 3.

Palmore, E.B. 1998. "Ageism." In D.E. Redburn and R.P. McNamara (eds.), *Social Gerontology.* Second edition. Westport, CT: Auburn House.

Pan American Health Organization. January 1997. *Workshop on Gender, Health and Development: A Facilitator's Guide.* Washington, DC: Pan American Sanitary Bureau, Regional Office of the World Health Organization.

Parry, J. 1986. "The Gift, the Indian Gift and the 'Indian Gift.'" *Journal of the Royal Anthropological Institute* 21.

Patterson, D., and K. Thompson. 1987. "Product Line Management: Organization Makes the Difference." *Health Care Financial Management* 41, 2.

Payne, M.E. 1997. "Counselling New Graduates to Find Jobs." *Recruitment, Retention & Restructuring Report* 10, 4.

Pedersen, R. 1998. "Obstetricians Halt Protest over Fees. *Calgary Herald,* November 17.

Pence, E. 1996. "Safety for Battered Women in a Textually Mediated Legal System." Unpublished doctoral thesis, University of Toronto, Toronto, ON.

Penrod, J.D., M.D. Finch and R.A. Kane. 1998. "Effects of Post-Hospital Medicare Home Health and Informal Care on Patient Functional Status." *Health Services Research* 3, 1.

Pettman, J. *Living in the Margins: Racism, Sexism and Feminism in Australia.* St. Leonards, NSW: Allen & Unwin.

Phillips, C. 1989. *Family-Centered Maternity and Newborn Care: A Basic Text.* St. Louis: Mosby.

Phillips, P., and E. Phillips. 1983. *Inequality in the Labour Market.* Toronto, ON: James Lorimer and Company.

Pilowsky, J.E. 1991. "A Population at Risk." *Healthsharing* 12.

Poliakoff, M. 1993. "Cancer and Cultural Attitudes." In R. Masi, L. Mensah and K.A. McLeod (eds.), *Health and Cultures: Exploring the Relationships, Programs, Services and Care.* Volume 2. New York: Mosaic Press.

Porter, M., and S. Sadli. 1997. "Is Global Feminism Possible? Developing 'Partnership' in a University Linkage Project." *Canadian Woman Studies Journal* 17, 2.

Pratt, R., G. Burr, B. Leelarthaepin, P. Blizard and S. Walsh. 1993. [Abstract]. "The Effects of All-RN and RN-EN Staffing on the Quality and Cost of Patient Care." *Australian Journal of Advanced Nursing* 10, 3.

Premier's Commission On Future Health Care for Albertans. December 1989. *The Rainbow Report: Our Vision For Health*. Edmonton, AB.

Prentice, A. 1985. "Themes in the Early History of the Women's Teacher's Association of Toronto." In P. Bourne (ed.), *Women's Paid and Unpaid Work: Historical and Contemporary Perspectives*. Toronto, ON: New Hogtown Press.

Prescott, P.A. 1993. "Nursing: An Important Component of Hospital Survival under a Reformed Health Care System." *Nursing Economics* 11, 4.

Provincial Health Council of Alberta. 1998. *1998 Report Card to the Minister of Health*. [http://www.healthcouncil.com].

Rabkin, M., and L. Avakian. 1992. "Participatory Management at Boston's Beth Israel Hospital." *Academic Medicine* 67, 5.

Rachlis, M., and C. Kushner. 1989. *Second Opinion*. Toronto, ON: Collins Publishers.

Ramsay, C., M. Walker and J. Alexander. 1999. "Alternative Medicine in Canada: Use and Public Attitudes" (Occasional Paper #21). Vancouver, BC: Public Policy Sources, Fraser Institute.

Rao, M.S. 1984. "An Interpretation of Holistic Health." *The British Homeopathic Journal* 76.

Raymond, J.G. 1993. *Women as Wombs: Reproductive Technologies and the Battle Over Women's Freedom*. San Francisco: Harper Collins.

Registered Nurses Association of Nova Scotia. 1996. *Report of Nova Scotia Graduate Employment Survey: Classes of 1990–95*. Halifax, NS.

Registered Nurses Association of Ontario (RNAO). 1995. "Nurses' Professional Association President Decries Replacement of Registered Nurses." *Press Release* (January 2).

Reid, E. 1992. "Gender, Knowledge and Responsibility." In J. Mann, D.J.M. Tarantola and T.W. Netter (eds.), *AIDS in the World: A Global Report*. Cambridge, MA: Harvard University Press.

Rekart, J. 1993. *Public Funds, Private Provision: The Role of the Voluntary Sector*. Vancouver, BC: University of British Columbia Press.

Richardson, E. 1990. "The Cambodians and Laotians." In N. Waxler-Morrison, J. Anderson and E. Richardson (eds.).

Roberts, J.V., and R.M. Mohr (eds.). 1994. *Confronting Sexual Assault: A Decade of Legal and Social Change*. Toronto, ON: University of Toronto Press.

Roberts, W. 1979. "Rocking the Cradle for the World: The New Woman and Maternal Feminism, Toronto 1877–1914." In L. Kealey (ed.), *A Not Unreasonable Claim: Women and Reform in Canada, 1880–1920s*. Toronto, ON: Women's Press.

Robinson, E. 1990. "Pregnancies, Deliveries and Perinatal Mortality in the James Bay Area, Québec, 1974–1984." In J. O'Neil and P. Gilbert (eds.).

Rock, A. 2000. "And the Beat Goes on: Rock Points Back to Witmer." *Toronto Star*, March 11.

Romalis, S. 1981. "An Overview." In S. Romalis (ed.), *Childbirth: Alternatives to Medical Control*. Austin, TX: University of Texas Press.

Ronayne, R. 1985. "Feelings and Attitudes during Early Convalescence following Vascular Surgery." *Journal of Advanced Nursing* 10, 5.

Rooney, B. 1998. "Low Birth Weight: Reducing the Risk." *Birthing,* Fall.

Rothman, B.K. 1989. *Recreating Motherhood.* New York: W.W. Norton.

Royal Commission on Aboriginal Peoples. 1996. *People to People, Nation to Nation: Highlights from the Report of the Royal Commission on Aboriginal Peoples.* Ottawa, ON: Ministry of Supply and Services Canada.

Rueschemeyer, D. 1983. "Professional Autonomy and the Social Contract of Expertise." In R. Dingwall and P. Lewis (eds.), *The Sociology of the Profession.* Hong Kong: Macmillan Press.

Rutledge, P.J. 1992. *The Vietnamese Experience in America.* Bloomington: Indiana University Press.

Ryten, E. 1997. *A Statistical Picture of the Past, Present and Future of Nursing in Canada.* Ottawa, ON: Canadian Nurses Association.

Salmon, J.W. 1984. "Defining Health and Reorganizing Medicine." In J.W. Salmon (ed.), *Alternative Medicines: Popular and Policy Perspectives.* New York: Tavistock Publications.

Sargent, C.F., and C.B. Brettell. 1996. *Gender and Health: An International Perspective.* Upper Saddle River, NJ: Prentice Hall.

Schellenberg, G. 1997. *The Changing Nature of Part-Time Work.* Social Research Series Report No. 4. Ottawa, ON: Canadian Council on Social Development.

Schutzenhofer, K. 1988. "The Problem of Professional Autonomy in Nursing." *Health Care for Women International* 9.

Scott, W., W. Forrest and B. Brown. 1976. "Hospital Structure and Postoperative Mortality and Morbidity." In S. Shortell and M. Brown (eds.), *Organizational Research in Hospitals.* Chicago: Blue Cross Association.

Sehdev, H.K. 1987. *Multiculturalism and Health Care: Culture Simulator Training for Health Care Professionals.* Ottawa, ON: Ministry of Citizenship, Government of Canada.

Shamian, J. June 1996. *Truths and Myths of the Cost of Professional Nursing Services.* Presentation at Mount Sinai Hospital, Toronto, ON.

Shamian, J., and E. Lightstone. 1997. "Hospital Restructuring Initiatives in Canada." *The Canadian Nurse* 94, 1.

Sharpe, M. 1997. "Ontario Midwifery in Transition: An Exploration of Midwives' Perceptions of the Impact of Midwifery Legislation in its First Year. In F.M.C. Shroff (ed.), *The New Midwifery: Reflections on Renaissance and Regulation.* Toronto, ON: Women's Press.

Sheikh, J.I., and J.A. Yesavage. 1986. "Geriatric Depression Scale (GDS): Recent Evidence and Development of a Shorter Version." In T.L. Brink (ed.), *Clinical Gerontology: A Guide to Assessment and Intervention.* New York: The Haworth Press.

Shindul-Rothschild, J. 1996. "Keynote Speech from the ONA Annual Meeting." *The ONA News* 3, 7 (February).

Shroff, F.M.C. 1991. "The Social Construction of AIDS, Heterosexism, Racism, and Misogyny: and the Challenges Facing Women of Colour." *Resources for Feminist Research* 20, 3/4.

——. 1996. "New Directions in Canadian Health Policy: Lessons from Holistic Medicine." Unpublished doctoral thesis, University of Toronto, Toronto,

ON.

Shua-Haim, J.R., M.E. Saba, E. Comsti and J.S. Gross. 1997. "Depression in the Elderly." *Hospital Medicine* 33, 7.

Shukla, R. 1983. "All-RN Model of Nursing Care Delivery: A Cost-Benefit Evaluation." *Inquiry* 20.

Schultz, M.A., G. van Servellen, B.L. Chang, D. McNeese-Smith and E. Waxenberg. 1998. "The Relationship of Hospital Structural and Financial Characteristics to Mortality and Length of Stay in Acute Myocardial Infarction Patients." *Outcomes Management for Nursing Practice* 2, 3.

Sibbald, B. 1998. "The Future Supply of Registered Nurses in Canada." *The Canadian Nurse* 94, 1.

Silvera, M. 1994. "Black Women Organize for Health: Interview with Erica Mercer." In E. Dua, M. Fitzgerald, L. Gardner, D. Taylor and L. Wyndels (eds.).

Singer, S.M., D.G. Willms, A. Adrien et al. 1996. "Many Voices: Sociocultural Results of the Ethnocultural Communities Facing AIDS Study in Canada." *Canadian Journal of Public Health* (Supplement 1).

Skelton-Green, J.M., and J.S. Sunner. 1997. "Integrated Delivery Systems: The Future for Canadian Health Care Reform?" *Canadian Journal of Nursing Administration* (September– October).

Smeltzer, S.C. 1992. "Women and AIDS: Sociopolitical Issues." *Nursing Outlook* 40.

Smith, D.E. 1987. *The Everyday World as Problematic: A Feminist Sociology.* Toronto, ON: University of Toronto Press.

——. 1990a. *The Conceptual Practices of Power: A Feminist Sociology of Knowledge.* Toronto, ON: University of Toronto Press.

——. 1990b. *Texts, Facts, and Femininity: Exploring the Relations of Ruling.* New York: Routledge.

——. 1999. *Writing the Social: Critique, Theory, and Investigations.* Toronto, ON: University of Toronto Press.

Smith, T., P. Leatt, P. Ellis and B. Fried. 1989. "Decentralized Hospital Management: Rationale, Potential, and Two Case Examples." *Health Matrix* VII, 1.

Social Services Department, City of Calgary. 1984. *Native Needs Assessment.* Calgary, AB.

Statistics Canada. 1994. *General Social Survey on Personal Risk.* (GSS-Cycle 8). Ottawa, ON.

——. 1996. *National Population Health Survey Overview 1994–1995.* Ottawa, ON.

——. 1997a. *Caring Canadians, Involved Canadians: Highlights from the 1997 National Survey of Giving, Volunteering and Participation.* [Catalogue No. 71-542-XPE]. Ottawa, ON.

——. 1997b. *A Portrait of Seniors in Canada.* Second edition. Ottawa, ON.

——. 1998a. *National Population Health Survey, Overview 1996–1997.* Ottawa, ON.

——. 1998b. *Registered Nurses 1997, Statistical Highlights.* Ottawa, ON.

Statutes of Ontario. 1994. *Regulated Health Professions Act 1991, C.18, as Amended By 1993, C.37.* Toronto, ON: Queen's Printer.

——. 1997. *Expanded Nursing Services for Patients Act 1997, An Act to Amend the Nursing Act 1991, C32.* Toronto, ON: Queen's Printer.

Stevens, S. 1993. "Newcomer Canadians and Mainstream Services." In R. Masi, L. Mensah and K.A. McLeod (eds.), *Health and Cultures: Exploring the Relation-*

ships, Programs, Services and Care. Volume 2. New York: Mosaic Press.

Stewart, M.J. (ed.). 1995. *Community Nursing: Promoting Canadians' Health.* Toronto, ON: W.B. Saunders.

Stimpson, L., and M.C. Best. 1991. *Courage above All: Sexual Assault against Women with Disabilities.* Toronto, ON: Disabled Women's Network.

Stingl, M., and D. Wilson (eds.). *Efficiency versus Equality: Health Reform in Canada.* Halifax, NS: Fernwood Publishing.

Storch, J.L. 1996. "Foundational Values in Canadian Health Care." In M. Stingl and D. Wilson (eds.).

Stuart, N., and H. Sherrard. 1987. "Managing Hospitals from a Program Perspective." *Health Management Review* 8, 1.

Sumrall, A.C., and D. Taylor (eds.). 1992. *Sexual Harassment: Women Speak Out.* Freedom, CA: The Crossing Press.

Swartz, D. 1998. "The Limits of Health Insurance." In D. Coburn, C. D'Arcy and G.M. Torrance (eds.).

Tiwari, M. 1995. *Ayurveda—A Life of Balance.* Rochester, VT: Healing Arts Press.

Terr, L. 1990. *Too Scared to Cry: How Trauma Affects Children and Ultimately Us All.* New York: Basic Books.

Tomm, W. 1995. *Bodied Mindfulness: Women's Spirits, Bodies and Places.* Waterloo, ON: Wilfrid Laurier University Press.

Torrance, G.M. 1998. "Socio-Historical Overview: The Development of the Canadian Health System. In D. Coburn, C. D'Arcy and G.M. Torrance (eds.).

Transken, S. 1995. *Reclaiming Body Territory.* Ottawa, ON: Canadian Research Institute for the Advancement of Women.

———. 1997. "Personal and Political Roles: Struggling with Empowerment and Burnout." In D. Hearne (ed.), *Equity and Justice.* Montreal, PQ: Université du Québec à Montreal.

Tripp-Reimer, T. 1989. "Cross-Cultural Perspective on Patient Teaching." *Nursing Clinics of North America* 24.

Tudiver, S. 1994. "Canadian Women's Health Network: One Step Back, Two Steps Forward." *Canadian Woman Studies Journal* 14, 3 (Summer).

Turkoski, B.B. 1985. "Growing Old in China." *Journal of Gerontological Nursing* 11.

Turner, B.S. 1995. "Aging and Identity: Some Reflections on the Somatization of the Self." In M. Featherstone and A. Wernick (eds.), *Images of Aging: Cultural Representations of Later Life.* London: Routledge.

United Way of York Region. 1996. *Fund Distribution: Community Initiatives Grants.* Markham, ON.

———. August 1998. *Fund Distribution Process: United Way of York Region 1999–2000.* Revised edition. Markham, ON.

Valverde, M. 1995. "The Mixed Social Economy as a Canadian Tradition." *Studies in Political Economy* 47.

Vega, W.A., B. Kolody, R. Valle and R. Hough. 1986. "Depressive Symptoms and their Correlation among Immigrant Mexican Women in the US." *Social Science & Medicine* 22.

Verhoef, M., and L. Sutherland. 1995. "Alternative Medicine and General Practitioners: Opinions and Behaviour." *Canadian Family Physician* 41 (June).

Verma, V. 1995. *Ayurveda: A Way of Life.* York Beach, ME: Samuel Weiser, Inc.

Wadel, C. 1979. "The Hidden Work of Everyday Life." In S. Wallman (ed.), *Social*

Anthropology of Work. Toronto, ON: Academic Press.

Wagner, M. 1994. *Pursuing the Birth Machine: The Search for Appropriate Birth Technology.* Australia: Ace Graphics.

Waldram, J., D.A. Herring and T.K. Young. 1995. *Aboriginal Health in Canada: Historical, Cultural and Epidemiological Perspectives.* Toronto, ON: University of Toronto Press.

Walker, G. 1995. "Violence and the Relations of Ruling: Lessons from the Battered Women's Movement." In M. Campbell and A. Manicom (eds.), *Knowledge, Experience, and Ruling Relation.* Toronto, ON: University of Toronto Press.

Walker, R. 1998a. "Pregnant Mom Petitions for Higher Obstetrician Fees." *Edmonton Journal,* July 27.

———. 1998b. "Post-Partum Care Concerns New Moms." *Calgary Herald,* August 15.

———. 1998c. "Preemies' Odds Improve but New Financial and Emotional Costs Emerge." *Calgary Herald,* December 17.

Walkom, T. 1998. "Hard Labour of Love." *Toronto Star,* October 31.

Waring, M. 1988. *If Women Counted: A New Feminist Economics.* San Francisco: Harper.

Waterfall, B. 1996. *The Practical Application of the Native Medicine Wheel Concept as an Assessment Tool in Direct Social Work Practice.* [Conference Handout.] Available From Barbara Waterfall, Department of Social Work, Laurentian University, Sudbury, ON.

Watkinson, A. 1999. "Personal Journey as a Result of Government Neglect." Paper presented at the Canadian Research Institute for the Advancement of Women Conference on Feminist Definitions of Caring Communities and Health Lifestyles, Sudbury, ON.

Watson, J. 1985. *Nursing: Human Science and Human Care — A Theory of Nursing.* Norwalk, CT: Appleton-Century-Crofts.

Waxler-Morrison, N. 1990. "Introduction." In N. Waxler-Morrison, J. Anderson and E. Richardson (eds.).

Waxler-Morrison, N., J. Anderson and E. Richardson (eds.). 1990. *Cross-Cultural Caring: A Handbook for Health Professionals in Western Canada.* Vancouver, BC: University of British Columbia Press.

Weiner-Davis, M. 1995. *Change Your Life and Everyone in It.* New York: Simon and Schuster.

Werner, D., and D. Saunders with J. Weston, S. Babb and B. Rodriguez. 1997. *Questioning the Solution.* Palo Alto, CA: Healthwrights.

Wertz, R., and D. Wertz. 1977. *Lying-in: A History of Childbirth in America.* New York: Free Press.

White, J.P. 1997. "After Total Quality Management, What?: Re-engineering Bedside Care." In P. Armstrong, H. Armstrong, J. Choiniere, E. Mykhalovskiy and J. White (eds).

Williams, A.P., J. Barnsley, J. Tanner and R. Cockerill. May 1997. "Political Conflict over the Future of Government Health Insurance in Ontario." Paper presented at the annual meeting of the Canadian Political Science Association, St. John's, NF.

Williams, C.C. 1999. *Ethnoracial Services Task Force Report to the Joint General Psychiatry Program Planning Committee.* Clarke Institute of Psychiatry, Toronto, ON.

Williams, H.A. 1990. "Families in Refugee Camps." *Human Organization* 49, 2.

Wizowski, L. 1994. *Nurses' Experience with the Transition from Compliance to Self-Management.* Unpublished masters' project, Brock University, St. Catharines, ON.

Women and Mental Health Association. April, 1987. *Women and Mental Health in Canada: Strategies for Change. Report Prepared by the Women and Mental Health Association National Office.* Toronto, ON.

Woollett, A., and N. Dosanjih-Mattwala. 1990. "Pregnancy and Antenatal Care: The Attitudes and Experiences of Asian Women." *Child: Care, Health and Development* 16.

Woollett, A., N. Dosanjih, P. Nicholson, H. Marshall, O. Dijhanbakhc and J. Harlow. 1995. "The Ideas and Experiences of Pregnancy and Childbirth of Asian and Non-Asian Women in East London." *British Journal of Medical Psychology* 68, 1.

World Health Organization (WHO). 1978a. *The Development of Traditional Medicine.* (Technical Report Series, No. 622). Geneva.

———. 1978b. *Health for All by the Year 2000.* Geneva.

Working Group on Health Care Services Utilization. June 1994. *When Less is Better: Using Canada's Hospitals Efficiently.* Report written for the Conference of Federal/Provincial/Territorial Deputy Ministers of Health. Toronto, ON.

Yeatman, A. 1994. *Postmodern Revisionings of the Political.* London: Routledge.

York Region Health Services. 1997. *York Region Health Status Report 1991–1996.* Toronto, ON.

Zack, N. 1994. "My Racial Self Over Time." In C. Camper (ed.), *Miscegenation Blues: Voices of Mixed Race Women.* Toronto, ON: Sister Vision.

Zimmerman, P. 1995. "Increased Use of Unlicensed Assistive Personnel: Pros and Cons." *Journal of Emergency Nursing* 21, 6 (December).

Index

Aboriginal Health Office 220

Aboriginal Health Policy 220

Aboriginal healers 283

Aboriginal peoples: Integrated community health care 199-218; Chippewas of Georgina Island 199-218; colonialism and, 91, 147, 200, 201, 202-4, 215; cutbacks to services for, 153, 191, 199-218, 219; health services for, 205-7, 210-15, 219-20; health status of, 17, 91, 200, 205, 206-7, 210-1; Royal Commission on Aboriginal Peoples 202, 219; traditional health and healing systems 91, 214-5, 283, 287, 292, 293

Aboriginal women (see First Nations women)

Abuse and violence: Brief Solution Focused therapy and, 23, 129, 131, 134, 143, 146-8; childhood sexual, 130, 146; recent immigrants and refugees and, 227, 234, 241; sexual violation 127-9, 131-4, 139, 142-4, 151, 294; (see also sexual assault treatment programs; sexual assault crisis centres)

Aging 18, 19, 249, 260

Aging women: cutbacks to services for, 44, 191, 207-10, 243-65, 267, 270; disabilities, 245; health care needs and 191, 207, 220, 255, 260; health reform and, 243-65; institutional-ized aging 255-6, 262, 265; network of shared caregiving, 24, 258-9; resistance and advocacy 24, 243-4 254-65, 269-70; traditional healing practices and 261; vulnerability of, 24, 191, 252, 255, 264, 268

Allopathy 87, 272-3, 274-5, 277, 278, 279, 282, 283, 294; consumer dissatisfaction with, 287; critique of, 274-5, 281, 294; definition of, 274, 294; holistic health care and, 24, 271-93; tension between traditional health and healing systems and, 214-5, 271-93 (see also biomedical model)

Allopathic medicine (see allopathy)

Alternative health care 275, 279-80 (see also complementary health care; holistic health care; traditional health and healing systems)

Alberta Association of Midwives 108, 119

Alberta Health 109-10, 118, 120-1, 123

Alberta Medical Asso-ciation 109-10

Alberta Association of Midwives 108, 119

Alberta Society of Obstetricians and Gynecologists 109, 126

Ayurveda 94, 274, 277, 285, 291-2; Parkinson's disease and, 285; pregnancy and, 94

B.C. Ministry of Health, 286

Biomedical model: (see also allopathy) absorption of tradi-tional care providers under, 87, 116; dominance of, 17, 22, 24, 50, 56, 67-70, 112, 116, 136, 209, 255, 271-2, 274-5, 277, 293, 294; midwifery and, 26-7, 87, 93, 116; support for, 94

Biomedical technology 15, 19, 27-8, 44, 47, 87, 221, 273, 284; child-birth and, 86, 107, 111-4, 115, 117, 119

Brief Solution Focused therapy 23, 129, 131, 134, 143, 146-8

Business paradigm: allocation of power and decision-making, 35-37, 45, 49-70, 107-26, 127-52, 177-97, 199-218; care providers, 23, 38-40, 42-3, 45-6, 49-70, 72-84, 85-106, 107-26, 127-52, 154-75, 177-97, 199-218, 222-41; caring encounters, 38-40, 85-106, 107-26, 127-52, 154-75, 177-97,

191, 199-218, 219;
minority women and,
21, 60, 61, 86, 99, 101,
144, 191-2, 196, 222-41;
patient outcomes and,
37-8, 45-7, 127, 133-4,
136, 138, 142-51, 177-8,
193-4, 196, 253, 272 ;
poor women and, 44,
191-2, 208-9; women's
greater vulnerability
to, 21, 60-2, 144, 151,
200, 207-9, 264, 268,
272

Cure-care paradigm 21,
25-6, 29-30, 33, 45; goal
of, 25-6; health reform
and, 25-47
Dentists and dentistry
51, 52, 69, 79, 248, 267;
patient attitudes
toward, 248, 267
Deskilling 26-7, 49, 50
Diagnosis Related
Groups 30
Diploma nurses 64-6
Disease prevention 16,
24,118, 205, 222, 231,
233, 236, 237, 275, 290,
292-3
DSM-IV 267
Disability: aging women
with, 245; caring for
family member with,
177, 191, 206, 211, 234,
235, 238; First Nations
women with, 211;
immigrants with, 232,
233-4; support for
women with, 194, 196,
211, 290; women with,
20, 144, 194, 196, 211,
232, 238, 245
Downloading caregiving
labour 33, 39, 62-4,
259; as return to
traditional community

values 210; benefits to
economy 20, 216;
burden for women,
191, 207-8, 216; from
hospital to home 13,
54, 19, 190-1, 206-7,
207-10, 233-6; from
paid to unpaid care
providers, 20, 54, 190-
1, 198, 206-7, 207-10; to
women 191, 206-7,
207-10, 216, 258-9
Elderly women (see
aging women)
Employment patterns
19-20, 37-8, 41-3, 45-6,
50-1, 54-70, 72, 74-5,
88-9, 114, 149,170-1,
208, 225-6
Empowerment 13, 40,
113, 118, 121-2, 128,
151, 194, 222, 227, 230-
1, 234, 236, 238, 254,
264, 287
Euro-Canadian 91, 103,
Evidence-based practice
13, 46-7, 292
Family as unpaid care
providers 14, 20, 21,
49, 54, 85, 92, 96, 101-
4, 177, 188-92, 195-7,
200, 205-8, 210-1, 220,
228, 230-1, 234-6, 294
Fee-for-service: com-
pared to fee for
course-of-care, 122;
midwives and, 56,
125; nurses and, 266;
obstetricians and, 109,
110-2, 115-6, 122, 125;
physicians and, 40,
111, 274; problem
with, 40, 111-2, 115,
125, 126, 274
First Nations women 85,
86, 91-2, 95-7, 147, 191,
202-4; addressing
needs of 116, 144, 153;

attitudes about
pregnancy and
childbirth 91-2;
childbirth 22, 91-2, 95-
7, 103, 116; concepts of
health 91-2; disabili-
ties, 211; interactions
with nurses 95-7;
racism and, 96-7;
resistance and advo-
cacy 15, 22, 103, 199-
218; sexual violation
and, 147
Flexible specialization
26, 28, 31, 32-3, 37-8,
41
Flexible workforce 50,
72, 74, 75-6, 79, 241
Free Trade Agreement
16, 166
Friends as unpaid care
providers 21, 99, 103-
4, 189, 207, 258
Fordism and post-
Fordist models of
management 26, 27-8,
31, 32, 35, 36, 37
Georgina Island First
Nations Reserve 218
Generic workers (see
unregulated care
providers)
Gender relations and
analysis 17-9, 21, 24,
26, 51, 60, 82, 86, 93,
105, 107, 119, 155, 157-
60, 164, 174, 207-8,
227, 264, 268, 271, 273,
274, 278-9
Globalization 16, 28, 33,
82, 217
Health: definitions of,
18, 91, 118, 142;
environment and, 91,
118, 236, 254-5, 275-6,
281-3, 286-8, 290, 293;
nutrition and, 123,
223, 224, 236, 270

health care 15, 22, 24, 90, 94, 96-8, 100-2, 222, 224-5, 227-9, 235-6, 241; of reform 13-4, 216, 217; of revolution 13-4; of social goals 117-9; linguistically and culturally appropriate services 15, 105, 144, 233, 236-7, 238-40
Lay-offs (see job displacement)
Licensed Practical Nurse 41-2; RNs working as, 75
Maguire Report 129, 148-50, 153
Management trends (see business model, re-engineering, product-line management, program management)
Mental health 20, 245, 291, 293; problems 141, 281, 287, 293; services 147, 228, 236, 238, 284, 293
Matrix model of care 46
Midwives: as safe, effective practitioners, 112, 119, 122; critique of medicalized childbirth, 86, 107, 112-4, 115, 117, 119; fee structure, 56, 115-6, 125; health insurance and, 120, 280; home births 114, 123; leaving profession, 124; normal, low-risk pregnancies and births and, 114, 122-3, 124: obstetricians' job action and, 107, 111-7, 124; occupational status within health care 86, 116, 119; on-

call status, 109; pregnant women and, 116-7; tension between obstetricians and, 86-7, 111-7, 124-6;
Midwifery: history of, 86-7, 93; holistic health care and, 113, 280, 292; measuring value of, 121-3; model of care, 86-8, 113-4, 116, 292; Rainbow Report and, 108, 117-20; regulation of, 50-3, 56, 70, 117, 119-21;
Mind-spirit-body connection: 91, 128, 143, 147-8, 151, 275-8, 286-7
Minority women: cutbacks and, 21, 59-61, 85-106, 192; working as UCPs, 59-60
Multi-skilling 28, 32, 37-8, 41-2
National Survey of Giving, Volunteering and Participation 155
Nursing: employment patterns, 54-7; flexible workforce, 72, 74, 75-6, 79, 241; occupational status within health care 37, 50, 51, 69-70; professionalization of nursing, 21, 50, 61-3, 68-9, 208, 215; replaced by volunteers, 17, 72, 170-1; Regulated Health Professions Act and 49-70
Nurse Practitioners 50, 56, 67-8; occupational status within health care 67-8
Nutrition 123, 223, 224,

236, 270
Obstetrical care, history of, 86-8
Obstetricians: dominance of, 50, 86-7, 107, 112, 116, 119, 124-6; high risk pregnancies and births and, 31, 112, 123-5; job action and, 107, 108-11, 124-6; leaving Alberta 124; normal, low risk pregnancies and births and, 111, 112, 113, 123-5; on-call status, 109; refusing to accept new patients, 56, 119; remuneration of, 109, 110-2, 115-6, 122, 125; tensions between midwives and, 86-7, 111-7, 124-6; use of technology 86, 107, 111-4, 115, 117, 119
Ontario Council of Hospital Unions 191
Ontario Hospital Insurance Plan 188, 193
Ontario Medical Association 56, 68
Ontario Ministry of Health 52, 56, 138, 178, 197, 205, 210-2, 214, 215-7, 220, 227, 270
Ontario Nurses' Association 55, 56, 59
Ontario Women's Directorate 135, 139
Organizational restructuring: community sector 106, 127-52, 177-97, 199-218; hospital sector 25-47, 49-70, 72-84, 85-106, 154-75
Palliative Care Services of York Region 210, 212-4, 215-7